M000294605

# IMPERIAL MEDICAMENTS

## —Medical Prescriptions Written for Empress Dowager Cixi and Emperor Guangxu with Commentary

*Edited by*
Professor Chen Keji, M.D.

FOREIGN LANGUAGES PRESS    BEIJING

First Edition 1996

Publisher's Note
The present volume is an English translation of the Chinese edition entitled
*Medical Prescriptions Written for Cixi and Guangxu with Commentary*,
published by the China Book Company, Beijing, in November 1981.

*English Translation by*: You Benlin

ISBN 7-119-01336-X
© Foreign Languages Press, Beijing, 1996
Published by Foreign Languages Press
24 Baiwanzhuang Road, Beijing 100037, China
Printed by Beijing Foreign Languages Printing House
19 Chegongzhuang Xilu, Beijing 100044, China
Distributed by China International Book Trading Corporation
35 Chegongzhuang Xilu, Beijing 100044, China
P.O. Box 399, Beijing, China
*Printed in the People's Republic of China*

# CONTENTS

CONTENTS

# INTRODUCTION

Traditional Chinese medicine (TCM), known worldwide, is a gem in the great cultural heritage of the Chinese nation. It has a unique theoretical system and rich legacy of practical experience. Over the past four decades academic studies have been greatly promoted concerning the carrying forward and development of TCM and its systematic research. But, as an important constituent of TCM treasure, the imperial medicine of the Qing Dynasty (1644-1911) drew little attention in medical circles. This was indeed a pity. The science of TCM dates back to remote antiquity and has survived throughout the generations. In the Qing Dynasty the school of febrile diseases arose, a milestone indicating unprecedented development in TCM. The extant medical archives of the Qing Dynasty truly mirrored the academic level of TCM practice of that period. A systematic study of such medical data will be of practical significance in TCM development, health care, and in-depth research into Qing Dynasty history.

A sizable number of imperial medical files and commonly used formulae of the Qing Dynasty are kept at the First History Archives of China. These files include first-hand information concerning the diagnosis and treatments carefully worked out for emperors, empresses, imperial concubines, eunuchs, ladies-in-waiting, princes and ministers. Such historical data are so valuable that they were rarely touched. In an attempt to carry forward and develop the essence of TCM and pharmacology to serve the ordinary people today and to enrich the legacy for future generations, Professor Chen Keji urgently brought forward the idea of carrying out systematic research in this field. As he spoke as a member of the TCM Group under the State Commission of Science and Technology and a consultant to the World Health Organization, his suggestion was given support by a number of eminent figures, among whom were Professor Ji Zhongpu, President of the China Academy of TCM; Professor Yue Meizhong, member of the Standing Committee of the Fifth National People's Congress, Vice-President of the All-China Medical Association, Vice-President of the All-China TCM Association, and also a well-known TCM doctor; and Dr. Zheng Xuewen, President of Beijing Xiyuan Hospital. Also, authorities from both the First History Archives of China and the Palace Museum. Specific arrangements concerning the compilation of the *Studies of the Imperial Medical Files of the Qing Dynasty (Qing Gong Yi An Yan Jiu)* and the *Studies of the Imperial Medical Formulae of the Qing Dynasty (Qing Gong Pei Fang Yan Jiu)* were made by the China Academy of TCM and the First History Archives of China. Professor Chen Keji, was in charge of organizing TCM experts, and those in the History Archives of the Qing Dynasty who were interested in the project to join in their efforts. Shan Shikui, an expert in the study of imperial archives of the Ming and Qing dynasties at the First History Archives of China, served as consultant. Also participating in its compilation were chief physician Zhou Wenquan, Doctor Jiang Youli, one of the first group of graduate students at the China Academy of TCM, and Xu Yipu, head of the Research Section of the First History Archives of China. Li Songling took responsibility for locating the files and making photo copies. Wang Tianjian assisted in checking the photocopied documents and the bookbinding. Illustrations were provided by the Photograph Section of the Central Laboratory at the China Academy of TCM.

*Studies of the Imperial Medical Files of the Qing Dynasty* and *Studies of the Imperial Medical Formulae* of the Qing Dynasty were compiled on the basis of detailed archives extant at the First History Archives of China. They involved the case-recording files of the Imperial Palace, handwritten files of the Imperial Household Department, original files on materia medica used for emperors and empresses, original files of imperial prescriptions, documents of the Imperial Pharmacy, daily life archives of emperors (including some of their consorts), Imperial Logistics Department files, and files on the use of medicines requiring the "red script" endorsement of emperors. These data provide a great deal of outstanding medical experience characterized by profound medical principles, close affinity to the TCM philosophy, unprecedented explanation in disease mechanism, and very concise syndrome differentiation. They also demonstrate precisely how prescriptions were formed in light of seeking the root cause of the diseases in the course of treatment. In those days priority was given to the ascending and descending mechanism in treatment, whereas the reinforcing principle was considered without neglecting the reducing. Both traditional and seasonal formulae were applied. Internal and external applications were adopted at the same time. Light-dose remedies were employed with flexibility while heavy doses with drastic effect were under strict monitoring. Therapeutic principles were chosen according to syndromes. Prescriptions were worked out from a wide range of references appended to both effective and empirical remedies. Most conventional formulae followed were modified, exhibiting their best qualities. Among them, the formulae for Emperor Guangxu and Empress Dowager Cixi constituted a larger number with special features. With overall planning, the book entitled *Imperial Medicaments—Medical Prescriptions Written for Empress Dowager Cixi and Emperor Guangxu with Commentary* was first compiled and published, offering a fine collection of commonly used prescriptions and remedies with objective comments. Those for longevity were general tonics, regulating menstruation, regeneration and miscellaneous diseases and ailments of internal organs and channels. The comments were also intended to present studies on the origins of some of the prescriptions, elaborations on the different uses of ingredients, and prescription-oriented discussions associated with the pulse files or comments based on modern science. It is expected to provide some valuable medical experience and to propose research projects in relation to TCM treatments for present-day diseases and illnesses encountered in the various departments, especially in the treatment of chronic illnesses and prevention of senile disorders. The Research Section of the Qing Dynasty Imperial Medical Files would also verify those empirical and effective prescriptions recorded in the Imperial Palace. In the meantime, modern scientific research will be conducted to study the therapeutic effect and mechanism.

In the compilation of this book, Hu Ximing, Deputy Director of TCM Bureau under the Ministry of Public Health and Vice-President of the All-China TCM Association, and Professor Deng Tietao, well-known TCM doctor and Vice-President of the Guangzhou College of TCM, also offered their warm support. Zheng Tianting, noted expert in the study of Qing Dynasty history and Vice-President of Nankai University in Tianjin; Professor Ren Yingqiu, member of the Invention Appraisal Committee under the State Commission of Science and Technology and Vice-President of the All-China TCM Association; and Professor Geng Jianting, well-known TCM doctor and Deputy Executive Member of the All-China Society of Medical History, contributed their foreword or preface for the book. Professor Huang Yongyu, famous painter, did the calligraphy of the Chinese book title and the cover design. Great support for the compilation of this book came also from the different sections of the First History Archives of China such as the Editorial Section, the Technical Section, the File Preserving Section, and the Manchu Language Section. The editor and his colleagues would hereby like to extend their gratitude and appreciation to them all.

Finally, our thanks and gratitudes should also go to Li Kan, the vice editor-in-chief, and to editors and the publishing staff from the China Publishing Bureau. Without their help this book would not have been so promptly in print to satisfy readers in China and abroad.

# PREFACE

## by President Ji Zhongpu

TCM is a crystallization of the wisdom of the Chinese people. Proud of having such an invaluable heritage, we should carry it forward and develop it. Carrying forward is the foundation, while developing is the purpose. Without carrying forward, developing TCM would be a rootless tree or water without a spring. Similarly, medicine would have no further prosperity without its own development.

Any branch of science involves inheriting, in one way or another, the knowledge of the past. In the course of TCM development as well as its integration with modern medicine, priority should be given to carrying forward the science of TCM.

Systematic research in the imperial medicine of the Qing Dynasty is highly significant in carrying forward TCM experience. We believed it a very good idea as soon as it was suggested by Professor Chen Keji. Contact was immediately made with Peng Yan, Deputy President of the Palace Museum. He said that the archives of both the Ming and Qing dynasties under the administration of the State Archives Bureau were now kept at the First History Archives of China, with whose cooperation the China Academy of TCM soon listed the research as a project for implementation and the institutions worked together in systematically researching the imperial medicine of the Qing Dynasty.

At the Science Conference of the China Academy of TCM in 1978, the noted TCM doctor Yue Meizhong stressed the importance of carrying forward TCM. He warned us against superficial efforts in exploring ancient TCM knowledge, mentioning the example of digging deeper in the mine in search of more gold. His comment was enlightening in our efforts to carry TCM forward. While endeavouring to dig deeper for the treasure of TCM, we should also work more widely and not be satisfied only with minor achievements. We should contribute every effort to find the essence from the treasure house of TCM, cast out the unnecessary, maintain the real and delete the unreal. Only in this way can we achieve sustained progress in carrying forward and developing TCM.

Thanks to the efforts of Professor Chen Keji and his working group some progress has been made in systematic studies of the Qing Dynasty imperial medicine. However, much remains to be done before the TCM experience that served only emperors and empresses can benefit the general public. A lot of work needs to be done not only in sorting out and publishing, but also in laboratory research and proof of therapeutic effects by clinical application. Only by so doing can there be both carrying forward and development of TCM.

Modern science and technology are developing at a rapid pace, as are the changes in man's social and natural environment. In order to hasten the development of TCM we need to draw on any positive force, not only from the ancients but also from the present, not only from China but also from abroad, so that they can mutually permeate and promote. Meanwhile, we should carry these forces forward in a critical manner, to discover and experiment, making the ancient serve the present and the foreign serve China.

We believe that efforts in sorting out and research into the imperial medical experience of the Qing Dynasty will definitely make a significant contribution to the development of TCM. We advocate the down-to-earth manner in carrying forward TCM, and hope that the various research departments concerned in the China Academy of TCM will devote even greater effort in such projects as systematic sorting out and research into imperial medical experience of the Qing Dynasty.

March 29, 1981
China Academy of TCM

# PREFACE

## by professor Yue Meizhong

In early autumn of 1980 I was hospitalized at Xiyuan Hospital when Professor and Doctor Chen Keji, Vice-President of the hospital, visited me. He told me that he was working together with doctors Zhou Wenquan and Jiang Youli as well as some experts in the history of the Ming and Qing dynasties at the First History Archives of China to sort out and study the imperial medical files of the Qing Dynasty. Their work was really a courageous effort that would be greatly valued in history. People used to say, "It is difficult to write the history of the Qing Dynasty." The sorting out and research of imperial medical experience of the Qing Dynasty is an arduous and tough job even though it pertains to the profession of medical science and technology. It was different from the straightening out of the Qing Dynasty chronicles. Case histories and the use of formulae, both abundant and profound, require much patient analysis.

It is generally believed that many of the imperial prescriptions were mild in action. But I do not hold that view. In older times TCM practitioners in present-day Beijing tended towards prescriptions initiated by Wang Mengyin, Wu Jutong and Ye Tianshi. Formulae handed down from the school of Zhang Zhongjing were sometimes ignored. Very often prescriptions containing Herba Ephedra, Ramulus Cinnamomi, Radix Bupleuri and Radix Puerariae or those containing Natrii Sulphas, Radix Rhei, Rhizoma Anemarrhenae and Gypsum Fibrosum were not considered suitable for clinical use. According to extant TCM files of the Qing Dynasty, both conventionally popular and empirical remedies were applied in the Imperial Palace. This was really an extraordinary thing.

Several emperors of the Qing Dynasty understood some TCM. In the early 1960s, Puyi, the last emperor of the Qing Dynasty, together with his wife visited me at my home for medical consultations. He mentioned that he not only read TCM books; he had studied them in his early youth. Having some knowledge of TCM, he was able to formulate herbal prescriptions. On many an occasion after consultations, we would discuss the medical mechanism and prescription experience of TCM in connection with actual cases. In 1962, I was sent by the government to Indonesia to treat the Indonesian president for urinary lithiasis. When I returned, Puyi visited me again and presented me with a copy of his book, *The First Half of My Life (Wo De Qian Ban Sheng*, its English edition being first published by the Foreign Languages Press in 1964 under the title *From Emperor to Citizen*), which included some discussions on TCM that may be used for reference.

In 1909, the first year of Emperor Xuantong, I was just over ten years old.

The whole country was mourning the death of Empress Dowager Cixi and Emperor Guangxu. My memories are still fresh about those days. For three months, no one was allowed to get a hair-cut, wear colourful clothes or attend any traditional entertainments such as Peking opera. It was not allowed to slaughter any pigs or sheep. Hearsay was that Emperor Guangxu, who had been ill for a considerable length of time, had been murdered by Empress Dowager Cixi and the eunuch Li Lianying. Others believed that he had not received proper medical treatment. The fairly complete collection of Emperor Guangxu's pulse files may help to solve the puzzle. It was also said that Emperor Tongzhi had died of syphilis. But Professor Chen Keji said that neither the pulse files of Emperor Guangxu nor the diary of Weng Tonghe, the emperor's tutor, supported the rumour. It is apparent that the sorting out and study of the imperial medical files of the Qing Dynasty is necessary indeed. Such efforts will yield some realistic significance in carrying forward TCM knowledge and medical experience of the Qing Dynasty as well as in the study of Qing Dynasty history. I am hereby happy to contribute this preface, because I believe that the old imperial medical files offer us some new knowledge.

March 1981
Beijing

# PREFACE

## by Professor Zheng Tianting

More than two thousand years ago (28-25 B.C.) Liu Xiang and Liu Xin headed the editing of books in the Imperial Palace. They completed *Seven Concise Medical Versions (Qi Lue)*, comprising a collection of medical experience of 7 schools in a total of 216 volumes, and 11 schools of classical prescriptions in 274 volumes. All those books were proof-read by the well-known TCM practitioner of the time, Li Zhuguo. Six hundred years later "A Collection of Ancient Classics" in the *History of the Sui Dynasty (Sui Shu·Jing Ji Zhi)* was compiled. There was a collection of 256 groups of formulae in a total number of 4,511 volumes. Yet prescriptions for gynecological and obstetric conditions were excluded, for they were listed under the category of the five elements. Of course, these figures may not be precisely accurate. Medical versions popular among the common people may not have all been put into those collections. However, they clearly indicate that TCM studies and practice had started a very long time ago. Both became more and more developed as time passed by.

Similarly, the commencement of TCM diagnosis and treatment serving the general public is traced to many centuries ago. In the Western Han Dynasty there arose private TCM practitioners of family traditions and those officially employed according to "Recordings of Literature and Art" in the *History of the Han Dynasty (Han Shu·Yi Wen Zhi)*, and imperial physicians according to "Recordings of Literature and Art" in the *History of the Sui Dynasty (Sui Shu·Yi Wen Zhi)*. In the Eastern Han Dynasty there began the system of appointing special medical officials according to "Biography of Huatuo from Wei State Recordings" in the *History of the Three Kingdoms (San Guo Zhi·Wei Zhi·Hua Tuo Zhuan)*. Down to the Sui and Tang dynasties, the Imperial Palace had one medical department with a total of two hundred staff. There were also medicinal herb farmers, registered TCM doctors, massagists and teaching assistants besides veterinary surgeons according to "Official Ranks" in the *History of the Sui Dynasty (Sui Shu·Bai Guan Zhi Xia)*, indicating widespread involvement in the medical profession with an increase in social demand, plus other aspects of TCM development.

In the Qing Dynasty TCM underwent substantial development. The "Category of Medicine Under the Different Schools" in the *Complete Library of the Four Treasuries of Knowledge (Si Ku Quan Shu Zong Mu·Zi Bu·Yi Jia Lei)* consists of 96 medical volumes in 1,743 chapters, 94 items in 681 chapters, and 6 indexes in 26 parts. Yet the number of medical files that failed to be included was enormous.

The Qing Dynasty had its official Imperial Hospital, an independent sector under the direction of the Protocol Department, "in charge of issuing medical law papers and monitoring medical affairs." The Imperial Hospital made all decisions by itself except its enrolling of new staff, which required the endorsement of the director of the Protocol Department. The professional staff of the Imperial Hospital, known as medical officials, included the director, the deputy director, 15 imperial physicians, 30 administrators, 40 live-in doctors and 30 nurses.

The Imperial Hospital also had a teaching unit. Two imperial physicians or administrators with "high professional attainment and superb personality" were selected as teaching officials to conduct lectures. All who served the imperial medical profession and their offspring were required to receive professional study and training there. The director and deputy director might order them to sit for an examination at any time. Their medical textbooks, known as *The Three Books (San Shu)* made official in the early years of Emperor Yongzheng, consisted of *Comments on the Classified Medical Classics (Lei Jing Zhu Shi), Compendium of Materia Medica (Ben Cao Gang Mu)* and *Treatise on Febrile Diseases (Shang Han Lun).* These were adapted for literature courses as well. *Comments on the Classified Medical Classics* had been compiled by the physician Zhang Jingyue of the Ming Dynasty.

All medical staff of the Imperial Hospital from the director to the nurses were required to be on duty according to their professional positions in the palace. The duties were divided into internal and external. The former was on duty outside of the palace, known as palace duty. The latter was on duty at the East Pharmacy, known as the sixth duty.

In the early period of the Qing Dynasty, the Imperial Hospital had 11 departments, i.e. Major Pulse Department, Minor Pulse Department, Febrile Disease Department, Gynecological Department, Carbuncle and Furuncle Department, Acupuncture and Moxibustion Department, Ophthalmological Department, Dental Department, Throat Department, Bone-setting Department and Smallpox Department. In time the Smallpox Department was included in the Minor Pulse Department while the Throat Department merged with the Dental Department. In the mid-dynasty the Febrile Disease and Gynecological departments were included in the Major Pulse Department, while the original department for furuncles and carbuncles was renamed the External Therapy Department and the bone-setting and acupuncture departments closed. *The Official Decree of Guangxu Era (Hui Dian Shi Li)* says, "There exist now five departments, namely, Major Pulse, Minor Pulse, External Therapy, Ophthalmological and Dental departments." Such a restructuring of the Imperial Hospital was only a reflection of change in the number of different cases and in no way affects our present research.

According to the official decree of the Qing Dynasty, all medicines proposed for the emperor must first of all be presented in written prescription. Then, two doses of the same ingredients were decocted under the direct supervision of the deputy director of the hospital. When the decoctions were poured separately into two utensils, both the director and deputy director of the hospital first tasted the medicine before it was given to the emperor. The procedures were strict and formal, and the prescriptions were made with great caution. This procedure was followed even when the emperor was out on inspection tours around the country. Further, officials in charge of administering medical supplies for the imperial examinations, for soldiers on the front line, and for prisoners of war were also sent by the Imperial Hospital.

The work of the Qing Dynasty Imperial Hospital was arduous and strict. Physicians serving there had outstanding skills and rich practical experience, and the general public therefore showed great interest and respect for the imperial physicians' prescriptions. However, very strict discipline and penalties made it almost impossible for the prescriptions to be known in society. Over centuries few of these invaluable TCM experiences were known to ordinary Chinese people. Any attempt to sort them out and study them was unimaginable.

Recently, Chen Keji, Zhou Wenquan and Jiang Youli of Beijing's Xiyuan Hospital, and Shan Shikui and Xu Yipu of the First History Archives of China discovered piles of medical files of the Qing Dynasty Imperial Hospital while sorting out historical data of the Qing Dynasty. Upon systematizing these files, they compiled three books, i.e. *Studies of the Imperial Medical Files of the Qing Dynasty (Qing Gong Yi An Yan Jiu), Studies of the Imperial Medical Formulae of the Qing Dynasty (Qing Gong Pei Fang Yan Jiu)*, and *Commentary on Prescriptions for Empress Dowager Cixi and Emperor Guangxu (Cixi Guangxu Yi Fang Xuan Yi)*. I am very happy to know about those. Although my profession does not directly involve TCM I have great concern for the sorting out of the Qing Dynasty medical files, believing that data of older times can still in one way or another serve the present.

Medical knowledge is the common heritage of all races of the world, and medical studies in China have a very long history. TCM has been practised through millennia. The mechanism of TCM is profound and complex, requiring a special approach to understand it. The progression of TCM is inseparable from the accumulation of practical experience. Throughout history, many difficult diseases have remained unexplained, while detailed court medical files of the Qing Dynasty have been rarely seen. The publishing of this book will make a great contribution to the development of TCM.

Studies of the imperial medical files of the Qing Dynasty carried out by Professor Chen Keji and his working group will not only promote the development of TCM but will also help clarify various historical disputes. Even nowadays, people are not very clear whether Emperor Guangxu died of illness or of murder. Also, who died first, Empress Dowager Cixi or Emperor Guangxu? The sorting out of these case files will probably provide clues to some of these unsettled issues.

June 10, 1981

# PREFACE

## by Professor Ren Yingqiu

The establishment of medical departments in the Imperial Palace had been very formal since the early period of the feudal society down to the prime of the Qing Dynasty. *Zhou Dynasty Ethics and Principles (Zhou Li)* states, "The medical administrator was in charge of medical affairs and the collecting of materia medica. At the end of the year he would inspect the work done by practitioners to decide their salaries. A ten-point grading system was adopted to examine their annual practice. Ten was excellent, nine good, eight above average, seven average and six bad.

In order to prolong their life expectancy, feudal rulers made very exacting demand on medicine. The imperial medical files of the Qing Dynasty proved such a demand. Medicine itself is a branch of science maintaining both the health and prosperous regeneration of mankind. Xu Baisha in the Song Dynasty once said, "How vast and profound the medical principles are! They help people keep healthy, make the physical body fit and strong, prolong life expectancy, and benefit the mass population and future generations."

Medical science is shared by all and in the service of all. But in feudal society it was devoted to a few nobles. Ordinary people could barely survive poverty and disease. Living now in a socialist country, people enjoy the right to medical care. Both TCM and modern medicine are now practised in China. And the practice of TCM herbal medicine fits the country's economic situation and is therefore well accepted. Over the last few thousand years, TCM has made tremendous contributions to the development and prosperity of the Chinese nation. To further develop TCM the search and sorting-out of the priceless treasure of TCM and pharmacology, the integration of TCM and modern medicine, and TCM study by means of modern science and technology have become an urgent task. Such efforts will make TCM better serve the cause of socialist construction. The First History Archives of China keeps a large number of imperial medical files of the Qing Dynasty. To sort out these data and make them known to the public as proposed by Professor Chen Keji, will be highly significant. It means making the medicine that used to serve feudal rulers return to serve ordinary people.

Formulae officially recognized by the feudal dynasties or used in the imperial hospitals were generally reliable. For example, more than 700 formulae published in Imperial Grace Formulary of the Taiping Era *(Tai Ping Hui Min He Ji Ju Fang)* were selected and verified by famous Imperial Hospital doctors of the time. Then, based on those formulae, patent medicines were made and sold. At the same time, hand-engraved recipes were handed down for future generations. Traditionally proved and effective remedies such as Greatest Treasure Special Pill (Zhi Bao Dan), Heart-heat Clearing Pill (Qing Xin Wan), Four Substances Decoction (Si Wu Tang), and Four Gentlemen Decoction (Si Jun Zi Tang) are still used. Mistakes did occur in copying them so many times through the ages. Bezoar Pill to Clear Heart (Niu Huang Qing Xin Wan), for instance, was taken for Rhizoma Dioscoreae Pill (Shan Yao Wan) and vice versa. Misinterpreted medicinal properties have not yet been corrected. Worth mentioning was the strictness exercised by Empress Dowager Cixi in her attitude towards herbal medicine. In an article by Princess De Ling entitled "The True Story of the Personal Life of Empress Dowager Cixi" published by *Shanghai Daily (Shen Bao)* in 1936 the section on the imperial physicians said that once when Empress Dowager Cixi was ill and summoned four imperial physicians to diagnose her, four separate prescriptions were written and handed in to the eunuch Li Lianying for Cixi's approval. Another eunuch in charge of medical books was then called in to double-check each ingredient used in the similar prescriptions from *Standards for Syndrome Differentiation and Treatment (Zheng Zhi Zhun Shen)* and *Compendium of Materia Medica (Ben Cao Gang Mu)*. A fifth prescription finally met her approval. Should anything unexpected happen, none of the four imperial physicians could shirk responsibility. The author De Ling was one of the princesses closest to the Empress Dowager, and some of the accounts could be from her personal experience and therefore largely reliable. All such prescriptions may also be in the files. Strict differentiation should be made in sorting out the data. Some 297 prescriptions approved in *Imperial Grace Formulary of the Taiping Era* by Chen Shiwen and Pei Zongyuan were very popular at the time when Zhu Danxi was also a noted TCM doctor. Zhu believed what they did was to "just take ancient formulae to deal with diseases while in reality they did not exactly fit even the old situation." Zhu Danxi meant those who only followed the ancient remedies blindly. He did not blame the book itself. Since now efforts will be made in sorting out the imperial medical files of the Qing Dynasty, we should first study the formation and composition of those prescriptions in order to find out whether they were worked out in line with TCM mechanisms. These prescriptions should then be applied in clinical practice to see if they were suitable. After repeated clinical proof of the therapeutic effects, some of the prescriptions could be recommended on a larger scale in clinical practice. I think this is the scientific way to do it.

Su Wenzhong said, long ago, "Prescriptions written by TCM doctors may not necessarily be their own, for most were formulated by their ancestors. However, they can be applied on a large scale provided they produce therapeutic effects in practice." The key to determining a prescription lies therefore mainly in the efforts made to observe its therapeutic effects. Xu Shuwei called the formulae books he had *Origin Tracing Books (Ben Shi Fang)*, meaning that his prescriptions traced back to original sources of therapeutic reference.

Sun Simiao also acknowledged, "Having read formulae books for three years, I started to believe that no disease was beyond my expertise to deal with. Yet, after spending three years in treating patients I came to understand there was no single prescription ready to be simply copied."

"It is easy to acquire a thousand prescriptions," he said, "but difficult to achieve a single cure." This view has been similar to those held by practitioners of TCM throughout history. The sorting out of imperial medical files of the Qing Dynasty by Professor Chen Keji and his colleagues will enable these ancient prescriptions to better serve the people today. The results of these outstanding prescriptions can be clearly stated in terms of their therapeutic mechanism and effect. This will be a project beneficial to the country, the professional domain of TCM and to patients.

April 1981
Beijing College of TCM

# PREFACE

## by Professor Deng Tietao

The feudal emperors, enjoying enormously the prosperity and wealth of the era, all wished to live forever. Much stress was laid on health care for the ruling house. TCM standards of the Imperial Palace were no doubt the highest of the time. However, serving as imperial physicians was like sleeping with tigers. In such extremely special circumstances, demonstrating an imperial physician's best healing talent depended on who he was and when he was practising. Li Shizhen once resigned as chief of the Imperial Hospital because he could not bear the life of an imperial physician. Liu Hejian was regarded noble for turning down three invitations by Emperor Zhangzong of the Jin Dynasty (1115-1234) to be an imperial physician.

It was said that the imperial physicians serving the Qing Dynasty were recommended by local governments. No local official would dare to recommend any ordinary candidate to serve as physician in the Imperial Palace. Thus TCM reached another golden age in the Qing Dynasty. It was only after the first Opium War, especially during the KMT regime, that TCM practice encountered discrimination and could not develop further until 1949. The efforts of Professor Chen Keji and his colleagues will make the imperial medical files at the First History Archives of China available to the public. The realization of this research project is extremely significant.

Presenting empirical prescriptions handed down in families to emperors was one way to gain royal favour. Secret prescriptions of the Imperial Palace have always attracted many people. The publishing of *Imperial Medicaments—Medical Prescriptions Written for Empress Dowager Cixi and Emperor Guangxu With Commentary (Cixi Guangxu Yi Fang Xuan Yi)* is to be followed by another two volumes, i.e. *Studies of the Imperial Medical Files of the Qing Dynasty (Qing Gong Yi An Yan Jiu)*, and *Studies of the Imperial Medical Formulae of the Qing Dynasty (Qing Gong Yi Fang Yan Jiu)*. These books present prescriptions for Empress Dowager Cixi and Emperor Guangxu, most of which were undoubtedly effective. With comments and corrections made by the editors on the origin and actions of these prescriptions they will be of invaluable help to readers and researchers.

The books may help readers understand the professional level and style of imperial physicians, reflect the health conditions of the imperial family, and medical requirements. They will also be useful for historians.

A large number of prescriptions for Empress Dowager Cixi were for treating aging conditions. These deserve further geriatric studies, which were greatly emphasized in the Qing Dynasty Imperial Palace.

Many prescriptions proposed for Emperor Guangxu were to treat his deficiency. Many emperors of older times led luxurious and unrestrained lives and relied heavily on TCM to maintain health. This is also an interesting subject in the study of imperial medicine.

All emperors had a rich life with good food and little physical exercise, giving rise to early decline in their cardiovascular functions. This book also suggests ways to cope with such problems. Apart from internal remedies, special attention was given to external treatment for diseases caused by a life of ease. In addition to hair-growth tonics, herbal baths and shampoos, the formulae for external application also deserve further study. External application therapy was to many imperial physicians a rather passive choice, for it involved less risk and safeguarded the imperial physicians. Sustained use and summarizing of the external applications promoted the therapy itself. Meanwhile, the indications for external application were more, another feature of the imperial medical practice.

Studies of the imperial medicine of the Qing Dynasty will be significant in TCM research. Hereby, I would like to contribute this preface for the book.

April 1981
Guangzhou

# PREFACE

## by Professor Gen Jianting

In the early 1980s, TCM research that would mark a page in history was the systematic sorting-out and laboratory proof of the imperial medical and pharmaceutical files of the Qing Dynasty. The work was headed by Professor Chen Keji. The systematic study and analysis of these TCM data will make possible their continued service, though now in the health care of ordinary people. This will be a major event not only at the China Academy of TCM, but nation-wide. The studies will inevitably contribute historically to TCM academics.

Since the birth of New China in 1949 a spate of old medical data and objects have been unearthed. Moreover, the imperial medical files of the Qing Dynasty, sealed for decades and of unprecedented number and quality, are now open to the public. Throughout history all imperial palaces established imperial medical departments whose documents were never included in the histories of feudal dynasties but were forbidden to be released outside the palaces. Ordinary people knew almost nothing about them. There might well have been certain rumours or anecdotes, but these were not in the official history. They neither reflect the situation of imperial medical files nor stand for any credibility. The imperial medical files of the Qing Dynasty were enormous in number from the early emperors Shunzhi and Kangxi to the later emperors Guangxu and Xuantong. The medical data for emperors Tongzhi, Guangxu and those for Empress Dowager Cixi are particularly complete, and it is therefore imperative to carry them forward.

It was believed that Emperor Shunzhi died of smallpox. Emperor Kangxi was crowned because he survived the disease. From then on greater attention was paid to developing imperial medicine. In the era of Yongzheng and Qianlong there appeared a version of *Golden Mirror of the Medical Tradition (Yi Zong Jin Jian)* revised by the medical department of the Imperial Palace. The book also included some of the prescriptions used there.

Life in the Imperial Palace was different from that led by the man on the street. Herbal medicines used in the palace were of better quality than those ordinarily used, and such a difference should be recognized. Imperial physicians had family traditions of practising TCM. Those who were promoted as imperial physicians must be outstanding in theory and practice besides standing high in literary attainment. In differentiation and treatment they must demonstrate logical consideration in therapeutic principle and method, plus appropriate writing of prescriptions, especially in treating chronic illnesses.

Medicines stored at the imperial pharmacy were cautiously selected. Much emphasis was given to the place of collection and quality. Written records were also available concerning the specific doses and strict preparation of the medicines in addition to actual samples for reference. Eight different substances were used to check the accuracy of the scales.

The design of this research project is not simply to carry out systematic studies and produce academic papers. It is more important to make clinical studies and collect cases in order to summarize therapeutic effects. In this way dead TCM data can serve the living, and successful experience can be widely applied in clinical practice, thus "weeding through the old to bring forth the new" and "making the ancient serve the present," as Mao Zedong put it.

April 1981
China Academy of TCM

## Part One
# MEDICAL PRESCRIPTIONS WRITTEN FOR EMPRESS DOWAGER CIXI WITH COMMENTARY

## I. LONGEVITY PRESCRIPTIONS

### I.1. HEART-NOURISHING LONGEVITY PILL

The prescription for Heart-nourishing Longevity Pill (Yang Xin Yan Ling Yi Shou Dan) was prepared by imperial physicians Zhuang Shouhe and Li Dechang on the 9th of the 11th month of the lunar calendar in 1875.

*Ingredients*

| | |
|---|---|
| Radix Poria (Fu Shen) | 15 g |
| Semen Biotae (Bai Zi Ren) | 12 g |
| Radix Codopsis Pilosulae (Dan Shen) | 12 g |
| Radix Paeoniae Lactiflorae (Bai Shao) | 12 g |
| Cotex Moudan Radicis (Dan Pi) | 12 g |
| Radix Angelicae Sinensis (Quan Dang Gui) | 15 g |
| Rhizoma Ligustici Chuanxiong (Chuan Xiong) | 6 g |
| Radix Rehmanniae (Sheng Di Huang) | 12 g |
| Unidentified | |
| Unidentified | |
| Fructus Gardeniae (Shan Zhi Zi) | 9 g |
| Radix Scutellariae (Huang Qin) | 9 g |
| Pericarpium Citri Reticulatae (Chen Pi) | 9 g |
| Rhizoma Atractylodis Macrocephalae (Bai Zhu) | 6 g |
| Fructus Aurantii (Zhi Ke) | 12 g |
| Semen Ziziphi Spinosae (Suan Zao Ren) | 12 g |

According to original records, the Semen Biotae, Rhizoma Actractylodis Macrocephalae, Fructus Aurantii and Semen Ziziphi Spinosae should be roasted before use. The Radix Angelicae Sinensis should be roasted with millet wine. The Radix Rehmanniae (dried) should be washed in millet wine. And the Rhizoma Atractylodis Macrocephalae should be the wild variety.

The above ingredients were processed into fine powder and made in pill form with refined honey in the size of mung beans. Nine grams of Cinnabari-coated pills were taken with boiled water each time.

*Comments*

Heart-nourishing Longevity Pill was prepared by imperial physicians on the basis of modifying ingredients in Semen Biotae Heart-nourishing Pill (Bai Zi Yang Xin Wan) as recorded in *Compilation of Materials of Benefit to the Body (Ti Ren*

*Hui Bian*), written by Peng Yongguang of the Ming Dynasty (1368-1644), and ingredients in Cinnabari Tranquilizing Pill (Zhu Sha An Shen Wan) first processed by Li Jinzhi. It acts to nourish the heart, calm the heart and mind, and reinforce kidney Yin. It was used in the treatment of insomnia, poor memory, palpitation and dream-disturbed sleep due to over-strain and stress or blood deficiency. Today it has remarkable effects in treating neurasthenia.

Although Empress Dowager Cixi was aged 40 in 1875, the cruel reality, such as the untimely death of Emperor Tongzhi and attendance to state affairs, had definitely aggravated the above symptoms and signs. According to the existing health record of Empress Dowager Cixi, she suffered from chronic "deficiency of the heart and spleen," "emaciation with occasional lack of energy and weakness of the whole body," "weakening voice during much talking," "low spirits that caused difficulty in falling asleep," and heart and kidney Yin deficiency manifested by "feverish sensation in the lumbar region and soles at night," "dryness in the throat," and "occasional sore throat." This prescription is good for nourishing the heart and is also highly recommended for extending life span.

## I.2. GREAT LONGEVITY PILL

The prescription for Great Longevity Pill (Yan Ling Yi Shou Dan) was carefully prepared by imperial physician Li Dechang on the 18th day of the first month of the lunar calendar in 1880.

### Ingredients

| | |
|---|---:|
| Radix Poria  (Fu Shen) | 15 g |
| Radix Polygalae  (Yuan Zhi) | 9 g |
| Radix Paeoniae Lactiflorae  (Bai Shao) | 12 g |
| Radix Angelicae Sinensis  (Dang Gui) | 15 g |
| Radix Codonopsis Pilosulae  (Dang Shen) | 12 g |
| Radix Astragali seu Hedysari  (Huang Qi) | 9 g |
| Rhizoma Atractylodis Macrocephalae  (Bai Zhu) | 12 g |
| Poria  (Fu Ling) | 15 g |
| Pericarpium Citri Reticulatae  (Ju Pi) | 12 g |
| Rhizoma Cyperi  (Xiang Fu) | 12 g |
| Radix Auchlandiae  (Mu Xiang) | 9 g |
| Fructus Amomi  (Sha Ren) | 9 g |
| Arillus Longan  (Gui Yuan) | 9 g |
| Semen Ziziphi Spinosae  (Suan Zao Ren) | 12 g |
| Rhizoma Acori Graminei  (Shi Chang Pu) | 9 g |
| Radix Glycyrrhizae  (Gan Cao) | 6 g |

According to original records, roasted Radix Paeoniae Lactiflorae collected in Hangzhou should be used. Both the Radix Angelicae Sinensis and Radix Astragali seu Hedysari should be roasted until seared yellow. Also, wild Rhizoma Atractylodis Macrocephalae should be used, as should the Fructus Amomi and Radix Auchlandiae collected from Guangdong.

The above ingredients were processed into fine powder and made in Cinnabari-coated, honeyed pills in the size of mung beans. Eight grams of the pill were taken with boiled water each time.

### Comments

Great Longevity Pill was prepared on the basis of modifying ingredients in the Spleen-governing Pill (Gui Pi Wan) recorded in *Formulae for the Living* (Ji Sheng Fang) by Yan Yonghe of the Song Dynasty (960-1279). It was then prescribed for the treatment of poor function of the spleen in governing blood or thinking too much affecting both the heart and spleen. The clinical manifestations include poor appetite, poor memory, loose stools, anxiety, palpitation and insomnia. It was also recommended for the treatment of irregular menstruation and leukorrhea in women.

In the prescription, Radix Codonopsis Pilosulae, Radix Astragali seu Hedysari, Rhizoma Atractylodis Macrocephalae, Radix Glycyrrhizae, Poria and Radix Poria reinforce the spleen because of their common warming property and sweet flavour. Radix Angelicae Sinensis, Radix Polygalae, Semen Ziziphi Spinosae and Arillus Longan moisten and nourish the heart. Rhizoma Acori Graminei and Rhizoma Cyperi aid in promoting the mechanism of *qi* (vital energy) in addition to the use of Radix Auchlandiae. It is therefore believed to be a highly useful remedy in extending women's life expectancy.

The health records of Empress Dowager Cixi in 1880 contain many such symptoms as "poor digestion after food intake and loose pasty stools," "poor appetite," "general weakness of the body," "general lassitude," and "chronic deficiency of the heart and spleen." This prescription was specially prepared for the above-mentioned conditions.

## I.3. ETERNAL SPRING LONGEVITY PILL

Eternal Spring Longevity Pill (Chang Chun Yi Shou Dan) was presented for imperial use on the fifth day of the second month of the lunar calendar in 1880.

### Ingredients

| | |
|---|---|
| Radix Asparagi  (Tian Men Dong) | 60 g |
| Radix Ophiopogonis  (Mai Men Dong) | 60 g |
| Radix Rehmanniae Praeparatae  (Shu Di Huang) | 60 g |
| Rhizoma Dio  (Shan Yao) | 60 g |
| Radix Achyranthis Bidentatae  (Niu Xi) | 60 g |
| Radix Rehmanniae  (Sheng Di Huang) | 60 g |
| Cortex Eucommiae  (Du Zhong) | 60 g |
| Fructus Corni  (Shan Zhu Yu) | 60 g |
| Poria  (Fu Ling) | 60 g |
| Radix Ginseng  (Ren Shen) | 60 g |
| Radix Auchlandiae  (Mu Xiang) | 60 g |
| Semen Biotae  (Bai Zi Ren) | 60 g |
| Fructus Schisandrae  (Wu Wei Zi) | 60 g |
| Radix Morindae Officinalis  (Ba Ji Tian) | 60 g |
| Pericarpium Zanthoxyli  (Chuan Jiao) | 30 g |
| Rhizoma Alismatis  (Ze Xie) | 30 g |
| Rhizoma Acori Graminei  (Shi Chang Pu) | 30 g |

| Radix Polygalae  (Yuan Zhi) | 30 g |
| Semen Cuscutae  (Tu Si Zi) | 120 g |
| Herba Cistanchis  (Rou Cong Rong) | 120 g |
| Fructus Lycii  (Gou Qi Zi) | 45 g |
| Fructus Rubi  (Fu Pen Zi) | 45 g |
| Cortex Lycii Radicis  (Di Gu Pi) | 45 g |

The original recipe calls for the kernel of the Radix Asparagi and Radix Ophiopogonis to be removed before use. Neither the Radix Rehmanniae Praeparatae nor the Radix Rehmanniae should be processed in iron utensils. The Pericarpium Zanthoxyli should be roasted, and the oily substance from the Semen Biotae should be separated out.

The above ingredients were processed in fine powder and mixed with honey and made into pills the size of the Chinese umbrella tree seeds. On starting the course of treatment, only 50 pills were taken each time. One month later the dosage was increased to 60 pills. After 100 days the dosage was further increased to 80 pills. When the effect of the remedy was observed, it was suggested to be taken early in the morning with salty water before breakfast.

### Comments

Eternal Spring Longevity Pill was prepared by modifying the ingredients in the ancient prescription for Yang's Rejuvenating Pill (Yang Shi Huan Shao Dan) and Hua Tuo's Beating the Youngest Son Pill (Da Lao Er Wan). The words "Eternal Spring" were added to the nomenclature of the remedy. It was believed to be related to the fact that Empress Dowager Cixi lived in the Eternal Spring Palace. Ingredients in this prescription greatly reinforce the heart, kidney and stomach, strengthen bones and tendons, and nourish Yin and Yang. It was recorded that long-time use of the pill helped blacken the hair, invigorate the spirit, and strengthen the lower limbs. It was therefore prescribed for weakness of the body, lumbar soreness and general lassitude.

Some of the ingredients in the prescription were originally in Beating the Youngest Son Pill. The pill was thus named because it was related to a folk tale which goes like this: A centenarian woman had to beat her youngest son for his reluctance to take a kind of herbal pill that was supposed to be good for curing his illness, and so was later named Beating the Youngest Son Pill. Another name for the pill was Sorceress Beating Her Youngest Son Pill (Xian Gu Da Lao Er Wan). Women may also take it for its effect in warming the uterus and adding luster to the face by moistening the skin.

## I.4.  LONGEVITY OINTMENT

The prescription for Longevity Ointment (Yi Shou Gao) was formulated by the imperial physician Li Hongzao on the 24th day of the fifth month of the lunar calendar in 1881.

### Ingredients

| Radix Aconiti Praeparatae  (Fu Zi) | 90 g |
| Cortex Cinnamomi  (Rou Gui) | 90 g |

| | |
|---|---|
| Rhizoma Pinelliae Praeparatae (Fa Ban Xia) | 30 g |
| Pericarpium Citri Reticulatae (Chen Pi) | 30 g |
| Sheep kidney (Yang Yao) | 3 pairs |
| Os Tigris (Hu Gu) | 240 g |
| Fructus Evodiae (Wu Zhu Yu) | 30 g |
| Pericarpium Zanthoxyli (Chuan Jiao) | 30 g |
| Rhizoma Typhonii Gigantei (Bai Fu Zi) | 30 g |
| Fructus Foeniculi (Xiao Hui Xiang) | 30 g |
| Rhizoma Atractylodis Macrocephalae (Bai Zhu) | 90 g |
| Rhizoma Atractylodis (Cang Zhu) | 60 g |
| Folium Artemisiae Argyi (Ai Rong) | 30 g |
| Radix Angelicae Sinensis (Dang Gui) | 90 g |
| Fructus Psoraleae (Po Gu Zhi) | 60 g |
| Rhizoma Cyperi (Xiang Fu) | 45 g |
| Rhizoma Ligustici Chuanxiong (Chuan Xiong) | 45 g |
| Cortex Eucommiae (Du Zhong) | 120 g |
| Radix Scrophulariae (Xu Duan) | 60 g |
| Radix Morindae Officinalis (Ba Ji Tian) | 30 g |
| Radix Astragali seu Hedysari (Huang Qi) | 45 g |
| Radix Codonopsis Pilosulae (Dang Shen) | 45 g |
| Rhizoma Cyperi Praeparatae (Zhi Xiang Fu) | 45 g |
| Rhizoma Dio (Shao Yao) | 30 g |
| Cortex Acanthopanacis Radicis (Wu Jia Pi) | 45 g |
| Fructus Alpiniae Oxyphylla (Yi Zhi Ren) | 30 g |
| Fructus Tribuli (Ji Li) | 45 g |
| Fructus Meliae Toosendan (Chuan Lian Zi) | 30 g |
| Ramulus Cinnamomi (Gui Zhi) | 30 g |
| Sulphur (Liu Huang) | 90 g |
| Cervi Taille (Lu Wei) | 3 |
| Semen Trigonella (Hu Lu Ba) | 30 g |
| Radix Aconiti (Chuan Wu) | 30 g |
| Cornu Cervi (Lu Jiao) | 240 g |
| Poria (Fu Ling) | 60 g |
| Rhizoma Dioscoreae Septemlobae (Bi Xie) | 30 g |
| Semen Myristicae (Rou Dou Kou) | 45 g |
| Semen Cuscutae (Tu Si Zi) | 30 g |
| Rhizoma Zingiberis (Gan Jiang) | 30 g |
| Herba Artemisiae Capilaris (Yin Chen) | 30 g |
| Semen Juglandis (Hu Tao Rou) | 60 g |
| Flos Syzygii Aromatici (Gong Ding Xiang) | 30 g |
| Rhizoma Zingiberis Recens (Sheng Jiang) | 90 g |
| Fructus Schisandrae (Wu Wei Zi) | 30 g |
| Fructus Lycii (Gou Qi Zi) | 60 g |
| Fructus Allii Fistulosi (Da Cong Tou) | 90 g |
| Fructus Amomi (Sha Ren) | 30 g |
| Radix Glycyrrhizae (Gan Cao) | 30 g |

According to original records, the Fructus Evodiae and Cortex Eucommiae should be roasted with salty water. The Radix Angelicae Sinensis should be washed in millet wine, and the sulphur should be ground into fine powder in a mortar.

These ingredients were well fried in 7.2 kg of sesame oil. After separating out the herbal residue, the remaining oil was further concentrated until the oil drops appeared like drops of water in freezing weather. This was followed by mixing the oil with 2.7 kg of powdered red lead that had been prepared in water.

On the 22nd day of the third month of the lunar calendar in 1885, an imperial edict was issued to change the name of this prescription prepared by the imperial physician Li Hongzao into Longevity Ointment.

### Comments

Ingredients in this prescription add up to a total of 50, most of which act to warm and reinforce kidney Yang. Many produce tremendous therapeutic effects. The chapter "Body Energy Communicating with Heaven in *Plain Questions* (Su Wen Sheng Qi Tong Tian Lun) says, "Yang of the body is like the sun and heaven. Man's life expectancy will be shortened when such energy is reduced." The gist of Yin-Yang is that "the body will be firm and strong when Yang *qi* is rich." The above record clearly indicates the importance of Yang energy in the body. Kidney *qi*, also known as inborn energy, has drawn the attention of physicians of traditional Chinese medicine throughout history. Kidney Yin and Yang are also called primary Yin and Yang. Reinforcing the energy of the kidney, therefore, helps strengthen the body's constitution.

Referring to the use of Longevity Ointment prepared by the imperial physician Li Dechang on the 20th day of the leap fourth month of the lunar calendar in 1887 on the basis of modifying the prescription for Longevity Syrup made by another imperial physician, Li Hongzao, it is clear that such a herbal plaster was applied externally to the lumbar region and umbilicus to treat lumbar and abdominal pain, leukorrhea and menstrual disorders. Empress Dowager Cixi had menstrual complaints even during her youth (refer to Cixi's Menstruation-regulating Pill). Similar descriptions were found in her health records when she was middle-aged. For instance, the record on the first day of the ninth month of the lunar calendar in 1880 states, "*Qi* deficiency of the heart and spleen and liver-*qi* stagnation caused soreness and pain in the lumbar region, legs and knees during menstruation, plus general lassitude after meals." In fact she suffered from chronic back pain and poor digestion, and this prescription was suitable in her case.

## I.5. LONGEVITY OINTMENT PLUS

The specific date for the preparation of this Longevity Ointment Plus (Yi Shou Gao You Fang) remains unknown.

### Ingredients

| | |
|---|---|
| Radix Aconiti Praeparatae  (Zhi Fu Zi) | 30 g |
| Cortex Cinnamomi  (Rou Gui) | 30 g |
| Rhizoma Pinelliae Praeparatae  (Fa Ban Xia) | 10 g |
| Pericarpium Citri Reticulatae  (Chen Pi) | 10 g |
| Rhizoma Typhonii Gigantei  (Bai Fu Zi) | 10 g |
| Sheep kidney  (Yang Yao) | 1 pair |
| Os Tigris  (Hu Gu) | 80 g |

Fructus Evodiae  (Wu Zhu Yu)                                    10 g
Pericarpium Zanthoxyli  (Chuan Jiao)                            10 g
Fructus Foeniculi  (Xiao Hui Xiang)                            10 g
Rhizoma Atractylodis Macrocephalae  (Bai Zhu)                  30 g
Rhizoma Atractylodis  (Cang Zhu)                               20 g
Folium Artemisiae Argyi  (Ai Rong)                            10 g
Radix Angelicae Sinensis  (Dang Gui)                          30 g
Fructus Psoralae  (Po Gu Zhi)                                 20 g
Rhizoma Cyperi Praeparatae  (Zhi Xiang Fu)                    15 g
Rhizoma Ligustici Chuanxiong  (Chuan Xiong)                   15 g
Cortex Eucommiae (Du Zhong)                                   40 g
Radix Dipsaci  (Xu Duan)                                      20 g
Radix Scrophulariae  (Ba Ji Tian)                            10 g
Radix Astragali seu Hedysari  (Huang Qi)                      15 g
Radix Codonopsis Pilosulae  (Dang Shen)                       15 g
Radix Paeoniae Lactiflorae  (Bai Shao)                        10 g
Sulphur  (Liu Huang)                                          30 g
Fructus Alpiniae Oxyphylla  (Yi Zhi)                          10 g
Cervi Taille  (Lu Wei)                                           1
Fructus Melliae Toosendan  (Chuan Lian Zi)                    10 g
Ramulus Cinnamomi  (Gui Zhi)                                  10 g
Cortex Acanthopanacis Radicis  (Wu Jia Pi)                    15 g
Poria  (Fu Ling)                                              20 g
Semen Trigonella  (Hu Lu Ba)                                  10 g
Radix Aconiti  (Chuan Wu)                                     10 g
Cornu Cervi  (Lu Jiao)                                        80 g
Fructus Tribuli  (Ji Li)                                      15 g
Rhizoma Dioscoreae Seplemobae  (Bi Xie)                       10 g
Semen Myristicae  (Rou Dou Kou)                               15 g
Semen Cuscutae  (Tu Si Zi)                                    10 g
Rhizoma Zingiberis  (Gan Jiang)                               10 g
Herba Artemisisae Capillaris  (Yin Chen Hao)                  10 g
Semen Juglandis  (Hu Tao Rou)                                 20 g
Flos Syzygii Aromatici  (Gong Ding Xiang)                     10 g
Rhizoma Zingiberis Recens  (Sheng Jiang)                      30 g
Fructus Schisandrae  (Wu Wei Zi)                              10 g
Fructus Lycii  (Gou Qi Zi)                                    20 g
Fructus Allii Fistulosi  (Da Cong Tou)                        30 g
Fructus Amomi  (Sha Ren)                                      10 g
Radix Glycyrrhizae  (Gan Cao)                                 10 g

According to original records, the Fructus Evodiae and Cortex Eucommiae should be roasted with salty water. The Radix Angelicae Sinensis should be washed in millet wine, and the sulphur should be ground into fine powder in a mortar.

These ingredients were well fried in 2.4 kg of sesame oil. After separating out the herbal residue the remaining oil was further concentrated until its drops fell like drops of water in freezing weather. This was followed by mixing it with 0.9 kg powdered red lead that was also prepared in water. This remedy was recommended for patients of different ages.

*Comments*

Compared with the composition of the last remedy, Longevity Ointment Plus leaves out only the ingredient Rhizoma Cyperi. The amount of each ingredient is about a third of the previous one. Yet it is quite similar to Longevity Ointment in terms of actions and indications.

## I.6. VITAL ENERGY-PRESERVING LONGEVITY PILL

The prescription for Vital Energy-preserving Longevity Pill (Bao Yuan Yi Shou Dan) was carefully prepared by the imperial physicians Zhuang Shouhe, Li Dechang and Wang Yinrui on the 26th day of the 11th month of the lunar calendar in 1882.

*Ingredients*

| | |
|---|---|
| Radix Ginseng  (Ren Shen) | 9 g |
| Rhizoma Atractylodis Macrocephalae  (Bai Zhu) | 9 g |
| Poria  (Fu Ling) | 15 g |
| Radix Angelicae Sinensis  (Dang Gui) | 12 g |
| Radix Paeoniae Lactiflorae  (Bai Shao) | 6 g |
| Radix Rehmanniae  (Sheng Di Huang) | 12 g |
| Pericarpium Citri Reticulatae  (Chen Pi) | 4.5 g |
| Fructus Amomi  (Sha Ren) | 3 g |
| Radix Bupleuri  (Chai Hu) | 3 g |
| Rhizoma Cyperi  (Xiang Fu) | 6 g |
| Radix Platycodi  (Jie Gen) | 6 g |
| Cortex Eucommiae  (Du Zhong) | 12 g |
| Ramulus Mori  (Sang Zhi) | 12 g |
| Fructus Oryzae Germinature  (Gu Ya) | 12 g |
| Semen Coicis  (Yi Yi Ren) | 15 g |
| Radix Glycyrrhizae  (Gan Cao) | 3 g |

According to original records, the Rhizoma Atractylodis Macrocephalae, Radix Paeoniae Lactiflorae, Cortex Eucommiae, Semen Coicis and Fructus Oryzae Germinature should be roasted, and the Radix Bupleuri prepared with vinegar, while processed Rhizoma Cyperi and Radix Glycyrrhizae should be used.

The above ingredients were ground into powder for internal use, and 4.5 grams of the powder were taken orally each time with congee made from the former year's rice.

*Comments*

After careful study for eight months on the 1882 health records of Empress Dowager Cixi it is clear that she suffered from chronic deficiencies of *qi* and blood and constitutional spleen. "Poor appetite, light sleep at night, slow digestion, occasional dizziness, belching and discomfort in the stomach at night, lack of energy and general lassitude, and loose stools with abdominal distention" are some of her complaints. This prescription was modified on the basis of Eight Treasures Pill (Ba Zhen Wan) in an attempt to nourish *qi* and blood, soothe the liver, and regulate the spleen and stomach. Dealing with both symptomatic (Biao) and root cause (Ben), it was administered to build up the source of *qi* and blood.

# I.7. LONGEVITY-PRESERVING OINTMENT

The prescription for Longevity-preserving Ointment (Yan Nian Yi Shou Gao) was prepared by the imperial physician Li Dechang on the 20th day of the leap fourth month of the lunar calendar in 1887. It was first prepared by Li Hongzao, who included natural sulphur in the recipe.

This ointment was made for dealing with cold-damp in the channels and collaterals, relaxing tendons and activating blood, reinforcing Yang, and nourishing Yin. It was used for the various types of deficiencies such as aversion to cold and cold feet with dampness retention, Wei and Bi syndromes, lumbar soreness, painful legs and joints, traumatic injuries, and damaged tendons and bones due to falling from a horse. It was also used in treating various types of chronic trauma, congenital deficiency and acquired malnutrition, deficiency cold in the spleen and kidney manifested as lack of energy, weak legs, tinnitus, pale complexion, emaciation, abdominal distention, edema, deficiency conditions manifested by irregular menstruation and disfunctional uterine bleeding. The plaster was for external use only, on the lumbar region or in the umbilicus. During its application the patients should avoid overstrain, overstress and exposure to cold.

*Comments*

The explanation of the prescription says that it could be applied in the treatment of "irregular menstruation, leukorrhea and disfunctional uterine bleeding." As a matter of fact it may also be taken into consideration for the treatment of other types of endogenous and exogenous diseases seen in clinical practice.

# I.8. VITAL ENERGY-REINFORCING LONGEVITY OINTMENT

The Old Buddha's (Emperess Dowager Cixi's) Vital Energy-reinforcing Longevity Ointment (Lao Fo Ye Pei Yuan Yi Shou Gao) was prepared on the second day of the fourth month of the lunar calendar in 1904.

*Ingredients*

| | |
|---|---|
| Sulphur (Liu Huang) | 18 g |
| Radix Aconiti (Fu Zi) | 15 g |
| Pericarpium Zanthoxyli (Chuan Jiao) | 30 g |
| Radix Rehmanniae Praeparatae (Shu Di Huang) | 30 g |
| Fructus Litseae Cubebae (She Chuan Zi) | 18 g |
| Semen Allii (Jiu Cai Zi) | 18 g |
| Radix Polycopi (Yuan Zhi) | 12 g |
| Radix Angelicae Sinensis (Dang Gui) | 18 g |
| Semen Sesami (Hei Zhi Ma) | 30 g |
| Semen Cuscutae (Tu Si Zi) | 15 g |
| Radix Achyranthis Bidentatae (Niu Xi) | 15 g |
| Os Tigris (Hu Gu) | 15 g |
| Rhizoma seu Radix Notopterygii (Qiang Huo) | 12 g |
| Rhizoma Atractylodis (Cang Zhu) | 18 g |
| Radix Scrophulariae (Xu Duan) | 12 g |
| Ramulus Mori (Sang Zhi) | 30 g |
| Caulis Aristolochia Debilis (Tian Xian Teng) | 15 g |

| Rhizoma Curcumae Longae  (Jiang Huang) | 15 g |
| Cortex Cinnamomi  (Rou Gui) | 15 g |
| Cornu Cervi Pantotrichum  (Lu Rong) | 15 g |
| Moschus  (She Xiang) | 3 g |

According to original records, the Cortex Cinnamomi, Cornu Cervi Pantotrichum and Moschus should be ground into fine powder and added after the other ingredients were processed.

The above ingredients were immersed in 3.84 kg of sesame oil for 10 days. This was followed by frying them until they became yellow. After separating out the herbal residue, the remaining oil was further concentrated until its drops fell like water drops in zero weather. It was ready then to put 600 grams of red lead into the highly concentrated oil. The previously prepared Cortex Cinnamomi, Corni Cervi, Pantotrichum and Moschus in powder form were added while it was still warm. A willow or Chinese scholar tree branch was used for stirring the mixture until it was ready for external application.

### Comments

Most of the ingredients in the formula warm the liver and kidney, strengthen tendons and bones, and remove obstruction from channels and collaterals. The amount of each of the ingredients was quite large. It was used externally as plasters only on the lumbar region, in the umbilicus or in the joints to help reinforce the vital energy and cure the illness. The health records of Empress Dowager Cixi say that she had facial paralysis which became worse on the second day of the fourth month of the lunar calendar in 1904. At that time she used Wind-eliminating and Facial Moistening Powder (Qing Feng Run Mian San). She also took the internal Syrup for Eliminating Liver-heat and Promoting *Qi* and Blood Circulation (Qing Re Yang Gan Huo Luo Gao). The remedy introduced here was for external use only.

## I.9. CHRYSANTHEMUM LONGEVITY SYRUP

On the fourth day of the 11th month of the lunar calendar in 1905, the imperial physicians Zhang Zhongyuan and Yao Baosheng carefully prepared Old Budda's Chrysanthemum Longevity Syrup. (Lao Fo Ye Ju Hua Yan Ling Gao).

### Ingredient

Fresh chrysanthemum leaves

The fresh chrysanthemum leaves were well boiled in water before they were removed from the decoction, which was further reduced before refined honey was added to form a syrup. Three or four grams of the syrup were taken with hot water each time.

### Comments

The health records of Empress Dowager Cixi on the second day of the eleventh month of the lunar calendar in 1905 say, "Empress Dowager Cixi had a wiry and rapid pulse in the liver region and a full but slippery pulse in the lung area. There was heat retention in the liver channel, and phlegm-heat in the lung and stomach, manifested by poor flow of *qi*, dry eyes, and occasional discomfort in the chest and diaphragm." In addition to this prescription, the Pill for Vision-brightening and Life-extending (Ming Mo Yan Ling Wan), a remedy for clearing fire from the liver channel and brightening the vision, was also applied.

Chrysanthemum Longevity Syrup (Ju Hua Yan Ling Gao), containing only the fresh chrysanthemum leaves, produces strong effects in clearing heat from the liver channel, promoting the vision and eliminating wind. The chrysanthemum enters into the lung and liver channels. *Complete Record of Sacred Benevolence (Shen Ji Zong Lu)* states that dried chrysanthemum leaves were ground together with Radix Glycyrrhizae into fine powder for treating eye congestion, dizziness and vertigo. *Prescriptions for Emergency Cases (Jiu Ji Fang)* says that chrysanthemum leaves were ground together with cicada shells into fine powder for the treatment of post illness nephelium. The above-mentioned remedies are very effective in treating eye conditions in the aged. Modern studies also prove that chrysanthemum has obvious effects in dilating coronary vessels, increasing blood flow in the coronary arteries, relieving tachycardia and strengthening cardiac systole, helping to extend life expectancy. *A Collection of Additional Topics (Mu Shu Xian Tan)* states "Cultivated chrysanthemum helps extend life expectancy while the wild plant helps sedate fire. Similarly, Rhizoma Polygonati extends life expectancy, while the herb known as Gouwen is toxic." Such remarks seem to be somewhat convincing.

## I.10. EARTHLY IMMORTAL AND GOLDEN MARROW PILL

A specific date for the preparation of Earthly Immortal and Golden Marrow Pill (Wu Zhi Dian Xian Jin Sui Dan) was not recorded.

Ingredients in this prescription, functioning to reinforce *qi*, produce fluid, regulate the spleen and stomach and increase appetite, help nourish brain energy and brighten the vision. The pill was used for clearing heat from the head and eyes and eliminating deficiency heat. After taking the pill for some hundred days the energy of the five Zang organs was invigorated and the skin lustrous. The literature advises that the pills be prepared and processed in the middle or on the first day of the Jiazi cycle (a period of 60 days in the ancient Chinese calendar).

### Ingredients

| | |
|---|---|
| Radix Ginseng (Ren Shen) | 60 g |
| Rhizoma Atractylodis Macrocephalae (Bai Zhu) | 60 g |
| Poria (Fu Ling) | 90 g |
| Flos Chrysanthemi (Ju Hua) | 60 g |
| Fructus Lycii (Gou Qi Zi) | 60 g |
| Radix Rehmanniae Praeparatae (Sheng Di Huang) | 180 g |
| Radix Ophiopogouis (Mai Dong) | 90 g |
| Pericarpium Citri Reticulatae (Chen Pi) | 60 g |
| Radix Peuriariae (Ge Gen) | 60 g |
| Fructus Viticis (Man Jing Zi) | 60 g |
| Massa Fermentata Medicinalis (Shen Qu) | 60 g |

The above ingredients were ground into fine powder and processed in pill form in the size of mung beans. Nine grams of the pills were taken each time with hot water.

### Comments

This prescription was formed on the basis of modifying ingredients in Four Gentlemen Decoction (Si Jun Zi Tang), Decoction of Three Noble Ingredients (San Cai Tang), Marvelous Effect Powder (Yi Gong San) and Decoction for Increasing Body Fluid (Zeng Ye Tang). Fructus Lycii and Radix Rehmanniae Praeparatae were used to nourish kidney Yin. Flos Chrysanthemi clears the brain and brightens the vision. The Wind-eliminating ingredients contained promote the circulation of liver *qi*. The combination of all these ingredients helps reinforce the energy of the five Zang organs, while regular use of the pill may prolong life expectancy. The so-called Wuzhi Dixian, meaning the five rare ingredients and earthly magic components, suggests that the remedy appears magical in extending life expectancy and making the body more agile.

Although the ingredients were used for reinforcing the five Zang organs, they were more for nourishing the kidney. The underlining principle is that the kidney dominates bones and produces marrow. The human brain is also known as the sea of marrow. Reinforcing the kidney may therefore help replenish energy in the brain to communicate with the eye system, thus the Chinese term Jinsui, meaning golden marrow, was adopted in the nomenclature of this patent remedy.

# II. TONIC PRESCRIPTIONS

## II.1. EIGHT TREASURES CAKE

The prescription for Eight Treasures Cake (Ba Zhen Gao) was carefully prepared by the imperial physician Li Deli on the 13th day of the ninth month of the lunar calendar in 1880.

### Ingredients

| | |
|---|---:|
| Poria  (Fu Ling) | 60 g |
| Semen Nelumbinis  (Lian Zi) | 60 g |
| Semen Euryales  (Qian Shi) | 60 g |
| Semen Dolichoris  (Bian Dou) | 60 g |
| Semen Coicis  (Yi Yi Ren) | 60 g |
| Noduls Nelumbinis Rhizomatis  (Ou Fen) | 60 g |
| Unidentified | 150 g |
| Unidentified | .... |

The original records say that the pits of the Semen Nelumbinis should be removed before use. The above ingredients were prepared in extremely fine powder, mixed with refined sugar, and made into cakes of some 30 grams each.

### Comments

This prescription was a modified version of the Eight Treasures Cake (Ba Zhen Gao) from *True Lineage of External Medicine (Wai Ke Zheng Zong)* by Chen Shigong of the Ming Dynasty (1368-1644), which strengthened the spleen, nourished the stomach and reinforced *qi* of the Middle Jiao. It was originally suggested for poor function of the spleen and stomach, indigestion, poor appetite, abdominal distention, sallow complexion, emaciation, and loose stools or diarrhea due to spleen deficiency. Empress Dowager Cixi's pulse record on the 13th day of the ninth month of the lunar calendar in 1880 was "a slightly large and slippery pulse in the spleen region and a slightly wiry one in the liver region. The pulse appeared quite normal in other regions. The stagnation of liver *qi* and deficient spleen caused dampness retention leading to anorexia, poor digestion, distention in the hypochondriac region, sore throat, nausea and loose stools. The Decoction for Regulating the Spleen and Dissolving Damp-Yin (Li Pi Hua Shi Yin) was prepared to cope with the condition." The imperial physician Li Deli thus prepared Eight Treasures Cake usually for infants but in no way contradicted in the Empress' case. The sweet and flavourful taste of the herbal cake overcame its herbal flavour so that while being used to treat diseases it served as refreshment as well. Giving this type of small medicinal cake to adult patients was indeed a superb idea.

## II.2.  VITAL ENERGY-PRESERVING OINTMENT

The prescription for Vital Energy-preserving Ointment (Bao Yuan Gu Ben Gao) was carefully prepared by the imperial physicians Xue Fuchen, Wang Shouzheng, Zhuang Shouhe, Li Dechang and Dong Wenbin on the 21st day of the fifth month of the lunar calendar in 1881.

*Ingredients*

| | |
|---|---:|
| Radix Codonopsis Pilosulae  (Dang Shen) | 45 g |
| Rhizoma Atractylodis Macrocephalae  (Bai Zhu) | 45 g |
| Cornu Cervi  (Lu Jiao) | 45 g |
| Radix Angelicae Sinensis  (Dang Gui) | 45 g |
| Rhizoma Cyperi  (Xiang Fu) | 45 g |
| Rhizoma Ligustici Chuan Xiong  (Chuan Xiong) | 30 g |
| Radix Aconiti Praeparatae  (Fu Zi) | 30 g |
| Radix Angelicae Pubescentis  (Du Huo) | 30 g |
| Rhizoma Zingiberis  (Gan Jiang) | 30 g |
| Pericarpium Zanthoxyli  (Chuan Jiao) | 30 g |
| Cortex Eucommiae  (Du Zhong) | 30 g |
| Carapax Trionycis  (Bie Jia) | 30 g |
| Fructus Piperis Longi  (Bi Bo) | 30 g |
| Fructus Tsaoko  (Cao Guo) | 30 g |
| Radix Paeoniae Lactiflorae  (Bai Shao) | 30 g |
| Radix Astragali seu Hedysari  (Huang Qi) | 45 g |

The above ingredients were fried in 900 grams of sesame oil until they became golden yellow. This was followed by separating the residue from the oily liquid which was further concentrated until it formed instant drops upon falling. Then 360 grams of red lead were mixed into the liquid before nine grams each of Cortex Cinnamomi, Lignum Aquilariae Resinatum and Flos Caryophylli were added. This mixture was ground into fine powder. After the powder became completely cold, it was made into balls of 120 grams each. After three days, when the frying smell was completely gone, they could be spread onto the umbilicus.

### Comments

Ingredients in this prescription had the effect of nourishing both the kidney and spleen, and treating both kidney Yin and kidney Yang. Reinforcing both the congenital and acquired causes were considered in drawing up the prescription. This external remedy was made at that time for Empress Dowager Cixi for her gastrointestinal dysfunction resulting from deficiency of both the spleen and kidney. Fructus Piperis Longi, Cortex Cinnamomi, Lignum Aquilariae Resinatum and Flos Caryophylli, ingredients of fragrant flavours and dispersing properties, were added to direct the therapeutic effect of the other ingredients deeper into the body in order to preserve the vital energy.

## II.3.  ALL-INCLUSIVE GREAT TONIFYING PILL

The prescription for All-inclusive Great Tonifying Pill (Shi Quan Da Bu Wan) was taken from *A Collection of Recommended Prescriptions* (Liang Fang Ji Cheng), but prepared in half doses for the Empress Dowager by the imperial physician Yang Deqing on the 16th day of the fifth month of the lunar calendar in 1884.

### Ingredients

| | |
|---|---|
| Radix Ginseng  (Ren Shen) | 7.5 g |
| Rhizoma Atractylodis Macrocephalae  (Bai Zhu) | 15 g |
| Radix Angelicae Sinensis  (Dang Gui) | 15 g |
| Rhizoma Ligustici Chuan Xiong  (Chuan Xiong) | 15 g |
| Radix Paeoniae Lactiflorae  (Bai Shao) | 15 g |
| Radix Astragali seu Hedysari  (Huang Qi) | 30 g |
| Poria  (Fu Ling) | 30 g |
| Cortex Cinnamomi  (Rou Gui) | 30 g |
| Radix Rehmanniae Praeparatae  (Shu Di) | 30 g |
| Radix Glycyrrhizae  (Gan Cao) | 7.5 g |

According to the original records, the Rhizoma Atractylodis Macrocephalae should be roasted with earth and the Radix Astragali seu Hedysari should be prepared with honey. The above ingredients were ground into fine powder and made with water into pills the size of Chinese umbrella tree seeds. One to two grams of the pills were taken each time with boiled water.

### Comments

The prescription for All-inclusive Great Tonifying Pill was originally from Volume V of *Imperial Grace Formulary of the Taiping Era* (Tai Ping Hui Min He Ji Ju Fang). Its prototype was a decoction containing Radix Auchlandiae and Lignum Aquilariae Resinatum, but no Radix Astragali seu Hedysari or Cortex Cinnamomi. Li Gao selected Radix Astragali seu Hedysari instead of Radix Auchlandiae in order to reinforce *qi*, and Cortex Cinnamomi instead of Lignum Aquilariae in order to warm the blood. The remedy was indicated in poor body constitution, general lassitude, weakness in the lumbar region and knees and general sexual deficiency, as it reinforces Yin, Yang, *qi* and blood, and was appropriate for Cixi. This prescription is actually the combination of three formulae, i.e. the Four Gentlemen Decoction (Si Jun Zi Tang), Four Ingredients Decoction (Si Wu Tang), and Huang's Middle Jiao Reinforcing Remedy (Huang Shi Jian Zhong Fang). It is in fact useful in preserving vital energy and acting as a general tonic.

## II.4. VITAL ENERGY-BUILDING AND MIDDLE JIAO PACIFYING SYRUP

The prescription for Vital Energy-building and Middle Jiao Pacifying Syrup (Fu Yuan He Zhong Gao) was prepared on the 13th day of the ninth month of the lunar calendar, with no mention of the year.

*Ingredients*

| | |
|---|---|
| Radix Angelicae Sinensis  (Dang Shen) | 45 g |
| Rhizoma Atractylodis Macrocephalae  (Bai Zhu) | 30 g |
| Poria  (Fu Ling) | 30 g |
| Fructus Amomi  (Sha Ren) | 12 g |
| Radix Angelicae Sinensis  (Dang Gui) | 30 g |
| Cortex Eucommiae  (Du Zhong) | 30 g |
| Rhizoma Cyperi  (Xiang Fu) | 18 g |
| Radix Astragali seu Hedysari  (Huang Qi) | 30 g |
| Fructus Oryzae Germinature  (Gu Ya) | 30 g |
| Endothlium Corneum Gieriae Galli  (Ji Nei Jin) | 30 g |
| Rhizoma Pinelliae  (Ban Xia) | 24 g |
| Herba Eupatorii  (Pei Lan) | 18 g |
| Rhizoma Zingiberis Recens  (Sheng Jiang) | 18 g |
| Fructus Ziziphi Jujubae  (Hong Zao) | 20 |

The original records require the Poria and Fructus Amomi to be ground before use, while the Rhizoma Atractylodis Macrocephalae, Cortex Eucommiae, and Fructus Oryzae Germinature should be roasted. The Radix Angelicae Sinensis should be roasted with earth, while the Rhizoma Cyperi should be prepared before use. The Rhizoma Pinelliae should be prepared with ginger juice, while the Endothlium Corneum Gieriae Galli should be griddled dry before use.

The above ingredients were soaked in water and well decocted before the residue was separated out. This was followed by further concentration of the liquid before 60 grams of sugar were added to make the syrup. Three grams of the syrup were taken daily together with boiled water.

*Comments*

This prescription was formulated by modifying the ancient remedy Powder for Pacifying the Middle Jiao (He Zhong San) and making it into a syrup. It is effective for poor appetite due to spleen deficiency, sensation of fullness in the chest, dryness in the mouth, nausea and discomfort in the epigastric region, and poor digestion in patients with chronic illness. The vital energy-building here refers to reinforcing *qi* of the spleen and kidney.

## II.5.  MODIFIED VITAL ENERGY-BUILDING AND MIDDLE JIAO PACIFYING SYRUP

The prescription for Modified Vital Energy-building and Middle Jiao Pacifying Syrup (Jia Jian Fu Yuan He Zhong Gao) was carefully prepared for Empress Dowager Cixi by the imperial physicians Wang Shouzheng, Li Deli and Zhuang Shouhe on the first day of the 11th month of the lunar calendar, with no mention of the year.

*Ingredients*

| | |
|---|---:|
| Radix Codonopsis Pilosulae  (Dang Shen) | 45 g |
| Rhizoma Atractylodis Macrocephalae  (Bai Zhu) | 30 g |
| Poria  (Fu Ling) | 30 g |
| Fructus Amomi  (Sha Ren) | 12 g |
| Radix Angelicae Sinensis  (Dang Gui) | 30 g |
| Radix Dipsaci  (Xu Duan) | 30 g |
| Rhizoma Cyperi  (Xiang Fu) | 18 g |
| Radix Astragali seu Hedysari  (Huang Qi) | 30 g |
| Fructus Oryzae Germinature  (Gu Ya) | 30 g |
| Endothelium Corneum Gieriae Galli  (Ji Nei Jin) | 30 g |
| Rhizoma Pinelliae  (Ban Xia) | 24 g |
| Herba Eupatorii  (Pei Lan) | 12 g |
| Rhizoma Zingiberis Recens  (Sheng Jiang) | 24 g |
| Radix Rehmanniae  (Shu Di Huang) | 18 g |
| Fructus Ziziphi Jujubae  (Hong Zao) | 20 |

The original records require the Radix Angelicae Sinensis and Rhizoma Atractylodis Macrocephalae to be roasted with earth. The Poria should be ground into powder. The Rhizoma Cyperi and Rhizoma Pinelliae were prepared in ginger juice. The Radix Dipsaci was to be roasted in millet wine and the Endothelium Corneum Gieriae Galli should be dry griddled. The Fructus Oryzae Germinature and Radix Rehmanniae should be roasted before use.

The above ingredients were well decocted in water before their residue was separated from the liquid, which was then further concentrated. That was followed by adding rock sugar to make a syrup for oral administration. Three grams of the syrup were taken daily with boiled water.

*Comments*

Compared with the previous prescription, the amount of Rhizoma Zingiberis Recens was increased while that of Herba Eupatorii was decreased. Radix Dipsaci was used instead of Cortex Eucommiae. Moreover, Radix Rehmanniae was added to further reinforce the liver and kidney.

## II.6.  VITAL ENERGY-BUILDING AND YIN-REINFORCING SYRUP

The prescription for Old Buddha's Vital Energy-building and Yin-reinforcing Syrup (Lao Fo Ye Fu Yuan Yi Yin Gao) was prepared on the 19th day of the seventh month of the lunar calendar, with no mention of the year.

*Ingredients*

| | |
|---|---:|
| Radix Codonopsis Pilosulae (Dang Shen) | 30 g |
| Rhizoma Atractylodis Macrocephalae (Bai Zhu) | 30 g |
| Poria (Fu Ling) | 30 g |
| Radix Paeoniae Lactiflorae (Bai Shao) | 30 g |
| Radix Angelicae Sinensis (Dang Gui) | 30 g |
| Cortex Lycci Radicis (Di Gu Pi) | 30 g |
| Cortex Moudan Radicis (Dan Pi) | 18 g |
| Fructus Amomi (Sha Ren) | 12 g |
| Radix Stellariae (Yin Chai Hu) | 9 g |
| Folium Perillae (Su Ye) | 3 g |
| Herba Menthae (Bo He) | 3 g |
| Colla Cornu Cervi (Lu Jiao Jiao) | 15 g |
| Rhizoma Cyperi (Xiang Fu) | 18 g |

The original records say that the Rhizoma Atractylodis Macrocephalae should be roasted and the Poria and Fructus Amomi ground into powder. The Radix Paeoniae Lactiflorae should be roasted with millet wine. The pits from the Cortex Moudan Radicis should be discarded. The Radix Angelicae Sinensis should be roasted with earth. The Colla Cornu Cervi should be melted into the concentrated liquid and the Rhizoma Cyperi should be processed.

The above ingredients were well decocted in water before their residue was separated from the liquid which was further concentrated. The Colla Cornu Cervi was then melted in and all were mixed with refined honey to make a syrup for oral administration. Three grams of the syrup were taken daily with boiled water.

*Comments*

The vital energy-building here refers to strengthening spleen *qi* and warming kidney Yang. Reinforcing Yin refers to nourishing Yin by cooling blood so as to reinforce the liver and kidney. The involved mechanism was to reinforce both the congenital and acquired deficiencies, while tonifying *qi* and blood. The formulation of this remedy implied Multi-function Powder of Five Flavours (Wu Wei Yi Gong San) and The Carefree Pill (Xiao Yao Wan) with slight modification. The former was adopted here to reinforce spleen *qi*, while the latter was for regulating the spleen and liver. The Colla Cornu Cervi was added to warm kidney Yang, and the Cortex Moudan Radicis to clear heat and cool the blood. The use of the Radix Stellariae instead of Radix Bupleuri was believed to drive away the low-grade fever caused by Yin deficiency. This prescription was quite balanced, characterized by the fact that general reinforcing was achieved without giving rise to any stagnation of *qi* or retention of pathogenic factors in the body.

## II.7. MODIFIED OLD BUDDHA'S VITAL ENERGY-BUILDING AND YIN-REINFORCING SYRUP

The prescription for Modified Old Buddha's Vital Energy-building and Yin-reinforcing Syrup (Lao Fo Ye Jia Jian Fu Yuan Yi Yin Gao) was prepared on the 29th day of the seventh month of the lunar calendar, with no mention of the year.

*Ingredients*

| | |
|---|---|
| Radix Codonopsis Pilosulae  (Dang shen) | 60 g |
| Rhizoma Atractylodis Macrocephalae  (Bai Zhu) | 60 g |
| Poria  (Fu Ling) | 30 g |
| Rhizoma Dio  (Shan Yao) | 30 g |
| Radix Angelicae Sinensis  (Dang Gui) | 60 g |
| Fructus Ligustri Lucidi  (Nu Zhen Zi) | 30 g |
| Radix Paeoniae Lactiflorae  (Bai Shao) | 24 g |
| Cortex Moudan Radicis  (Dan Pi) | 18 g |
| Fructus Amomi  (Sha Ren) | 12 g |
| Colla Cornu Cervi  (Lu Jiao Jiao) | 15 g |
| Rhizoma Cyperi  (Xiang Fu) | 18 g |
| Radix Stellariae  (Yin Chai Hu) | 9 g |

The original records require the Rhizoma Atractylodis Macrocephalae to be roasted. The Poria and Fructus Amomi should be ground into powder. The Radix Paeoniae Lactiflorae was to be roasted with vinegar and the Radix Angelicae Sinensis roasted in powdery earth. The Rhizoma Cyperi should be processed and then ground before application. The Colla Cornu Cervi should later be melted into the concentrated decoction.

The above ingredients were well decocted in water before their residue was separated out. The liquid was then concentrated, followed by melting in the Colla Cornu Cervi and refined honey to make the syrup for oral administration. Four grams of the syrup was taken daily with boiled water.

*Comments*

This prescription was actually modified on the basis of the previous one by leaving out Herba Menthae and Cortex Lycci Radicis, and adding Rhizoma Dio and Fructus Ligustri Lucidi. Its purpose was to strengthen the effect of the remedy to reinforce the spleen and kidney. Also, according to the analysis of the original manuscript and date recorded, there was only an interval of 10 days between the administration of these two prescriptions. It might be related to the fact that the previous one was on the greasy side, and therefore ingredients for balancing the greasiness were added so as to make a revised prescription for the same condition.

## II.8. CHEWING GINSENG

In the ninth month of the lunar calendar in 1901, an inquiry was submitted to Rong Bayue, the director of Longevity and Health Palace Pharmacy, concerning the habitual chewing of ginseng by Empress Dowager Cixi. The regular supply of ginseng began on the 23rd day of the 11th month of the lunar calendar in 1900 and ended on the 28th day of the ninth month of the lunar calendar in 1901, a total of 331 days. Altogether 993 grams of ginseng for chewing were prescribed. Rong Bayue said that one gram of ginseng for chewing was prepared daily for the Empress Dowager. The package was prepared according to the daily dosage, handed to Guo Yongqing, the head of General Logistics, and then to the eunuch Qin Shangyi for delivery. This was the reply to the inquiry.

*Comments*

Chewing a slice of ginseng to promote body constitution and prevent illness is a method widely known and practised among the people. The practice is also followed abroad. According to the *Compendium of Materia Medica (Ben Cao Gang Mu)* by Li Shizhen, "Ginseng corrects various deficiency conditions in men and women." Ginseng is listed as medicinal material of superior quality in *Shen Nong's Materia Medica (Shen Nong Ben Cao Jing)*. It is recorded as having such functions as "nourishing the five Zang organs, calming the mind, easing fright and palpitation, eliminating pathogenic factors, promoting eyesight, strengthening cardiac function, and promoting intelligence. Regular use of ginseng may help invigorate the body and prolong life expectancy."

Studies done by present-day professionals prove that ginseng can raise work efficiency, reduce strain and fatigue, strengthen human adaptation to varying difficult environments, regulate the function of the reticuloendothelial system, and strengthen human adaptation to weather changes. Experiments conducted on adult female mice in Japan showed that ginseng exerted a similar action in promoting the sexual gland hormones, extending the ovulation period. These experiments further showed that saponin in ginseng had a certain effect in promoting sexual gland hormonal activity.

Empress Dowager Cixi took ginseng as a general tonic, a practice later affirmed to have a scientific basis. In order to guarantee ginseng supply for the Empress Dowager, original prescriptions for her include Emperor Guangxu's inquiries whether Cixi's ginseng supply was sufficient. He thus showed how much concern ginseng drew from the Emperor while on routine courtesty calls on her.

# III. LUSTROUS HAIR-MAINTAINING PRESCRIPTIONS

## III.1. HAIR GROWTH REMEDY

Two portions of Hair Growth Remedy (Ling Fa Yi Zhang Fang) were prescribed with no information given as to the date.

### Ingredient
Radix Ziziphi Jujubae  (Zao Shu Gen)                                    1 metre

The original records state that the jujube tree root growing eastward was used. Fresh Radix Ziziphi Jujubae was placed on an old roof tile and steamed until liquid oozed from both ends. It was this liquid that was collected for external application to stimulate hair growth.

### Comments
Human hair is produced by blood. The use of Radix Ziziphi Jujubae is noted in both *Compendium of Materia Medica (Ben Cao Gang Mu)* and *A Collection of Commentary Notes of Canon in Materia Medica (Ben Cao Jing Ji Zhu)*. Bland and sweet in flavour and non-toxic, it activates blood and clears wind and heat, thus promoting hair growth.

## III.2. HAIR GROWTH REMEDY PLUS

*Ingredients*

Folium Mori (Sang Ye)
Folium Cannabis Sativa (Ma Ye)

Suitable amounts of the above ingredients were decocted in water for shampoo. Washing the hair with this seven times produced substantial growth in the hair.

*Comments*

Folium Mori, bitter, sweet and cold, has the action of clearing wind-heat, cooling blood and brightening the vision. Its powder form can be used as tea. It was believed to be good for promoting human intelligence. It was known as the magic leaf according to the *Illustrated Materia Medica (Ben Cao Tu Jing)*. Folium Cannabis Sativa has a detoxicating effect. It can be mixed into tobacco for the treatment of asthma. Records concerning the use of the two for promoting hair growth were respectively seen in *Prescriptions Worth a Thousand Gold in Emergencies (Bei Ji Qian Jin Yao Fang)* and *A Collection of Classified Prescriptions (Yi Fang Lei Ji)*. "Washing the hair seven times made the hair grow several decimetres" was more than a simple exaggeration.

## III.3. REMEDY FOR STOPPING HAIR LOSS

Two doses of Remedy for Stopping Hair Loss were submitted on the 12th day of the 10th month of the lunar calendar, with no mention of the year.

*Ingredients*

| | |
|---|---|
| Semen Torreyae (Fei Zi) | 3 |
| Juglandis (He Tao) | 2 |
| Cacumen Biotae (Ce Bai Ye) | 30 g |

The above ingredients were mashed and soaked in melted-snow water to be used in combing the hair. On the 17th day of the same month, the same dose was repeated. On the 19th day of that same month another two doses were used. The treatment stopped on the 23rd day of the same month after one more dose was prescribed.

*Comments*

Hair loss can be caused by such conditions as heat retention in blood, weak body constitution, or lack or over-abundance of succorrhea of the scalp. The Semen Torreyae in this prescription, bland and sweet, moistens the skin and cures fungi infection. The Juglandis was used to nourish the hair and skin. The Cacumen Biotae, astringent and bitter, was to cool the blood, remove blood stasis, and especially to disperse wind. The use of the three combined could prevent hair loss. It has been reported that people today soak fresh Cacumen Biotae in 60% alcohol for about one week and then rub it on the area with alopecia areata. This is believed to have both therapeutic and preventive effects.

# III.4. HAIR FRAGRANCE POWDER

The prescription for Old Buddha's Hair Fragrance Powder (Lao Fo Ye Xiang Fa San) was recorded on the fifth day of the seventh month of the lunar calendar in 1905.

There was succorrhea of the scalp, and the hair should not simply be washed with water. The Hair Fragrance Powder was spread on the fine-toothed comb used for combing Cixi's hair and it cleaned the suborrhea. Regular application of this procedure made lost hair grow again and remain black even in advanced age.

*Ingredients*

| | |
|---|---|
| Herba Lysimachia  (Ling Ling Cao) | 30 g |
| Flos Magnoliae  (Xin Yi) | 15 g |
| Flos Rosae Rugosae  (Mei Gui Hua) | 15 g |
| Lignum Santali  (Tan Xiang) | 18 g |
| Radix Rhei  (Da Huang) | 12 g |
| Radix Glycyrrhizae  (Gan Cao) | 12 g |
| Cortex Moudan Radicis  (Mu Dan) | 12 g |
| Rhizoma Kaempferiae  (Shan Nai) | 9 g |
| Flos Syzygii Aromaticis  (Gong Ding Xiang) | 9 g |
| Herba Asari  (Xi Xin) | 9 g |
| Resina Liquidanbar Orientalis  (Su He You) | 9 g |
| Radix Angelicae Dahuricae  (Bai Zhi) | 90 g |

The above ingredients were prepared in fine powder, mixed with Resina Liquidanbar Orientalis and dried without exposure to the sun. It was then made into extremely fine powder to be used in fine combing of the hair.

*Comments*

Most of the ingredients in this remedy are of warming properties and strong aroma. The underlying mechanism was to relieve obstruction, clean and nourish the hair. It was believed to enrich the hair and prevent it from turning gray. Among the ingredients, Herba Lysimachia was called the "steaming" plant in *Classic of Mountains and Seas (Shan Hai Jing)*, and the "fragrant plant" in *Materia Medica of the Northern Song Dynasty (Kai Bao Ben Cao)*. According to *Transactions of Famous Physicians (Ming Yi Bie Lu)* it was a deodorant. According to *Compendium of Materia Medica (Ben Cao Gang Mu)*, "Rhizoma Kaempferiae grows in the mountains and is also cultivated in fields. Its leaves and roots look like those of ginger. Its fragrant smell is often used instead of that from camphorwood." *Transactions of Famous Physicians* says, "Flos Magnoliae makes the hair grow." Lignum Santali, Herba Asari and Radix Angelicae Dahuricae were all used because of their fragrances. The reason why Radix Rhei and Cortex Moudan Radicis were used was probably to avoid excessive dryness from other ingredients.

# IV. OPHTHALMOLOGICAL PRESCRIPTIONS

## IV.1. EPIDEMIC HEAT-PREVENTING POWDER FOR BRIGHTENING VISION

The prescription of Epidemic Heat-preventing Powder for Brightening Vision (Bi Wen Ming Mu Qing Shang San) was for inhalation only. It was prepared by the imperial physician Yang Jihe on the 18th day of the fifth month of the lunar calendar in 1887.

### Ingredients

| | |
|---|---|
| Herba Menthae (Bo He) | 15 g |
| Radix Angelicae Dahuricae (Bai Zhi) | 15 g |
| Radix Rhei (Da Huang) | 18 g |
| Rhizoma Qsmundae (Guan Zhong) | 36 g |
| Folium Isatidis (Da Qing Ye) | 36 g |
| Herba Chloranthus Spicatus (Zhu Lan Cha) | 36 g |
| Lignum Dalbergiae Odoriferae (Jiang Xiang) | 12 g |
| Realgar (Xiong Huang) | 9 g |
| Cinnabari (Zhu Sha) | 6 g |
| Borneoleum Syntheticum (Bing Pian) | 3 g |

The original records say that the realgar should be ground in water into powder. The first nine ingredients were prepared in dry powder form, followed by further grinding together with Borneoleum syntheticum to produce an extremely fine powder, until no more grinding sound was heard.

### Comments

Most of the ingredients in this prescription are fragrances for preventing epidemic invasion and clearing toxic heat. Sniffing of the powder helped clear wind-heat in the head to treat congestion and pain in the eyes, aversion to light and poor eyesight. It is an effective prescription in the treatment of Empress Dowager Cixi's eye condition because it includes many other ophthalmological formulae, e.g. Eight Treasures Brightening Powder (Ba Bao Guang Ming San) that consisted of Moschus, Cinnabari, agate, coral and Borneoleum; Blue Cloud Powder (Bi Yun San) which included Indigo Naturalis and Radix Angelicae Dahuricae; Vision-brightening Powder with Resina Murrhea and Resina Draconis (Ming Mu Mo Jue San) that contained Radix Rhei, and Heat-cooling and Vision-protecting Powder (Bao Guang Qing Liang San) and Eye-brightening Powder (Ming Mu San). The last two medicines contained Natrii Sulphas Exsiccatus.

## IV.2. EYEWASH

Old Buddha's Eyewash (Lao Fo Ye Xi Mu Fang) was recorded on the 26th day of the fourth month on the lunar calendar in 1902.

### Ingredients

| | |
|---|---|
| Fructus Viticis (Man Jing Zi) | 9 g |
| Herba Schizonepetae (Jing Jie) | 6 g |
| Fructus Tribuli (Ji Li) | 6 g |

Folium Mori, frosted  (Shuang Sang Ye)                                 6 g
Cortex Fraxini  (Qin Pi)                                               3 g

The above ingredients were boiled in water and used while still warm for washing the face.

### Comments

Having the effect of dispersing wind-heat, sedating the liver and brightening the vision, this prescription must have been effective in the treatment of congestion and pain in the eye due to exogenous wind-heat invasion. In this prescription the bitter and cool Folium Mori was especially good for dispersing wind-heat and brightening the vision. It was called Folium Mori and Sesame Pill (Sang Ma Wan) when combined with black sesame and applied in the treatment of dizziness and blurring of vision due to flaring-up of liver fire resulting from liver-Yin deficiency. Cortex Fraxini, bitter, astringent and cold, has usually been known for its effect in treating diarrhea. However, its effect in congestion and pain in the eye due to liver heat has been known as empirical. Both Fructus Viticis and Fructus Tribuli have the effect of dispersing wind and brightening the vision. Herba Schizonepetae clears toxins from the blood and is effective in treating sore throat and congestion in the eyes resulting from heat retention in the blood. The prescription was formulated by the imperial physician Xu Benlin and on the same day another external application was also prepared for Empress Dowager Cixi. The Semen Phaseoli Radiatus, Periostracum Cicadae, Herba Schizonepetae, Herba Lycopi, Cortex Fraxini, Spica Prunellae, Fructus Forsythiae, Radix Angelicae Dahuricae and Fructus Viticis were prepared in extremely fine powder to be mixed with light honey water for external application.

## IV.3. EYE-BRIGHTENING AND LONGEVITY PILL

Prescription of Old Buddha's Eye-brightening and Longevity Pill (Lao Fo Ye Ming Mu Yan Ling Wan) was carefully worked out by the imperial physician Zhang Zhongyuan on the 27th day of the seventh month of the lunar calendar in 1905.

### Ingredients

Folium Mori, frosted  (Shuang Sang Ye)                                 6 g
Flos Chrysanthemi  (Ju Hua)                                            6 g

The above ingredients were ground into fine powder and mixed with refined honey to be made into pills the size of Semen Phaseoli Radiatus. Two grams of the pills were taken orally with boiled water each day.

### Comments

Folium Mori and Chrysanthemi have actions in clearing heat, eliminating wind, soothing the liver and brightening the eyes. Regular and prolonged use of the pill is recommended. For the treatment of headache and congestion in the eyes, the two should be combined with Fructus Tribuli Terrestris; and for blurring of vision due to flaring up of liver Yang, they should be combined with Fructus Lycii and Concha Haliotidis.

## IV.4.  EYE-BRIGHTENING AND LONGEVITY PILL PLUS

Old Buddha's Eye-brightening and Longevity Pill Plus (Lao Fo Ye Ming Mu Yan Ling You Fang) was carefully prepared by the imperial physician Yao Baosheng on the seventh day of the eighth month of the lunar calendar in 1905.

*Ingredients*

| | |
|---|---:|
| Folium Mori, frosted  (Shuang Sang Ye) | 6 g |
| Flos Chrysanthemi  (Ju Hua) | 6 g |
| Cornu Antelopis  (Ling Yang Jiao) | 4.5 g |
| Radix Rehmanniae  (Sheng Di) | 6 g |
| Fructus Ligustri Lucidi  (Nu Zhen Zi) | 6 g |
| Flos Buddlejae  (Meng Hua) | 4.5 g |
| Concha Ostreae  (Mu Li) | 6 g |
| Rhizoma Alismatis  (Ze Xie) | 6 g |
| Radix Paeoniae Lactiflorae  (Bai Shao) | 4.5 g |
| Fructus Aurantii  (Zhi Ke) | 4.5 g |

The original records say that the Fructus Ligustri Lucidi should be ground into powder, and the Fructus Aurantii roasted before use. The above ingredients were ground into fine powder and mixed with refined honey to be made into small pills. Two grams of the pills were to be taken daily with boiled water.

*Comments*

This prescription bears the same nomenclature as the previous one but contains more ingredients. Here the top part of Cornu Antelopis was used. It was more appropriate for eye congestion due to excessive liver fire. Cornu Antelopis enters the liver channel and has the effect of "clearing the nephelium and brightening the vision" according to *Compendium of Materia Medica (Ben Cao Gang Mu)*. Quite a few eye remedies contained Cornu Antelopis, e. g. Cornu Antelopis Decoction (Ling Yang Jiao Tang) in the book entitled *A Complete Record of Sacred Benevolence (Sheng Ji Zong Lu)*, and Cornu Antelopis Powder in *Sacred and Benevolent Prescriptions (Sheng Hui Fang)*. *Shen Nong's Materia Medica (Shen Nong Ben Cao)* also claimed that Cornu Antelopis "was indicated in brightening the vision." Salty and cold with no toxicity, it was fairly appropriate to prescribe it for Empress Dowager Cixi, for she had chronic liver heat.

## IV.5.  MULBERRY LEAF EYEWASH

Frosted Folium Mori Eyewash (Shuang Sang Ye Xi Mu Fang) was recorded on the 16th day of the first month of the lunar calendar. No lunar year was given.

*Ingredient*

| | |
|---|---:|
| Folium Mori, frosted  (Shuang Sang Ye) | 9 g |

The frosted Folium Mori, boiled in water, was used to wash the eyes every day after washing the face. Then, on the 17th day of each month six grams of Flos Chrysanthemi were added to the prescription.

*Comments*

Folium Mori has been mentioned as having the effect of clearing wind-heat.

Using it to "wash the eyes after washing the face" agreed with the hygienic principles.

## IV.6. EYEWASH FOR BRIGHTENING VISION AND NOURISHING YIN

| | |
|---|---|
| Flos Chrysanthemi  (Ju Hua) | 9 g |
| Folium Mori, frosted  (Shuang Sang Ye) | 9 g |
| Herba Menthae  (Bo He) | 3 g |
| Cornu Antelopis  (Ling Yang Jiao) | 4.5 g |
| Radix Rehmanniae  (Sheng Di) | 9 g |
| Spica Prunellae  (Xia Ku Cao) | 9 g |

The original records say the top part of the Cornu Antelopis should be used. All the above ingredients were decocted in water for eye steaming, to be followed by eyewashing.

*Comments*

To the previous prescription were added Spica Prunellae (9 g), Radix Rehmanniae (9 g), Herba Menthae (3 g) and Cornu Antelopis (4.5 g). Spica Prunellae, pungent, bitter and cold, enters the liver channel of the gallbladder channel and so is appropriate in treating eye conditions due to flaring up of liver fire. *Compendium of Materia Medica (Ben Cao Gang Mu)* says: "According to the book entitled *Handbook of Simple Remedies (Yi Jian Fang)* by Li Jushi, 'Spica Prunellae was soaked in sandy sugar water overnight and given orally for treating eye conditions. Used in this way, it dispersed internal fire and relieved liver fire.'" Lou Quanshan wrote, "Spica Prunellae produces incredible effects in stopping eye pain which worsens at night. It also has remarkable effects when used to ease eye pain due to the external application of bitter and cold remedies.... Spica Prunellae, receiving pure Yang-*qi* from the earth, reinforces blood in the liver channel. This is why it produces such remarkable effects in using Yang to treat Yin." Spicae Prunellae was also often used in TCM external therapy in treating scrofula, goiter, protuberance of the abdomen, mastitis, and breast carcinoma, according to *A New Compilation of Materia Medica (Ben Cao Cong Xin)*.

## IV.7. EYE-BRIGHTENING AND LONGEVITY SYRUP

Old Buddha's Eye-brightening and Longevity Syrup (Lao Fo Ye Ming Mu Yan Ling Gao) was carefully prepared by the imperial physician Zhang Zhongyuan on the 17th day of the seventh month of the lunar calendar. No lunar year was given.

*Ingredients*

| | |
|---|---|
| Folium Mori, frosted  (Shuang Sang Ye) | 30 g |
| Flos Chrysanthemi  (Ju Hua) | 30 g |

The above ingredients were well decocted before their residue was separated from the decoction. This was followed by concentration of the decoction and mixing in a small amount of refined honey to make a syrup for oral administration. Three grams of the syrup were taken daily with boiled water.

*Comments*

This remedy was prepared in syrup form though it bore the same ingredients as in IV.3. The choice between pills and syrup made it easier for patients to accept and persist in the treatment.

## IV.8. FOOT BATH FOR BRIGHTENING EYES AND ELIMINATING DAMPNESS

One standard portion of Foot Bath for Brightening Eyes and Eliminating Dampness (Ming Mu Chu Shi Yu Zu Fang) was ordered on the 20th day of the fifth month of the lunar calendar, with no mention of the year.

*Ingredients*

| | |
|---|---:|
| Flos Chrysanthemi  (Ju Hua) | 9 g |
| Folium Mori  (Sang Ye) | 15 g |
| Fructus Chaenomelis  (Mu Gua) | 15 g |
| Radix Achyranthis Bidentatae  (Niu Xi) | 15 g |
| Radix Stephaniae Tetrandrae  (Fang Ji) | 12 g |
| Rhizoma Atractylodis Macrocephalae  (Bai Zhu) | 15 g |
| Cortex Phellodendri  (Huang Bai) | 9 g |
| Radix Glycyrrhizae  (Gan Cao) | 9 g |

The above ingredients were boiled in water for foot bathing.

*Comments*

This prescription, with the effect of brightening the vision, stopping itching and removing dampness, consisted of Flos Chrysanthemi and modified Three Wonders Powder (San Miao San), intended originally to treat dampness in the Lower Jiao, while here it was applied for brightening the eyesight. The prescription was probably applied according to the underlying mechanism of treating an upper body condition by treating the Lower Jiao. Or, dampness may have been manifested in both Lower Jiao and foot simultaneously, a situation not known for sure.

## IV.9. DECOCTION FOR SEDATING LIVER FIRE AND CLEARING NEBULAE

Empress Dowager Cixi suddenly developed white spots appearing like nebulae over her left pupil. She also felt a foreign body sensation and pain in the eye. This was caused by the rising of damp-heat out of stagnant heat in the liver channel. One course of Live Fire Sedating and Nebulae-clearing Decoction (Yi Huo Qing Gan Tui Yi Tang) was therefore prescribed to deal with the condition.

*Ingredients*

| | |
|---|---:|
| Cornu Antelopis  (Ling Yang Jiao) | 4.5 g |
| Herba Equiseti Hiemalis  (Mu Zei Cao) | 9 g |
| Fructus Tribuli  (Ji Li) | 9 g |
| Pericarpium Citri Reticulatae Viride  (Qing Pi) | 9 g |
| Rhizoma Alismatis  (Ze Xie) | 6 g |
| Flos Buddlejae  (Meng Hua) | 6 g |
| Periostracum Serpentis  (She Tui) | 4.5 g |

| | |
|---|---|
| Concha Haliotidis  (Shi Jue Ming) | 9 g |
| Radix Ledebouriellae  (Fang Feng) | 6 g |
| Radix Glycyrrhizae  (Gan Cao) | 3 g |

The original directions say that the Fructus Tribuli should be prepared in powder form, and the Concha Haliotidis (raw) be ground into fine powder before use.

## Comments

This prescription has the effect of sedating liver fire and clearing nebulae, apparently to treat acute conjunctivitis. This editor is not quite sure. Cornu Antelopis, Flos Buddlejae, Fructus Tribuli, Periostracum Serpentis and Herba Equiseti Hiemalis have strong effects in clearing liver fire. According to *Materia Medica of Emperor Jiayou's Era (Jia You Ben Cao)*, Herba Equiseti Hiemalis was indicated in congestion of the eyes and for nebulae. *Essence of Materia Medica (Ben Cao Qiu Zhen)* claimed Herba Equiseti Hiemalis as the main ingredient for clearing nebula. Periostracum Cicadae and Flos Eriocauli might also be included in this prescription besides Periostracum Serpentis.

# V.  PRESCRIPTIONS FOR NASAL CONDITIONS

## V.1.  SNUFFBOX REPLACEMENT REMEDY

Old Grandpa Gao (a palace eunuch) conveyed the order for the preparation of the Snuffbox Replacement Remedy (Dai Bi Yan Fang) on the 16th day of the fourth month of the lunar calendar with no mention of the year.

### Ingredients

| | |
|---|---|
| Herba Centipedae  (E Er Bu Shi Cao) | 6 g |
| Herba Asari  (Xi Xin) | 1.8 g |
| Radix Angelicae Dahuricae  (Bai Zhi) | 6 g |
| Scorpio  (Quan Xue) | 18 g |
| Herba Menthae  (Bo He) | 3 g |
| Rhizoma Ligustici Chuanxiong  (Chuan Xiong) | 1.5 g |
| Indigo Naturalis  (Qing Dai) | 3 g |

The above ingredients were prepared in fine powder form to replace snuffbox contents, with 240 grams of Bulbus Fritillariae Cirhosae ground into fine powder. Three doses were made.

### Comments

This prescription was modified on the basis of the Blue Cloud Powder (Bi Yun San) that was first recorded in *Standards for Syndrome Differentiation and Treatment (Zheng Zhi Zhun Shen)* by Wang Kentang. The formula was made to treat headache, sticky eye secretion and lacrimation, and also used to treat nasal obstruction and itching due to wind disturbance. The Empress Dowager Cixi used it to treat her eye and nasal conditions. The original ingredients of Blue Cloud Powder included the following in powder form: Herba Centipedae, Indigo Naturalis, Rhizoma Ligustici Chuanxiong, Herba Asari and Spina Gleditsiae. Extremely fine powder was used to treat both nasal discharge and eye secretion. In this prescription, Herba Centipedae was the principal one, pungent and warm, for wiping away nebulae and clearing nasal obstruction. The *Compendium of Materia Medica (Ben Cao Gang Mu)* says that Herba Centipedae was indicated in "nasal obstruction and dispersing boils. Administered into the nasal cavity it could remove a polyp." Today, extremely fine powder is used to treat allergic rhinitis and is often administered into the nasal cavity several times daily. It can also be applied on a piece of wet cotton inserted into the nasal cavity for half an hour once daily. Or, it can be made into an ointment for insertion into the nasal cavity on cotton rolls. The whole plant of Herba Centipedae contains many kinds of triterpenes. According to *Materia Medica on Diet Therapy (Shi Xing Ben Cao)*, another name for Herba Centipedae is Shihusui.

## V.2. BLUE CLOUD POWDER

The prescription for Blue Cloud Powder (Bi Yun San) was carefully prepared by the imperial physician Li Deli on the 18th day of the tenth month of the lunar calendar in 1877.

*Ingredients*

| | |
|---|---|
| Herba Centipedae  (E Er Bu Shi Cao) | 9 g |
| Herba Asari  (Xi Xin) | 4.5 g |
| Herba Menthae  (Bo He) | 9 g |
| Indigo Naturalis  (Qing Dai) | 9 g |

The original directions are to grind the Indigo Naturalis into powder in water. All ingredients were ground into extremely fine powder and sealed in two bottles of 15 grams each.

*Comments*

As has been mentioned previously, this prescription deals with both eye and nasal conditions. It should also be possible to add Spina Gleditsiae into the powder for the treatment of eye conditions.

# VI.  EAR PRESCRIPTION

## VI.1.  TEA REPLACEMENT FOR CLEARING LIVER HEAT

The prescription for Tea Replacement for Clearing Liver Heat (Ping Gan Qing Re Dai Cha Yin) was carefully prepared by the imperial physician Ai Shixin.

The Empress Dowager's blocking sensation in the right ear was caused by flaring up of liver heat and so the method used for soothing the liver and clearing liver heat was applied.

*Ingredients*

| | |
|---|---|
| Radix Gentianae  (Long Dan Cao) | 1.8 g |
| Radix Bupleuri  (Chai Hu) | 1.8 g |
| Rhizoma Ligustici Chuanxiong  (Chuan Xiong) | 1.8 g |

Flos Chrysanthemi  (Ju Hua)                                               3 g
Radix Rehmanniae  (Sheng Di)                                             3 g

According to the original records, the Radix Bupleuri was prepared with vinegar and all the above ingredients were decocted and taken as Chinese tea early each afternoon.

## Comments

This prescription was proposed for the blocking sensation in the ear due to excessive heat retention in the liver and gallbladder. Radix Gentianae was taken as the main ingredient. According to *Compendium of Materia Medica (Ben Cao Gang Mu)*, "Lodging of sinister fire in the liver and gallbladder should only be reduced without any reinforcement. Therefore, Radix Gentianae was applied to regulate *qi* of the liver and gallbladder because of its effect in relieving the heat retention from the liver and gallbladder." Radix Gentianae may also be applied in eye disorders due to heat retention. *The Enlightenment and Origin of Medicine* (Yi Xue Qi Yuan) says, "Radix Bupleuri must be used as the principal ingredient and Radix Gentianae the secondary in formulae suggested for the treatment of eye conditions."

# VII.  LIP CONDITION PRESCRIPTION

## VII.1.  DAMP-HEAT AND WIND CLEARING OINTMENT

The prescription for this ointment (Qing Re Chu Shi Qu Feng Gao) was carefully prepared by the imperial physician Luan Fuqing on the 20th day of the fifth month of the lunar calendar in 1878.

This ointment was specially prepared for conditions due to retention of damp-heat in the spleen channel, and manifested by itchiness, ulcers or swollen lips. External application of the ointment was to deal with such symptoms and signs.

### Ingredients

Rhizoma Coptidis  (Huang Lian)                                           6 g
Cortex Phellodendri  (Huang Bai)                                         9 g
Radix Rehmanniae  (Sheng Di)                                            9 g
Herba Psirodelae  (Fu Ping Cao)                                          9 g
Radix Angelicae Dahuricae  (Bai Zhi)                                    9 g
Radix Ledebouriellae  (Fang Feng)                                       9 g
Cortex Dictamni Dasycarpi Radicis  (Bai Xian Pi)                        6 g
Radix Angelicae Sinensis  (Dang Gui)                                    9 g
Rhizoma Bletillae Striatae  (Bai Ji)                                     6 g
Bombyx Batryticatus  (Jiang Can)                                         6 g
Flos Mume (Mei Hua)                                                     0.9 g

The original directions call for roasting the Bombyx Batryticatus, while the Flos Mume was ground into fine powder and added in. The above ingredients were made into a coarse powder and decocted, then the residue was separated out. This was followed by concentration of the liquid into an ointment for external application.

**Comments**

Itching, ulcers and swelling of lips are all common conditions due to retention of heat in the spleen channel. This prescription has the action of clearing damp-heat and wind. Its external application is convenient and therapeutic effects may be even stronger in relieving the inflammation if Caculus Bovis is added.

# VIII.  DENTAL CONDITION PRESCRIPTIONS

## VIII.1.  TOOTH POWDER FOR STRENGTHENING TEETH

The prescription of Tooth Powder for Strengthening Teeth (Gu Chi Shua Ya San) was carefully prepared by the imperial physicians Li Deli and Zhong Shouhe on the first day of the 11th month of the lunar calendar in 1880.

**Ingredients**

| | |
|---|---:|
| Sea Sal  (Qing Yan) | 60 g |
| Pericarpium Zanthoxyli  (Chuan Jiao) | 60 g |
| Herba Ecliptae  (Han Lian Cao) | 60 g |
| Alumen  (Ku Bai Fan) | 30 g |
| Refined Sal  (Bai Yan) | 120 g |

The Herba Ecliptae and Pericarpium Zanthoxyli were first decocted to one cup of pure decoction without the residue. To this was added the Sea Sal, Alumen and Refined Sal to be roasted into powder, which was ground into extremely fine powder for tooth brushing. This was believed to protect against dental disease.

**Comments**

This prescription was made for brushing and strenghening the teeth. Herba Ecliptae, reinforcing kidney Yin, is often used for loose teeth or prematurely gray hair due to kidney Yin deficiency. Its tannic substance, astringent in taste, has styptic properties. Alumen, also antiseptic and astringent, helps eliminate damp-ness and toxic heat. Pericarpium Zanthoxyli is bactericidal and analgesic. Herba Ecliptae and sea sal are also ingredients of a similar formula for strengthening the teeth known as Superb Treasure Powder (Zhi Bao Dan) in the book *Complete Works on Surgical Diseases (Yang Yi Da Quan)* by Gu Shicheng.

## VIII.2.  PRESCRIPTION FOR BRIGHTENING EYES AND STRENGTHENING TEETH

The Prescription for Brightening Eyes and Strengthening Teeth (Gu Chi Ming Mu Fang) was carefully prepared by the imperial physicians Zhang Zhon-gyuan and Yao Baosheng on the ninth day of the 11th month of the lunar calendar in 1905.

**Ingredient**

| | |
|---|---:|
| Sea Sal  (Qing Yan) | 960 g |

The salt should be cleaned before dissolving it in water that has been boiled continuously for a long time. The clean salty liquid was then poured into a silver utensil and boiled again until the salt crystallized out. This salt was then ground very fine and stored in a porcelain container.

Each morning three grams of the powder were used for rubbing and rinsing the teeth. The fingers of both hands were used to move the salty saliva in the mouth to wash the inner and outer canthuses. The eyes were then closed for some 15 minutes. Finally, the face was washed with clean water. The vision was thus "extended to more than 500 kilometres."

### Comments

Sea salt, salty and cold, clears fire and cools blood. It was used for treating gum bleeding, sore throat and nebulae in the eyes. *Amplification of Materia Medica (Ban Cao Yan Yi)* says, "Whenever there is some bleeding from gums, rinse the mouth with salt water and the bleeding will soon stop. This is the experience dealing with gum bleeding." Using salty water to rinse the teeth and mouth, and to wash eyes was recorded in many ancient books such as *Ren Zhai Zhi Internal Medicine Formula* (Ren Zhai Zhi Zhi Fang) and *Everlasting Categorization of Seal Formulas* (Yong Lei Qian Fang). The statement, "The vision was thus extended to more than 500 kilometres," is indeed an exaggeration.

## VIII.3. EMPIRICAL REMEDY FOR STRENGTHENING TEETH

Empirical Remedy for Strengthening Teeth (Gu Chi Mi Fang) was presented by the imperial physician Chun Hai on the second day of the seventh month of the lunar calendar in 1896.

### Ingredients

| | |
|---|---|
| Rhizoma Rhei  (Da Huang) | 30 g |
| Rhizoma Rhei Praeparatum  (Shu Da Huang) | 30 g |
| Gypsum Fibrosum  (Shi Gao) | 30 g |
| Gypsum Fibrosum Praeparatum  (Shu Shi Gao) | 30 g |
| Rhizoma Drynariae  (Gu Sui Bu) | 30 g |
| Cortex Eucommiae  (Du Zhong) | 30 g |
| Sea Sal  (Qing Yan) | 30 g |
| Table Sal  (Shi Yan) | 30 g |
| Alumen  (Ming Fan) | 15 g |
| Dried Alum  (Ku Fan) | 15 g |
| Radix Angelicae Sinensis  (Dang Gui) | 15 g |

The above ingredients were ground into fine powder which was first scattered around the gums every morning for rubbing, then applied to the face for similar rubbing. This was followed by rinsing the mouth with clean water.

There are many prescriptions for strengthening the teeth, some countering others. Some may provide temporary relief without preventing future attacks. Some may be simply analgesics with no effect of strengthening the teeth. The prescription introduced here is an empirical remedy of the Huang family for generations, first handed down by the generation of my great grandfather. Those in my family who followed the instructions and used the remedy for teeth rinsing all lived past 70 without losing a single tooth. None complained of toothache.

Those of my relatives who used the remedy were equally free from tooth problems. My mother, now 80, has teeth as firm as ever, really incredible. Almost everyone in my locality has a copy of the remedy, and recently, more and more people who have heard about it are asking for it. Therefore, I am hereby willing to make it public for the benefit of more.

Yours sincerely,
Huang Youlong of Jiangyou
Summer of 1896

### Comments

The main actions of this remedy were to nourish blood, reinforce the kidney, kill bacteria and relieve toxic heat. Gypsum Fibrosum and Rhizoma Rhei were also added. This recipe was especially good for toothache due to stomach fire. The pity is that Huang's claims seem somewhat exaggerated too.

## VIII.4. GUM BRUSHING REMEDY

Gum Brushing Remedy (Cha Ya Gen Fang) was carefully prepared by the imperial physician Jilu on the 28th day of the fifth month of the lunar calendar in 1902.

### Ingredients

| | |
|---|---|
| Rhizoma Drynariae (Gu Sui Bu) | 30 g |
| Fructus Mori (Sang Shen) | 15 g |
| Table Sal (Shi Yan) | 15 g |
| Semen Juglandis (Hu Tao) | 24 g |

The original recipe calls for black Fructus Mori and for the Table Sal to be roasted before use. The Semen Juglandis should be peeled and wrapped and char-baked to dispel the oily substance. The above ingredients were ground into extremely fine powder for rubbing at the roots of the teeth.

### Comments

This is a remedy for reinforcing the kidney, strengthening the teeth, cooling blood and clearing fire. It should be effective for the treatment of gingivitis.

## VIII.5. RINSING REMEDY

Old Buddha's Rinsing Remedy (Lao Fo Ye Shu Kou Fang) was carefully prepared on the first day of the first month of the lunar calendar, with no mention of the year. 1.5 grams of the powder were used daily.

### Ingredients

| | |
|---|---|
| Lignum Cervis Chinensis (Zi Jin Pi) | 9 g |
| Radix Ledebouriellae (Fang Feng) | 6 g |
| Herba Menthae (Bo He) | 6 g |
| Gypsum Fibrosum (Sheng Shi Gao) | 12 g |
| Table Sal (Shi Yan) | 9 g |
| Radix Glycyrrhizae (Sheng Gan Cao) | 6 g |

The above ingredients were decocted and divided into five portions for oral rinsing.

On the 23rd day of the same month, the same prescription was followed with some modifications. The Radix Ledebouriellae was omitted, while Bombyx Batryticatus (6 g) and Squama Manitis (6 g) were added, both roasted and ground into powder to which was added 6 grams of Acacia Catechu.

Five portions of the decoction were sent to the Empress Dowager immediately. Then further instructions came to smash 120 grams of Bulbus Cremastrae for addition to the decoction.

*Comments*

This prescription was made especially for acute toothache or pain in the mouth. This could be assumed from the statement "Five portions of the decoction were sent immediately" from the original script on the 23rd of the same month. This prescription had the action of clearing wind-heat and cooling blood. Bombyx Batryticatus, Acacia Catechu and Bulbus Cremastrae were also used to relieve toxic heat and swelling. Experts nowadays have shown that Acacia Catechu and Bulbus Cremastrae have antifungal effect. They must therefore have been effective in treating mycotic infection in the mouth.

## VIII.6. RINSING REMEDY PLUS

Rinsing Remedy Plus (Shu Kou Fang You) was prepared on the 24th day of the same month.

The prescription was modified by omitting the Radix Glycyrrhizae while adding six grams of Fructus Forsythiae. A total of 90 grams of Fructus Forsythiae were requested.

*Comments*

The Fructus Forsythiae was added to strengthen the effect of the remedy in clearing toxic heat, relieving swelling and softening masses. The antiseptic effect of Fructus Forsythiae is generally known.

## VIII.7. TOOTHACHE EXTERNAL REMEDY

The original script gave no specific information regarding the date and name of the imperial physician who prepared the remedy.

*Ingredients*

| | |
|---|---|
| Radix Aconiti Kusneziffii (Cao Wu) | 4.5 g |
| Fructus Piperis Longi (Bi Bo) | 4.5 g |
| Pericarpium Zanthoxyli (Chuan Jiao) | 9 g |
| Herba Asari (Xi Xin) | 9 g |

The above ingredients were ground into extremely fine powder. A tiny portion of the powder was put onto the affected tooth or tooth cavity and the toothache was soon less. (However, the original text says, "In a moment the tooth would fall out spontaneously.") More of the powder was used in case the pain persisted.

*Comments*

Radix Aconiti Kusneziffii, Fructus Piperis Longi, Pericarpium Zanthoxyli and Herba Asari are all fragrant warming ingredients for pain relief. They were used here to treat swollen gums and pain related to tooth cavity. Its external application was effective. Toothache Laughing Powder (Ya Tong Shi Xiao San) contained Fructus Piperis Longi, Herba Asari and Borneoleum Syntheticum. Instant Tooth-ache Powder (Li Zhi Ya Tong San) consisted of Radix Aconiti Kusneziffii, Herba Asari and Realgar. The patent medicine for relieving toothache produced in Jinan in Shandong Province and Chengde in Hebei Province contained Frutucs Piperis Longi, Rhizoma Alpiniae Officinalis, Herba Asari and Pericarpium Zanthoxyli. The herbal mechanism was more or less the same. In the original script, "Tooth would fall out spontaneously," actually meant that the toothache would be relieved. The above ingredients could also be soaked in alcohol for external application.

# IX. PRESCRIPTIONS FOR FACIAL NERVE SPASM

## IX.1. MODIFIED JADE COSMETIC POWDER

On the 20th day of the fourth month of the lunar calendar in 1888, Qian Xiang, the minor eunuch, told the imperial physicians Li Dechang and Wang Yonglong to prepare Modified Jade Cosmetic Powder (Jia Jian Yu Rong San).

*Ingredients*

| | |
|---|---|
| Radix Angelicae Dahuricae (Bai Zhi) | 45 g |
| Semen Pharbitidis (Bai Qian Niu) | 15 g |
| Radix Ledebouriellae (Fang Feng) | 9 g |
| Bai Ding Xiang | 30 g |
| Rhizoma Nardostachyos (Gan Song) | 9 g |
| Herba Asari (Xi Xin) | 9 g |
| Rhizoma Kaempferiae (Shan Nai) | 30 g |
| Semen Nelumbinis (Bai Lian Zhi) | 30 g |
| Lignum Santali (Tan Xiang) | 15 g |
| Bombyx Batryticatus (Bai Jiang Can) | 30 g |
| Rhizoma Bletillae Striatae (Bai Ji) | 9 g |
| Yin Tiao Bai | 30 g |
| Bai Jian (Radix Ampelopsis) | 9 g |
| Ge Tiao Bai | 30 g |
| Tuan Fen | 60 g |
| Rhizoma Typhonii Gigantei (Bai Fu Zi) | 30 g |

The above ingredients were ground into an extremely fine powder. Each time a tiny portion of the powder was put on the palm to be mixed with some water to make a paste which was rubbed on the face for some time before it was washed away with water. This was done two to three times daily.

*Comments*

Empress Dowager Cixi suffered from facial nerve spasm for many years, a condition known as facial wind syndrome in terms of traditional Chinese medicine. She had occasional rebounding pain in the lower eyelid to the cheek on the left side of the face. This was no doubt facial nerve spasm. At the age of 53 in 1888 her facial nerve spasm had already shown major improvement. Jade Cosmetic Powder (Yu Rong San) was originally described in *Golden Mirror of the Medical Tradition (Yi Zong Jin Jian)*. It was primarily prescribed for treating "dark gray facial complexion with wrinkles." The principle was to warm and promote the circulation of *qi* and blood in the channels and collaterals, and eliminate wind. Its external application was to moisten the skin. But here the original formula was modified by omitting Radix Notopterygii, Radix Angelicae Pubescentis, white Poria and Semen Dolichoris, and by adding Rhizoma Kaempferiae.

## IX.2. SCORPIO AND BOMBYX BATRYTICATUS EXTERNAL APPLICATION

The prescription for Scorpio and Bombyx Batryticatus External Application (Jiang Can Quan Xie Fu Zhi Fang) was carefully prepared by the imperial physician Zhuang Shouhe on the 24th day of the fourth month of the lunar calendar in 1902.

*Ingredients*

| | |
|---|---|
| Bombyx Batryticatus  (Jiang Can) | 9 g |
| Scorpio  (Quan Xie) | 2 |
| Bathing soap  (Xiang Zao) | 3 |

The original records say the Scorpio should be rid of poison before use. The three ingredients were mashed into an ointment for external application.

*Comments*

This prescription, having the effect of eliminating phlegm-wind and stopping spasm, was modified on the basis of the well-known Pulling to Normal Powder (Qian Zhen San). It was applied for facial nerve spasm and facial paralysis. In addition to its external application, it could be taken internally together with warm millet wine or warm boiled water. Referring to the pulse record of Empress Dowager Cixi on the 25th day of the fourth month of the lunar calendar in 1902, her liver pulse was "wiry and rapid, but her lung and spleen pulses were rapid and slippery. [There were] eyelid twitching and facial muscle rebounding, and blurred vision...," but no deviation of the mouth corner nor of the eyes. Her problem was no doubt facial nerve spasm.

## IX.3.  TWO REMEDIES FOR FACIAL NERVE SPASM

On the 24th day of the fifth month of the lunar calendar in 1902 Empress Dowager Cixi again complained of twitching of the lower eyelid in the left eye and muscular spasm in the left cheek. This was assumed to have been caused by liver *qi* stagnation and upward disturbance of dampness and wind. Therefore two external remedies were prepared together.

*Ingredients*

| | |
|---|---|
| Herba Schizonthemi  (Jin Jie Sui) | 6 g |

| | |
|---|---|
| Flos Chrysanthemi  (Ju Hua) | 4.5 g |
| Rhizoma Ligustici Chuanxiong  (Chuan Xiong) | 6 g |
| Rhizoma Gastrodiae  (Tian Ma) | 4.5 g |
| Radix Angelicae Dahuricae  (Bai Zhi) | 4.5 g |
| Folium Mori, frosted  (Shuang Sang Ye) | 12 g |
| Silkworm droppings | 30 g |

The first six ingredients above were decocted together with two boiled eggs with no shell. They were cooked for a long time to make sure the medicinal flavours pervaded the eggs. One egg was taken out for hot packing. When it became cool, the other egg was used for the hot pack. The silkworm droppings were fried together with millet wine and wrapped in a piece of silk cloth for frequent hot compress.

### Comments

Most of the ingredients in this prescription were for soothing the liver and clearing wind. The second contained only Bombyx Batryticatus that had the effect of eliminating wind and dampness and activating blood. Both the *Compendium of Materia Medica (Ben Cao Gang Mu)* and *Analytical Comments on Materia Medica (Ben Cao Jing Shu)* claimed that Bombyx Batryticatus could be used to treat patients for "windstroke" and "Bi syndrome with limited movement."

## IX.4.  HOT COMPRESS FOR CLEARING WIND AND ACTIVATING BLOOD

On the first day of the sixth month of the lunar calendar in 1902, the Imperial Pharmacy received an order to prepare three portions of Hot Compress for Clearing Wind and Activating Blood (Qu Feng Huo Luo Tang Fang).

### Ingredients

| | |
|---|---|
| Radix Ledeouriellae  (Fang Feng) | 9 g |
| Radix Dahuricae  (Bai Zhi) | 9 g |
| Squama Manitis  (Chuan Shan Jia) | 9 g |
| Spina Gleditsiae  (Zoa Jiao Ci) | 9 g |
| Herba Menthae  (Bo He) | 3 g |

The original records require that the Squama Manitis be prepared before use. The above ingredients were ground into fine powder and mixed with alcohol and water for steaming and external hot compress with the mixture in a silk bag.

### Comments

This prescription was primarily for clearing wind and dissolving phlegm in the channels and collaterals. But in the meantime, Squama Manitis was used to remove obstruction from the channels and collaterals, expel wind and eliminate dampness so as to strengthen the effect of the hot compress. According to the book entitled *Records of Heartfelt Medical Experience with Reference to the West (Yi Xue Zhong Zhong Can Xi Lu)*, Squama Manitis may "promote *qi* circulation of the Zang-Fu organs as well as the channels and collaterals. Its effect may reach even minor joints and organs." It may also "guide medicinal ingredients to act in the planned organs or areas."

## IX.5.  WHEAT-TRICHOSANTHIS CAKE

Wheat-Trichosanthis Cake (Gua Lou Da Mai Bing) was recorded on the second day of the sixth month of the lunar calendar in 1902.

### Ingredients

| | |
|---|---|
| Fructus Trichosanthis  (Gua Lou) | 960 g |
| Wheat Flour  (Mai Mian) | 180 g |

According to the original prescription, fresh Fructus Trichosanthis was squeezed for its juice to use as binder for the wheat flour and the making of small cakes which were steamed for hot packing. This compress should be stopped as soon as the discomfort passed. It was applied in treating deviation of mouth and eyes in facial paralysis.

### Comments

The main ingredient in this prescription was Fructus Trichosanthis, which is sweet, bitter and cold. Its medicinal effects such as moistening, clearing heat, dissolving phlegm and relieving hypochondriac pain due to stagnation of liver *qi* were achieved here in external therapy.

## IX.6.  HERBAL BATH FOR CLEARING WIND AND ACTIVATING CHANNELS

Herbal Bath for Clearing Wind and Activating Channels (Qu Feng Huo Luo Xi Yao Fang) was, as always, meticulously prepared by the imperial physicians Zhuang Shouhe, Fan Shaoxiang, Zhang Zhongyuan and Zhong Xun on the 21st day of the sixth month of the lunar calendar in 1902.

### Ingredients

| | |
|---|---|
| Radix Ledebouriellae  (Fang Feng) | 6 g |
| Radix Angelicae Dahuricae  (Bai Zhi) | 6 g |
| Rhizoma Typhonii Gigantei  (Bai Fu Zi) | 6 g |
| Bombyx Batryticatus  (Jiang Can) | 9 g |
| Herba Asari  (Xi Xin) | 1.8 g |
| Rhizoma Gastrodiae  (Tian Ma) | 4.5 g |
| Flos Chrysanthemi  (Ju Hua) | 6 g |
| Arisaema cum Bile  (Nan Xing) | 6 g |
| Retinervus Citri Grandis  (Ju Luo) | 6 g |
| Herba Menthae  (Bo He) | 3 g |

The above ingredients were boiled in water for compress and bathing.

### Comments

This prescription was formed by modifying the two formulae of Restoring to Normalcy Powder (Qian Zheng San) and Strange Wind Powder (Qi Feng San). The modified recipe has greater specific action in clearing wind and activating *qi* and blood circulation in the channels and collaterals. The dose of Bombyx Batryticatus was the largest because of its effect in quelling wind, dissolving phlegm and easing spasm. Modern studies prove that Bombyx Batryticatus is rich in the protein that stimulated the adrenal gland. The subject deserves further study to assess its effect in the treatment of facial neuritis and facial paralysis.

## IX.7. RESTORING TO NORMALCY PILL

This pill (Qian Zheng Wan) was carefully prepared by the imperial physicians Zhuang Shouhe and Zhang Zhongyuan on the fifth day of the eighth month of the lunar calendar in 1902.

### Ingredients
| | |
|---|---|
| Rhizoma Typhonii Gigantei  (Bai Fu Zi) | 15 g |
| Bombyx Batryticatus  (Jiang Can) | 15 g |
| Scorpio  (Quan Xie) | 12 g |

The original records stipulate that the poison should be removed from the Scorpio before use. The above ingredients were ground into fine powder and mixed with refined honey to make pills the size of mung beans. Six grams of the pills were taken daily with boiled water, while a small amount of wine could enhance the effect.

### Comments

Restoring to Normalcy Pill (Qian Zheng Wan) or Restoring to Normalcy Powder (Qian Zheng San) is a traditional patent remedy for the treatment of facial paralysis. Scorpio and Bombyx Batryticatus had strong actions in relieving spasm and tranquilizing the patient. Combining Scorpio and Scolopendrae made another patent remedy known as Spasm-relieving Powder (Zhi Jin San). Rhizoma Typhonii Gigantei, pungent, sweet and very warm, was used here to clear wind and phlegm. Both the inositol and ß— sterol in Rhizoma Typhonii Gigantei produce a tranquilizing effect which is even stronger after processing the raw ingredients. Rhizoma Typhonii Gigantei was used as the main ingredient in the Real Jade Powder (Zhen Yu San) according to *Orthodox Surgery (Wai Ke Zheng Zong)*. The powder was also believed to be effective in treating tetanus.

## IX.8. FACIAL SPASM ADJUSTING OINTMENT

Facial Spasm Adjusting Ointment (Zheng Rong Gao) was carefully prepared by the imperial physicians Zhuang Shouhe and Zhang Zhongyuan on the fifth day of the eighth month of the lunar calendar in 1902.

### Ingredients
| | |
|---|---|
| Semen Ricini  (Bi Ma Zi) | 15 g |
| Borneoleum syntheticum  (Bing Pian) | 1.8 g |

The original recipe says the Semen Ricini should be peeled before use, then two ingredients were ground to a paste for external application in the treatment of facial paralysis. The external application was made on the left side for facial paralysis on the right, and vice versa.

### Comments

Semen Ricini, sweet, pungent, bland and hot in nature, enters the liver, spleen and lung channels. *Compendium of Materia Medica (Ben Cao Gang Mu)* describes it as "having a wandering characteristic and clearing obstruction in its related channels. Therefore, it is often prescribed for aphasia, lock-jaw and deviation of the mouth corner and eye manifested in facial paralysis." Semen Ricini as an ingredient for external application in the treatment of facial paralysis was also recorded in the book *Compendium of Fine Prescriptions for Women (Fu Ren Liang Fang)*. The combination of Semen Recini with Borneoleum has the effect of removing obstruction of the five sense organs, thus the expression in the name facial spasm adjusting. It may be worthwhile to try it in practice. The paste can be applied at the mandible joint and mouth corner on the affected side and fixed in place by a bandage. The poultice is changed daily.

## IX.9. HERBAL PLASTER FOR CLEARING WIND AND ACTIVATING CHANNELS

Herbal Plaster for Clearing Wind and Activating Channels (Qu Feng Huo Luo Tie Yao Fang) was carefully prepared by the imperial physicians Zhuang Shouhe, Zhang Zhongyuan and Yao Baosheng on the 27th day of the first month of the lunar calendar in 1903.

*Ingredients*

| | |
|---|---:|
| Radix Ledebouriellae  (Fang Feng) | 9 g |
| Radix Angelicae Dahuricae  (Bai Zhi) | 9 g |
| Rhizoma Typhonii Gigantei  (Bai Fu Zi) | 6 g |
| Bombyx Batryticatus  (Jiang Can) | 9 g |
| Radix Gastrodiae  (Tian Ma) | 6 g |
| Herba Menthae  (Bo He) | 4.5 g |

The above ingredients were ground into fine powder and mixed with 180 grams of bath soap. This was well steamed and thus ready for external application at any time.

*Comments*

In fact, ingredients in this remedy were similar to those carried in Herbal Bath for Clearing Wind and Activating Channels (IX. 6.). The alternative of a poultice should be an improvement on the former.

## IX.10. CAULIS SPATHOLOBI PLASTER FOR CLEARING WIND AND ACTIVATING CHANNELS

Caulis Spatholobi Plaster for Clearing Wind and Activating Channels (Ji Xue Teng Qu Feng Huo Luo Tie Yao Fang) was recorded on the seventh day of the eighth month of the lunar calendar in 1903.

*Ingredients*

| | |
|---|---:|
| Caulis Spatholobi  (Ji Xue Teng) | 60 g |
| Spina Gleditsiae  (Da Jiao Zi) | 120 g |
| Bath soap  (Xiang Fei Zao) | 10 small bars |

The original records say that the Caulis Spatholobi should be prepared in powder form before use. The Spina Gleditsiae and the bath soap were melted in brown sugar syrup. Caulis Spatholobi powder was then added to form into balls of six grams each.

### Comments

Caulis Spatholobi activates and nourishes blood, its activating action being the more prominent. At the same time, it has the action of clearing wind from the channels and collaterals and is thus often applied in treating facial wind syndrome. Caulis Spatholobi was first seen in *The Supplement to Compendium of Materia Medica (Ben Cao Gang Mu Shi Yi)* published in 1805. It was also recorded in *Shunning County Chronicles (Shun Ning Fu Zhi)* in the era of Emperor Yong Zheng in 1725.

## IX.11. SEMEN RICINI PLASTER

Semen Ricini Plaster (Bi Ma Zi Gao ) was carefully prepared by the imperial physician Zhuang Shouhe on the 19th day of the third month of the lunar calendar in 1904.

Semen Ricini, pungent, sweet and hot, may flow through the channels and collaterals to clear pathogenic wind.

### Ingredient
Semen Ricini  (Bi Ma Zi)                                                       30 g

The Semen Ricini was peeled, mashed and spread onto a piece of cloth to make a plaster which was applied to the facial area affected by nerve spasm. The Semen Ricini seeds could also be mashed and mixed into face soap.

### Comments

Semen Ricini was also used in Facial Spasm Adjusting Ointment (Zheng Rong Gao) where it was combined with Borneoleum Syntheticum. However, only Semen Ricini was used in this remedy. The seeds were often used for external remedies either by mashing for single use or by mixing with other ingredients to relieve swelling and toxicity in the treatment of boils and furuncles. They were also used in the treatment of wind-Bi syndrome of the arms. Such application in empirical cases is recorded in *Compendium of Materia Medica (Ben Cao Gang Mu)*.

## IX.12. HERBAL PLASTER PLUS FOR CLEARING WIND AND ACTIVATING CHANNELS

Herbal Plaster Plus for Clearing Wind and Activating Channels (Qu Feng Huo Luo Tie Yao Fang You) was carefully prepared by the imperial physicians Zhuang Shouhe and Yao Baosheng on the third day of the sixth month of the lunar calendar in 1904.

### Ingredients
Rhizoma Typhonii Gigantei  (Bai Fu Zi)                                  15 g
Bombyx Batryticatus  (Jiang Can)                                         30 g

| | |
|---|---|
| Scorpio tails  (Xie Wei) | 15 g |
| Herba Menthae  (Bo Ho) | 90 g |
| Radix Ledebouriellae  (Fang Feng) | 30 g |
| Herba Schizonepetae  (Jing Jie Sui) | 30 g |
| Rhizoma Gastrodiae  (Tian Ma) | 30 g |
| Radix Glycyrrhizae  (Gan Cao) | 30 g |
| Rhizoma | No |
| opterygii  (Qiang Huo) | 15 g |
| Rhizoma Ligustici Chuanxiong  (Chuan Xiong) | 15 g |
| Radix Aconiti  (Wu Tou) | 15 g |
| Herba Agastachis  (Huo Xiang) | 15 g |

The above ingredients were made into powder first and mixed together with 40 pieces of Spina Gleditsiae, 20 bars of bath soap and brown sugar syrup for making lozenges weighing 60 grams each for external use.

On the fourth day of the sixth month, another 40 pieces of Spina Glegitsiae were added. And on the 24th day of the seventh month, 1.5 grams of Flos Magnoliae were added for each lozenge.

### Comments

This prescription was enriched by adding certain ingredients to Herbal Plaster for Clearing Wind and Activating Channels (Qu Feng Huo Luo Tie Yao Gao). Most important were the ingredients for activating blood and clearing wind, i. e. Rhizoma Notopterygii and Rhizoma Ligustici Chuanxiong. Studies done by experts at China Academy of Traditional Chinese Medicine in Beijing found that both had antithrombotic effects and could promote microcirculation. Herba Agastachis, fragrant and slightly warm, helped to clear obstruction without causing dryness in the body. This is how it differs from Radix Aconiti, which has a drastic effect in eliminating cold and phlegm.

## IX.13. FACIAL MOISTENING POWDER FOR CLEARING WIND

The Imperial Pharmacy was ordered to prepare five portions of Facial Moistening Powder for Clearing Wind (Qu Feng Run Mian San) on the 23rd day of the sixth month of the lunar calendar in 1904.

### Ingredients

| | |
|---|---|
| Powdered Semen Pasaeoli Radicis  (Lu Dou Bai Fen) | 1.8 g |
| Rhizoma Kaempferiae  (Shan Nai) | 1.2 g |
| Rhizoma Typhonii Gigantei  (Bai Fu Zi) | 1.2 g |
| Bombyx Batryticatus  (Jiang Can) | 1.2 g |
| Borneoleum syntheticum  (Bing Pian) | 0.6 g |
| Moschus  (She Xiang) | 0.3 g |

The above ingredients were ground into fine powder and sifted through silk cloth. The powder was then mixed with 120 grams of high-quality soap made from the pancreas of sheep or pigs.

### Comments

This was still a formula made by modifying the traditional remedy Restoring to Normalcy Powder (Qian Zheng San). Special mention should be made of the mutual effect of combining Moschus and powdered Semen Pasaeoli Radicis. The former, being fragrant and resuscitating, helped to remove obstruction from the channels and collaterals, disperse blood stasis and eliminate pathogenic factors from the body. The latter, sweet and detoxicating, moistened the muscle, making the two synergistic.

## IX.14. EXTERNAL REMEDY FOR ACTIVATING COLLATERALS

Old Buddha's External Remedy for Activating Collaterals (Lao Fo Ye Huo Luo Fu Yao Fang) was painstakingly prepared by the imperial physician Yao Baosheng on the 16th day of the intercalary fourth month of the lunar calendar in 1906.

### Ingredients

| | |
|---|---|
| Resina Olibani  (Ru Xiang) | 6 g |
| Resina Murrhae  (Mo Yao) | 6 g |
| Moschus  (She Xiang) | 0.3 g |

The original records stipulate that the oil in both the Resina Olibani and Resina Murrhae should be extracted before use while the Moschus should be used without processing. The above ingredients were ground into fine powder and mixed with some 60 grams of Spina Gleditsiae. This was applied externally to areas of strong pulsation.

### Comments

Stagnation of *qi* causes blood stasis with subsequent obstruction. In turn, obstructed blood circulation causes poor circulation of *qi*. The combination of Resina Olibani and Resina Murrhae tends to regulate the circulation of *qi* and blood and activate blood in the treatment of *qi* stagnation and blood stasis. Moschus was added to enhance the effect of promoting blood circulation and removing obstruction in the channels and collaterals. While oily substance in both the Resina Olibani and Resina Murrhae should be extracted according to the original records. In *Records of Heartfelt Medical Experience with Reference to the West (Yi Xue Zhong Zhong Can Xi Lu)*, however, Zhang Xichun states, "Resina Olibani and Resina Murrhae are fragrant ingredients for clearing obstruction, and are not likely to overconsume the anti-pathogenic *qi*. It would be most appropriate therefore to use them raw."

## IX.15. TYPHONII GIGANTEI EXTERNAL REMEDY

Typhonii Gigantei External Remedy (Bai Fu Zi Fang) for clearing wind and activating blood circulation was prepared on the 12th day of the sixth month of the lunar calendar in 1906.

### Ingredient

| | |
|---|---|
| Rhizoma Typhonii Gigantei  (Bai Fu Zi) | 9 g |

Nine grams of the Rhizoma Typhonii Gigantei were ground into fine powder and mixed with 60 grams of Spina Gleditsiae for making cakes of 30 grams each to be used externally.

## Comments

Rhizoma Typhonii Gigantei is a commonly used ingredient for clearing wind and phlegm, and activating channels and collaterals. In addition to being used in the ancient formula Restoring to Normalcy Powder (Qian Zheng San), it was also used in many other patent remedies, e.g. Scorpio and Typhonii Gigantei Powder (Xie Fu San) and Convulsion-relieving Powder (Ding Xu San) recorded in *Standard Reference for Syndromes and Treatments (Zheng Zhi Zhun Sheng)*, Soul Regaining Powder (Fan Hun Dan) formulated by Wang Haizang, The Eight Immortals Powder (Ba Xian Dan) formulated by Sheng Jinao, and Scorpio Powder (Quan Xie San) recorded in the book *Essentials of Infant Care ( Bao Yin Cuo Yao)* by Xue Kai. Rhizoma Typhonii Gigantei was also used in Jade and Gold Powder (Qing Jin Wan) as recorded in *Complete Collection of Patterns and Treatments in External Medicine ( Wai Ke Zheng Zhi Quan Sheng Ji)*. All these remedies are well-known in medical history. Most were prescribed for internal use, while the one introduced here is for external application.

## IX.16. HERBAL PLASTER FOR CLEARING WIND-HEAT

Herbal Plaster for Clearing Wind-Heat (Qing Re Qu Feng Tie Yao Fang) was prepared with the usual great care by the imperial physician Yao Baosheng for Empress Dowager Cixi on the 13th day of the seventh month of the lunar calendar in 1906.

### Ingredients

| | |
|---|---|
| Radix Ledebouriellae  (Fang Feng) | 6 g |
| Herba Menthae  (Bo He) | 2.4 g |

The above ingredients were ground into extremely fine powder and well mixed with 60 grams of Spina Gleditsiae for making the plasters for external use.

## Comments

According to *Analytical Comments on Materia Medica (Ben Cao Jing Shu)*, Radix Ledebouriellae was used in the "treatment of spasm due to wind disturbance in the blood." The book entitled *A Collection of Changsha Folk Recipes (Chang Sha Yao Jie)* says, "Radix Ledebouriellae promotes circulation of *qi* and blood in the channels and collaterals." It is apparent that the remedy has a mild effect in dispelling wind. It may also be that Radix Ledebouriellae differs from Rhizoma Notopterygii, Radix Bulpeuri and Radix Puerariae because of its warm and drying property. Radix Ledebouriellae is commonly believed to be good for acute convulsions due to wind invasion and may therefore be effective in improving vessel adaptation. Herba Menthae, pungent and cooling, helps dilate the capillary vessels so as to promote the use of the active ingredients by the body. In the latter half of the year 1906 Empress Dowager Cixi showed less facial muscle twitching than earlier, due no doubt to the application of the prescriptions introduced in this chapter.

# X. PRESCRIPTION FOR THROAT CONDITIONS

## X.1. PERLINGUAL REMEDY FOR CLEARING LUNG HEAT

Perlingual Remedy for Clearing Lung Heat (Qin Hua Shang Qing Wan) was prepared with care by the imperial physician Li Deli on the 26th day of the 11th month of the lunar calendar in 1876.

*Ingredients*

| | |
|---|---|
| Radix Platycodi  (Jie Gen) | 30 g |
| Radix Trichosanthis  (Hua Fen) | 30 g |
| Radix Puerariae  (Ge Gen) | 30 g |
| Herbal plant root  (Bai Yao Jian) | 30 g |
| Powder from the surface of dried persimmon  (Shi Zi Shuang) | 30 g |
| Flos Rosae Rugosae  (Mei Gui) | 30 g |
| Osmanthus Fragrans  (Mu Xi) | 30 g |
| Fructus Mume  (Wu Mei Rou) | 18 g |
| Radix Peucedani  (Qian Hu) | 18 g |
| Radix Glycyrrhizae  (Gan Cao) | 18 g |
| Herba Menthae  (Bo Ho) | 18 g |
| Radix Ophiopogonis  (Mai Dong) | 18 g |
| Semen Armenicacae  (Xin Ren) | 18 g |
| Borax  (Peng Sha) | 18 g |
| Lignum Santali  (Bai Tang Xiang) | 6 g |
| Sacchrum Sinensis  (Bing Tang) | 1,240 g |

The above ingredients were ground into fine powder and made in the form of water-bound pills the size of euryale seeds.

*Comments*

This prescription, acting to clear the voice, dissolve phlegm and relieve a sensation of fullness in the chest and diaphragm, was prepared for treating sore throat and ulceration of the mouth and tongue. The composition of this prescription was different from the Perlingual Remedy for Clearing Lung Heat (Qin Hua Shang Qing Wan) recorded in *The New Edition of Empirical Formulae* (Yan Fang Xin Bian) by Bao Xiangao. That prescription contained Calcitum and Indigo Naturalis, but not herbal plant root and Lignum Santali.

# XI. PRESCRIPTIONS FOR ANXIETY AND PALPITATION

## XI.1. CINNABAR TRANQUILIZING PILL

Cinnabar Tranquilizing Pill (Zhu Sha An Shen Wan) was carefully prepared for Empress Dowager Cixi on the 24th day of the eighth month of the lunar calendar in 1904.

*Ingredients*

| | |
|---|---|
| Radix Angelicae Sinensis  (Dang Gui) | 30 g |
| Radix Ophiophogonis  (Mai Dong) | 30 g |

⟩ Radix Asparagi  (Tian Dong) 30 g
Radix Scrophulariae  (Xuan Shen) 15 g
Radix Codopsis Pilosulae  (Dan Shen) 15 g
Radix Playgalae  (Yuan Zhi) 15 g
Poria  (Fu Ling) 15 g
Semen Biotae  (Bai Zi Ren) 30 g
Radix Ginsneg  (Ren Shen) 7.5 g
Radix Rehmanniae  (Sheng Di Huang) 60 g
Semen Ziziphi Spinosae  (Zao Ren) 30 g
Fructus Schisandrae  (Wu Wei Zi) 15 g

The Semen Ziziphi Spinosae should be roasted before use according to the original recipe. All the above ingredients were ground into extremely fine powder and made into honey-bound pills coated with cinnabar. Two grams of the pills were taken orally each time.

### Comments

The other name for the Cinnabar Tranquilizing Pill was Imperial Cinnabar Tranquilizing Pill (Gong Zhong Zhu Sha An Shen Wan). Its composition suggests that it was actually a modification of Biota Seed Pill for Nourishing the Heart (Bai Zi Yang Xin Wan). That pill was also coated with cinnabar and used for anxiety, palpitation and poor sleep quality due to deficiency of heart blood.

## XI.2. SIMPLIFIED CINNABAR TRANQUILIZING PILL

Simplified Cinnabar Tranquilizing Pill (Jian Wei Zhu Sha An Shen Wan) was prepared on the 18th day of the eighth month of the lunar calendar, with no mention of the year.

### Ingredients

Radix Angelicae Sinensis  (Dang Gui) 150 g
Radix Glycyrrhizae  (Gan Cao) 150 g
Radix Rehmanniae  (Sheng Di Huang) 150 g
Rhizoma Coptidis  (Huang Lian) 360 g

The above ingredients were ground into fine powder and made into pills the size of Semen Phaseoli Radiatus.

### Comments

This prescription was a simplified version of the Cinnabar Tranquilizing Pill (Zhu Sha An Shen Wan) formulated by the imperial physician Li Dongyuan. The original was coated with purified cinnabar though cinnabar was not considered appropriate. This pill was not coated with cinnabar, and therefore the constraining of floating deficient fire by using ingredients with tranquilizing effects was not achieved. Nor was the effect of eliminating heat with its cold property or its effect of producing fluid with sweet flavour retained. Only the effect of Radix Glycyrrhizae for relieving acute pain, that of Rhizoma Coptidis for clearing fire, that of Radix Angelicae Sinensis for nourishing and that of Radix Rehmanniae for reinforcing were retained for calming the heart and mind.

# XII.  PRESCRIPTIONS FOR ELIMINATING COUGH AND PHLEGM AND REGULATING PULMONARY *QI*

## XII.1.  PILL FOR CLEARING WIND AND STOPPING COUGH

Pill for Clearing Wind and Stopping Cough (Shu Feng Zhi Ke Wan) was carefully formulated by the imperial physicians Li Dechang and Quan Shun on the second day of the second month of the lunar calendar in 1891. It was based on an ancient prescription, with only one tenth of the original dosage being suggested. Folium Perillae was replaced by Ganlis Perillae. The pills were coated with cinnabar.

*Ingredients*

| | |
|---|---:|
| Ganlis Perillae  (Su Gen) | 15 g |
| Radix Ledebouriellae  (Fang Feng) | 9 g |
| Radix Pueraiae  (Gang Ge) | 9 g |
| Fructus Aurantii  (Zhi Ke) | 9 g |
| Radix Peucedani  (Qian Hu) | 9 g |
| Radix Platycodis  (Jie Geng) | 9 g |
| Folium Mori  (Sang Pi) | 9 g |
| Semen Armenicacae  (Xin Ren) | 9 g |
| Rhizoma Pinelliae  (Ban Xia) | 9 g |
| Poria  (Fu Ling) | 9 g |
| Pericarpium Citri Reticulatae  (Chen Pi) | 6 g |
| Bulbux Fritillariae Cirhosae  (Chuan Bei) | 6 g |
| Rhizoma Notopterygii  (Qiang Huo) | 6 g |
| Radix Scutellariae  (Huang Qin) | 6 g |
| Radix Glycyrrhizae  (Gan Cao) | 3 g |

The original records say the Fructus Aurantii is roasted, and the Rhizoma Pinelliae prepared before use. The pits of the Bulbux Fritillariae should be discarded before use, and all ingredients were ground into fine powder and made with honey into cinnabar-coated pills the size of mung beans. Nine grams of the pills were taken with boiled water each time.

*Comments*

This prescription was prepared on the basis of Stopping Cough Powder (Zhi Sou San) originally from *Medical Revelations (Yi Xue Xin Wu)*, and modified Double Cure Decoction (Er Chen Tang). It was effective for cough with excessive sputum due to invasion of exogenous pathogenic wind-cold, or cough with sputum difficult to expectorate. It was also effective for lingering cough with sputum as well as certain remaining superficial symptoms and signs. Its actions were to clear superficial wind, promote dispersing action by the lung, stop cough and dissolve phlegm.

## XII.2.  PILL FOR CLEARING PULMONARY FIRE AND RESOLVING PHLEGM

Pill for Clearing Pulmonary Fire and Resolving Phlegm (Qing Fei Yi Huo

Hua Tan Wan) was prepared exactly according to the recipe of Tong Ren Tang Pharmacy on the 12th day of the third month of the lunar calendar in 1891.

### Ingredients

| | |
|---|---|
| Pericarpium Citri Reticulatae  (Chen Pi) | 30 g |
| Rhizoma Pinelliae  (Ban Xia) | 30 g |
| Radix Peucedani  (Qian Hu) | 30 g |
| Radix seu Rhizoma Rhei  (Shu Da Huang) | 18 g |
| Fructus Gardeniae  (Zhi Zi) | 18 g |
| Radix Ophiopogonis  (Mai Dong) | 18 g |
| Radix Platycodis  (Jie Geng) | 18 g |
| Fructus Aurantii  (Zhi Ke) | 18 g |
| Radix Trichosanthis  (Hua Fen) | 18 g |
| Hai Shi | 21 g |
| Semen Armencacae  (Xin Ren) | 12 g |
| Radix Stemonae  (Bai Bu) | 12 g |
| Rhizoma Coptidis  (Huang Lian) | 9 g |
| Radix Glycyrrhizae  (Gan Cao) | 9 g |
| Semen Trichosanthis  (Gua Lou Ren) | 12 g |
| Radix Scutellariae  (Huang Qin) | 37.5 g |

The original records say that both the Fructus Gardeniae and Rhizoma Coptidis should be roasted with ginger, and that the Rhizoma Pinelliae should be prepared before use. The above ingredients were ground into fine powder and made into honey-bound pills the size of mung beans. Six grams of the pills were taken orally each time.

### Comments

Pill for Clearing Pulmonary Fire and Resolving Phlegm has been widely used in the Beijing area and still has a good sale in the market. It was modified on the basis of Decoction for Clearing Throat and Constraining Fire (Qing Yan Yi Huo Fang) recorded in *Achieving Longevity by Guarding the Source (Shou Shi Bao Yuan)*. Having the action of clearing excess heat from the lung and stomach, it was applied in the treatment of cough with production of yellow sputum, sore throat, dry tongue and constipation. It was also applicable for toothache and ulceration of the mouth and tongue.

## XII.3. PILL FOR CLEARING PULMONARY HEAT AND STRENGTHENING THE LUNG AND SPLEEN

Pill for Clearing Pulmonary Heat and Strengthening the Lung and Spleen (Qing Bu Li Fei Jian Pi Wan) was carefully formulated by the imperial physicians Zhuang Shouhe and Quan Shun on the fifth day of the eighth month of the lunar calendar in 1891.

### Ingredients

| | |
|---|---|
| Ginseng  (Ren Shen) | 4.5 g |
| Rhizoma Atractylodis Macrocephalae  (Bai Zhu) | 9 g |
| Poria  (Fu Ling) | 15 g |
| Radix Rehmanniae  (Sheng Di) | 12 g |

| | |
|---|---|
| Radix Angelicae Sinensis  (Dang Gui) | 12 g |
| Radix Paeoniae Lactiflorae  (Bai Shao) | 9 g |
| Pericarpium Citri Reticulatae Rubra  (Ju Hong) | 6 g |
| Radix Ophiopogonis  (Mai Dong) | 12 g |
| Radix Platycodis  (Jie Geng) | 9 g |
| Rhizoma Pinelliae Fermentata  (Ban Xia Qu) | 9 g |
| Bulbus Fritillariae Cirhosae  (Chuan Bei) | 15 g |
| Radix Glycyrrhizae  (Gan Cao) | 4.5 g |

According to the original records, the Radix Ginseng and Rhizoma Atracty-lodis Macrocephalae required special permission. The Pericarpium Citri Reticula-tae Rubra should be harvested from old trees. The above ingredients were ground into extremely fine powder and made into cinnabar-coated pills with honey the size of mung beans. Nine grams of the pills taken with boiled water were one dose.

### Comments

This prescription was formulated to deal with both the lung and spleen according to the principle of simultaneously clearing and reinforcing. It was modified on the basis of three traditional formulae, i.e. Eight Treasures Decoction (Ba Zhen Tang), Six Gentlemen Decoction (Liu Jun Zi Tang) and Double Cure Decoction (Er Chen Tang). It was appropriate for the damp-phlegm syndrome of Empress Dowager Cixi due to her constitutional spleen and stomach *qi* deficiency. It reinforces *qi*, nourishes blood and strengthens the spleen.

## XII.4. PILL FOR SOOTHING THE LIVER AND PROMOTING LUNG *QI*

Pill for Soothing the Liver and Promoting Lung *Qi* (Yi Qi Qing Fei Huan Gan Wan) was meticulously prepared by the imperial physician Zhang Zhongyuan on the second day of the eighth month of the lunar calendar in 1895.

### Ingredients

| | |
|---|---|
| Radix Pancis Quiquefloii  (Xi Yang Shen) | 18 g |
| Poria  (Fu Ling) | 18 g |
| Rhizoma Atractylodis Macrocephalae  (Bai Zhu) | 9 g |
| Radix Glycyrrhizae  (Gan Cao) | 4.5 g |
| Radix Rehmanniae  (Sheng Di) | 18 g |
| Radix Paeoniae Lactiflorae  (Bai Shao) | 9 g |
| Cortex Moudan Radicis  (Mu Dan Pi) | 12 g |
| Rhizoma Alismatis  (Ze Xie) | 9 g |
| Fel Ursi  (Xiong Dan) | 9 g |
| Cornu Rhinoceri Asiatici  (Xi Jiao) | 9 g |
| Radix Ophiopogonis  (Mai Dong) | 18 g |
| Fructus Amomi Kravanh  (Bai Kou Ren) | 6 g |
| Bulbus Fritillariae Thunbergii  (Zhe Bei) | 12 g |
| Radix Platycodis  (Jie Geng) | 9 g |
| Herba Dendrobii  (Shi Hu) | 9 g |
| Radix Curcumae  (Guang Yu Jin) | 18 g |

The original directions require the Poria to be prepared with cinnabar before use. The Radix Ophiopogouis pits should be included. The above ingredients were ground into fine powder and made into cinnabar-coated pills with honey the size of mung beans. Six grams of the pills were to be taken with boiled water in the morning and evening.

### Comments

The actions of this prescription are to reinforce *qi*, clear the lung and soothe the liver. It was in case Empress Dowager Cixi had high fever and nosebleed or any eye conditions due to heat. The principle for reinforcing *qi* was based on the Four Gentlemen Decoction (Si Jun Zi Tang). Radix Pancis Quiquefloii was used to reinforce *qi* and nourish Yin without causing dryness in the body. The principle for clearing heat in the blood was based on both Paeoniae Lactiflorae and Rehmanniae Decoction (Shao Yao Di Huang Tang) as recorded in *Handbook of Remedies (Xiao Pin Yao Fang)*, and Rhinoceri-Rehmanniae Decoction (Xi Jiao Di Huang Tang) as recorded in *Prescriptions Worth a Thousand Gold* (Qian Jin Yao Fang). Both were considered good for clearing heat, cooling blood and dispersing blood stasis. The Fel Ursi and Cornu Rhinoceri Asiatici were mainly applied to soothe the liver. Fel Ursi, bitter, cold, and entering the liver, gallbladder, spleen and stomach channels, helped clear heat, calm the patient, enhance vision and kill parasites. External application of Fel Ursi helped clear nebulae. Experimental studies show that Fel Ursi relieved muscle spasm and cleared toxins. Cornu Rhinoceri Asiatici, bitter, salty, cold, and entering the heart and liver channels, was very effective in clearing heat, calming the patient, cooling blood, dispersing toxins and soothing the liver.

## XII.5.   PILL FOR SOOTHING THE LIVER AND PROMOTING THE LUNG IN RESOLVING PHLEGM

Pill for Soothing the Liver and Promoting the Lung in Resolving Phlegm (Huan Gan Li Fei Hua Tan Wan) was carefully formulated by the imperial physician Zhang Zhongyuan on the 30th day of the ninth month of the lunar calendar in 1895.

### Ingredients

| | |
|---|---|
| Radix Rehmanniae  (Sheng Di) | 15 g |
| Radix Paeoniae Lactiflorae  (Bai Shao) | 9 g |
| Radix Ophiopogonis  (Mai Dong) | 9 g |
| Herba Dendrobii  (Shi Hu) | 12 g |
| Radix Curcumae  (Yu Jin) | 12 g |
| Radix Platycodis  (Jie Geng) | 9 g |
| Pericarpium Citri Reticulatae Rubra  (Ju Hong) | 6 g |
| Flos Farfarae  (Kuan Dong Hua) | 12 g |
| Bulbus Fritillariae Thunbergii  (Zhe Bei) | 12 g |
| Rhizoma Anemarrhenae  (Zhi Mu) | 9 g |
| Cortex Mori Radicis  (Sang Pi) | 9 g |
| Radix Glycyrrhizae  (Gan Cao) | 3 g |
| Poria  (Fu Ling) | 12 g |
| Cortex Moudan Radicis  (Mu Dan Pi) | 9 g |

| | |
|---|---|
| Radix Codopsis Pilosulae  (Dan Shen) | 9 g |
| Rhizoma Alismatis  (Ze Xie) | 9 g |

The above ingredients were ground into fine powder and made with honey into pills the size of mung beans and coated with cinnabar. Nine grams of the pills were taken with boiled water as one dose.

### Comments

The main purpose of this prescription was to soothe the liver, not to clear its fire. Therefore, Fel Ursi and Cornu Rhinoceri Asiatici were omitted. Radix Panacis Quiquefloii and Rhizoma Atractylodis Macrocephalae were also omitted because the aim of promoting rather than reinforcing lung *qi* was stressed. The prescription may help in convalescing from inflammation in the respiratory system.

## XII.6. ASPARAGI-OPHIOPOGONIS SYRUP WITH PYRUS

On the 30th day of the eighth month of the lunar calendar in 1899, the eunuch Qian He conveyed the order for the preparation of Asparagi-Ophiopogonis Syrup with Pyrus (Er Dong Gao Li Gao).

### Ingredients

| | |
|---|---|
| Radix Asparagi  (Tian Men Dong) | 240 g |
| Radix Ophiopogonis  (Mai Men Dong) | 240 g |
| Pyrus  (Ya Li) | 20 |

The ingredients were first decocted and their residue separated out. The decoction was then mixed with 60 grams of Bulbus Fritillariae Cirhosae, and further decocted with honey to make a syrup. The pits from the 20 Pyrus were removed and the fruit squeezed for addition to the mixture for still further decoction into the final syrup.

### Comments

Asparagi-Ophiopogonis Syrup (Er Dong Gao) was applied for dryness and heat in the lung and stomach manifested by cough and sputum difficult to expectorate. It was originally from *Comprehension to Medicine According to Master Zhang (Zhang Shi Yi Tong)*. The actions of this syrup were associated with the nomenclature of its ingredients. The middle name in the first two ingredients means Door, while the last characters mean Winter. In basic philosophy of traditional Chinese medicine winter is the season of storage and accumulation. A door functions in opening and closing an entrance. Any wind-cold invasion in winter first affects the lung, the entrance or the body's door. Asparagi-Ophiopogonis Syrup therefore helps moisten the lung and clear phlegm. Regular use of the syrup may have a reinforcing effect on the lung. There is now Asparagi-Ophiopogonis Syrup with Bulbus Fritillariae Cirhosae (Bei Mu Er Dong Gao) which was primarily made by adding both Bulbus Fritillariae Cirhosae and Sacchrum Sinensis to Asparagi-Ophiopogonis Syrup.

Pyrus Syrup or Snow Pear Syrup, having the action of moistening the lung and clearing lung heat, is indicated in stubborn dry cough with dry throat, hoarse voice, panting and blood in sputum. The syrup may also produce fluid and calm pulmonary fire, its effect being strengthened by adding fresh juice of radish, lotus, Rhizoma Imperatae, Radix Rehmanniae, persimmon cortex or Ophiopogonis.

## XII.7.  PILL FOR PROMOTING LUNG *QI* IN DESCENDING AND DISPERSING

On the 17th day of the 10th month of the lunar calendar in 1899, the Pill for Promoting Lung *Qi* in Descending and Dispersing (Tong Xuan Li Fei Wan) followed almost exactly the first one as recorded on the 22nd day of the sixth month of the lunar calendar in 1891.

*Ingredients*

| | |
|---|---|
| Radix Ginseng  (Ren Shen) | 15 g |
| Folium Perillae  (Su Ye) | 30 g |
| Radix Puerariae  (Ge Gen) | 25.5 g |
| Rhizoma Pinelliae  (Ban Xia) | 15 g |
| Pericarpium Citri Reticulatae  (Chen Pi) | 22.5 g |
| Radix Peucedani  (Qian Hu) | 22.5 g |
| Poria  (Fu Ling) | 15 g |
| Fructus Aurantii  (Zhi Ke) | 22.5 g |
| Radix Platycodi  (Jie Geng) | 30 g |
| Radix Glycyrrhizae  (Gan Cao) | 7.5 g |
| Radix Auchlandiae  (Mu Xiang) | 5.8 g |
| Radix Ephedrae  (Ma Huang) | 18.75 g |

The original records state that the Rhizoma Pinelliae was prepared, and the Fructus Aurantii was roasted before use. The above ingredients were ground into fine powder and made in honey-bound pills of nine grams each.

*Comments*

This patent Pill for Promoting Lung *Qi* in Descending and Dispersing was popular in northern and eastern China as it could eliminate persistent cough. It is often applied for fever with aversion to cold, nasal obstruction, headache with no sweating, and soreness and pain of the four limbs occurring in common cold attack due to wind-cold invasion. However, this patent medicine by the same name may consist of slightly different ingredients in different areas of China. The one introduced here contained ginseng which was prescribed for Empress Dowager Cixi for her exogenous type of cough related to her poor general health.

## XII.8.  SYRUP FOR MOISTENING THE LUNG AND SOOTHING THE LIVER

Syrup for Moistening the Lung and Soothing the Liver (Run Fei He Gan Gao) was painstakingly formulated by the imperial physician Zhang Zhongyuan on the 13th day of the ninth month of the lunar calendar in 1902.

*Ingredients*

| | |
|---|---|
| Radix Codonopsis Pilosulae  (Dang Shn) | 15 g |
| Semen Coicis  (Yi Yi Ren) | 30 g |
| Radix Ophiopogonis  (Mai Men Dong) | 24 g |

| | |
|---|---|
| Pericarpium Citri Reticulatae Rubra (Ju Hong) | 12 g |
| Folium Mori (Sang Ye) | 24 g |
| Folium Eriobotryae (Pi Pa Ye) | 24 g |
| Radix Paeoniae Lactiflorae (Bai Shao) | 18 g |
| Herba Dendrobii (Shi Hu) | 24 g |
| Radix Glycyrrhizae (Gan Cao) | 9 g |
| Fructus Aurantii (Zhi Ke) | 12 g |

According to the original records, the Pericarpium Citri Rectulatae Rubra from the fruits of old trees were to be used, and the Folium Eriobotryae prepared and packed during decocting. The above ingredients were first well decocted, followed by concentrating the decoction after the residue was separated out. The concentration was then mixed with refined honey to make the syrup. Nine grams of the syrup were taken with boiled water as one dose.

### Comments

In the health history of Empress Dowager Cixi there appeared on the 11th day of the ninth month of the lunar calendar in 1902 the following: "The circulation of *qi* of the liver and lung was abnormally rough, and she had occasional cough." This prescription was no doubt written with her specific condition in mind.The option of Radix Codonopsis Pilosulae instead of Radix Adenonhorae Strictae was probably related to her deficiency of lung *qi*.

# XIII.  PRESCRIPTIONS FOR SPLEEN AND STOMACH CONDITIONS

## XIII.1.  PILL FOR SOOTHING THE LIVER AND RESOLVING SPLEEN DAMPNESS

Pill for Soothing the Liver and Resolving Spleen Dampness (He Gan Xing Pi Hua Shi Wan) was carefully worked out by the imperial physicians Zhuang Shouhe and Li Dechang on the 30th day of the second month of the lunar calendar in 1879.

### Ingredients

| | |
|---|---|
| Radix Bupleuri (Qian Hu) | 9 g |
| Cortex Fraxini (Qing Pi) | 12 g |
| Rhizoma Cyperi (Xiang Fu) | 18 g |
| Radix Paeoniae Lactiflorae (Bai Shao) | 12 g |
| Herba Agastachis (Huo Xiang Geng) | 12 g |
| Cortex Magnoliae Officinalis (Hou Po) | 12 g |
| Pericarpium Citri Chachiensis (Xin Hui Pi) | 12 g |
| Rhizoma Atractylodis (Cang Zhu) | 12 g |
| Lignum Aquilariae Resinatum (Luo Shui Cheng) | 9 g |
| Rhizoma Atractylodis Macrocephalae (Bai Zhu) | 9 g |
| White Poria (Bai Fu Ling) | 18 g |
| Fructus Amomi (Sha Ren) | 9 g |
| Fructus Oryzae Germinature (Gu Ya) | 18 g |
| Radix Auchlandiae (Mu Xiang) | 9 g |

| | |
|---|---|
| Fructus Crataegi  (Shan Zha) | 24 g |
| Fructus Aurantii Immaturus  (Zhi Shi) | 12 g |

According to the original records, the Cortex Fraxini, Rhizoma Atractylodis, Fructus Oryzae Germinature and Fructus Aurantii Immaturus should be roasted before use. The Rhizoma Atractylodis Macrocephalae and Radix Paeoniae Lactiflorae should be roasted to a burnt-yellow colour. The Rhizoma Cyperi should be prepared before use. The above ingredients were ground into extremely fine powder and mixed with refined honey to make pills the size of mung beans and coated with cinnabar. One dose was 7.5 grams of the pills taken with boiled water.

### Comments

Empress Dowager Cixi liked to eat Peking duck, a dish that is typically fatty. In her later years she suffered from spleen and stomach conditions for which this Pill for Soothing the Liver and Resolving Spleen Dampness was formulated on the basis of Carefree Powder (Xiao Yao San), Calming Stomach Powder (Ping Wei San), and Awakening Spleen Powder (Xing Pi San) which first appeared in *Standards for Syndrome Differentiation and Treatment* (*Zheng Zhi Zhun Shen*). The use of Lignum Aquilariae Resinatum and Herba Agastachis enhanced its therapeutic effect in resolving dampness retained in the spleen.

## XIII.2. PILL FOR RESOLVING SPLEEN DAMPNESS AND NOURISHING YIN

The prescription for Pill for Resolving Spleen Dampness and Nourishing Yin (Yi Pi Yang Yin Chu Shi Wan) was carefully prepared by the imperial physicians Li Dechang and Yang Jihe on the sixth day of the seventh month of the lunar calendar in 1886.

### Ingredients

| | |
|---|---|
| Radix Ginseng  (Ren Shen) | 9 g |
| Rhizoma Atractylodis Macrocephalae  (Bai Zhu) | 15 g |
| Radix Poria  (Fu Shen) | 15 g |
| Pericarpium Citri Reticulatae Rubra  (Ju Hong) | 6 g |
| Radix Angelicae Sinensis  (Dang Gui) | 15 g |
| Radix Rehmanniae  (Di Huang) | 18 g |
| Radix Paeoniae Lactiflorae  (Bai Shao) | 9 g |
| Pericarpium Citri Reticulatae Viride  (Qing Pi) | 4.5 g |
| Radix Polygalae  (Yuan Zhi) | 6 g |
| Fructus Gardeniae  (Zhi Zi) | 9 g |
| Radix Auchlandiae  (Mu Xiang) | 4.5 g |
| Fructus Amomi  (Sha Ren) | 4.5 g |
| Radix Gentianae  (Long Dan Cao) | 9 g |
| Rhizoma Pinelliae  (Ban Xia) | 9 g |
| Rhizoma Alismatis  (Ze Xie) | 9 g |
| Radix Glycyrrhizae  (Gan Cao) | 3 g |

According to the original records the Radix Paeoniae Lactiflorae, Pericarpium

Citri Reticulatae Viride and Fructus Gardeniae should be roasted. The Radix Gentianae should be rinsed in millet wine. The Rhizoma Pinelliae should be prepared before use. The above ingredients were ground into extremely fine powder and mixed with nine grams of ginger powder and 20 dates in separate packings for decocting. The decoction with powdery substance was then mixed with refined honey to make pills the size of mung beans and coated with cinnabar. Six grams of the pills were taken with boiled water as one dose.

### Comments

This Pill for Resolving Spleen Dampness and Nourishing Yin was formed on the basis of Six Gentlemen Pill with Auchlandiae and Amomum (Xiang Sha Liu Jun Wan), plus ingredients for nourishing Yin, clearing liver heat and resolving dampness.

## XIII. 3. DECOCTION FOR RESOLVING SPLEEN DAMPNESS AND CLEARING LIVER HEAT

Decoction for Resolving Spleen Dampness and Clearing Liver Heat (Tiao Pi Qing Gan Li Shi Yin) was carefully prepared by the imperial physician Li Dechang on the 22nd day of the sixth month of the lunar calendar in 1889.

### Ingredients

| | |
|---|---|
| Poria (Fu Ling) | 9 g |
| Rhizoma Atractylodis Macrocephalae (Bai Zhu) | 4.5 g |
| Pericarpium Citri Reticulatae (Chen Pi) | 4.5 g |
| Fructus Amomi (Sha Ren) | 3 g |
| Semen Coicis (Yi Yi Ren) | 3 g |
| Rhizoma Alismatis (Ze Xie) | 6 g |
| Semen Dolichorii (Bian Dou) | 9 g |
| Radix Gentianae (Long Dan Cao) | 4.5 g |
| Radix Codopsis Pilosulae (Dan Shen) | 6 g |
| Radix Rehmanniae (Sheng Di) | 9 g |
| Cortex Dictamni Dasycarpi Radicis (Bai Xian Pi) | 6 g |
| Semen Plantaginis (Che Qian Zi) | 9 g |
| Fructus Kochiae (Di Fu Zi) | 9 g |

The original records state that the Poria should be prepared with cinnabar, and the Fructus Amomi ground before use. The Rhizoma Atractylodis Macrocephalae, Semen Coicis and Semen Dolichorii should be roasted before use. The Radix Gentianae should be prepared with millet wine, and the Semen Plantaginis packed before use.

This decoction was specially prescribed for clearing damp-heat retention in the spleen and stomach, or *qi* stagnation with dampness or poor function of the liver in maintaining free flow of *qi*, as well as damp-heat retention due to kidney Yin deficiency or to poor function of the urinary bladder in transforming *qi* conditions resulting from emotional depression. TCM classics state that the heart and small intestine are internally-externally related. The liver channel curves around the external genitalia and anus. Ascending, it distributes along both sides of the hypochondriac regions. The kidney and urinary bladder are internally-externally related and also enter the small intestine and distribute in the external genitalia for maintaining the *qi* transforming function of the urinary bladder.

Symptoms and signs included white turbid urinary discharge, scanty urine, acute pain in the lower lateral abdomen radiating towards the umbilicus, and dripping urine with pain. Lin syndrome was diagnosed, and prescriptions should be modified according to the six different types of Lin syndrome. Modifications were made according to whether there was painful urination, bloody urine, difficult urination or pain after urination. Should more than one of the above symptoms and signs appear, the prescription should be accordingly more comprehensive to cover them all.

*Comments*

A note following the prescription indicated that Empress Dowager Cixi suffered from urinary system inflammation causing painful urination and acute pain in the lower lateral abdomen. To regulate the spleen, clear heat from the liver and eliminate dampness from the urinary tract, this decoction also had anti-inflammatory action and promoted urination.

## XIII.4. ATRACTYLODIS MACROCEPHALAE AND AURANTII PILL FOR REGULATING THE SPLEEN AND REINFORCING *QI*

Atractylodis Macrocephalae and Aurantii Pill for Regulating the Spleen and Reinforcing *Qi* (Yi Qi Li Pi Zhi Zhu Wan) was carefully prepared by the imperial physician Zhang Zhongyuan on the 14th day of the eighth month of the lunar calendar in 1895.

*Ingredients*

| | |
|---|---|
| Radix Codonopsis Pilosulae  (Dang Shen) | 12 g |
| Poria  (Fu Ling) | 18 g |
| Radix Atractylodis Macrocephalae  (Bai Zhu) | 9 g |
| Radix Glycyrrhizae  (Gan Cao) | 4.5 g |
| Pericarpium Citri Reticulatae  (Chen Pi) | 9 g |
| Semen Coicis  (Yi Yi Ren) | 15 g |
| Fructus Hordei Germinature  (Mai Ya) | 30 g |
| Semen Arecae  (Bing Lang) | 9 g |
| Fructus Crataegi  (Shan Zha) | 18 g |
| Fructus Amomi  (Sha Ren) | 4.5 g |
| Fructus Aurantii  (Zhi Ke) | 9 g |
| Semen Dolichoris  (Bian Dou) | 15 g |
| Radix Paeoniae Lactiflorae  (Bai Shao) | 9 g |
| Semen Raphani  (Lai Fu Zi) | 15 g |
| Radix Curcumae  (Yu Jin) | 12 g |
| Herba Dendrobii  (Shi Hu) | 15 g |

The original records state that raw Semen Coicis and Radix Paeoniae Lactiflorae should be used. The Fructus Hordei Germinature, Semen Arecae, Fructus Crataegi, Fructus Aurantii, and Semen Dolichoris should be roasted before use.

The above ingredients were ground into extremely fine powder and mixed with honey to form into pills the size of mung beans. Nine grams of the pills were taken each time with boiled water.

### Comments

This prescription was formed by modifying Ginseng-poria and Atractylodis Macrocephalae Pill (Shen Ling Bai Zhu Wan) as recorded in *Imperial Grace Formulary of the Tai Ping Era* (*Tai Ping Hui Min He Ji Ju Fang*), and Immature Bitter Orange and Atractylodis Macrocephalae Pill (Zhi Zhu Wan). It had the action of reinforcing *qi* of the spleen, pacifying the stomach, relieving food retention, eliminating dampness and resolving phlegm. It was applied for treating retention of dampness and phlegm, poor appetite, general lassitude and loose stools. The prescription suited Empress Dowager Cixi's condition.

## XIII.5.  REINFORCED HARMONY-PRESERVING PILL

The ingredients of Reinforced Harmony-preserving Pill (Jia Wei Bao He Wan) were the same as those of Nanjing Tong Ren Tang Pharmacy, the only difference being that half of the original dosage was prepared on the 11th day of the second month of the lunar calendar in 1900.

### Ingredients

| | |
|---|---:|
| Radix Atractylodis Macrocephalae  (Bai Zhu) | 45 g |
| Massa Fermentata Medicinalis  (Shen Qu) | 45 g |
| Semen Raphani  (Lai Fu Zi) | 45 g |
| Pericarpium Citri Reticulatae  (Chen Pi) | 45 g |
| Fructus Forsythiae  (Lian Qiao) | 45 g |
| Rhizoma Pinelliae  (Ban Xia) | 45 g |
| Rhizoma Cyperi  (Xiang Fu) | 45 g |
| Poria  (Fu Ling) | 45 g |
| Radix Astragali seu Hedysari  (Huang Qin) | 45 g |
| Radix Coptidis  (Huang Lian) | 15 g |
| Fructus Crataegi  (Shan Zha) | 30 g |
| Cortex Magnoliae Officinalis  (Hou Po) | 30 g |
| Fructus Aurantii Immaturatus  (Zhi Shi) | 30 g |
| Fructus Hordei Germinatus  (Mai Ya) | 30 g |

The original recipe calls for roasting the Semen Raphani and Fructus Crataegi, while the Fructus Aurantii Immaturatus, Fructus Hordei Germinatus, and Radix Atractylodis Macrocephalae were to be roasted in earth before use. The Rhizoma Pinelliae, Rhizoma Cyperi and Cortex Magnoliae Officinalis should be prepared before use. The above ingredients were ground into powder and made with water into pills the size of mung beans. Nine grams of the pills were taken each time with boiled water.

### Comments

The Reinforced Harmony-preserving Pill was formulated on the basis of Harmony-preserving Pill formulated by Zhu Danxi, with Rhizoma Cyperi, Cortex Magnoliae Officinalis and Radix Astragali seu Hedysari added to it. This changing of ingredients was for the following reasons. In the original Harmony-preserving Pill, the use of Semen Raphani and Fructus Hordei Germinatus might possibly damage *qi* of the lung and stomach, and of the kidney. Fructus Aurantii Immaturatus and Rhizoma Cyperi were thus added to adjust the deviation so that neither the congenital nor the acquired vital energy would be affected. This prescription, having the action of promoting nourishing blood, was good for eliminating epigastric distention due to overeating or symptoms caused by over indulgence in alcohol. It was also effective in eliminating phlegmatic fluid, relieving a sensation of fullness in the chest, belching, nausea, acid regurgitation, and diarrhea. In terms of therapeutic principle, it effected both reinforcing and reducing, though reducing was apparently dominant.

## XIII.6. IMPERIAL GINSENG-PORIA AND ATRACTYLODIS MACROCEPHALAE PILL

Two doses of Imperial Ginseng-Poria and Atractylodis Macrocephalae Pill (Yu Zhi Shen Ling Bai Zhu Wan) were prepared on the third day of the 12th month of the lunar calendar in 1906.

### Ingredients

| | |
|---|---|
| Radix Ginseng  (Ren Shen) | 60 g |
| Rhizoma Atractylodis Macrocephalae  (Bai Zhu) | 15 g |
| Poria  (Fu Ling) | 60 g |
| Rhizoma Dio  (Shan Yao) | 60 g |
| Semen Dolichoris  (Bian Dou) | 60 g |
| Semen Coicis  (Yi Yi Ren) | 60 g |
| Semen Nelumbinis  (Lian Zi Rou) | 120 g |
| Pericarpium Citri Reticulatae  (Chen Pi) | 60 g |
| Fructus Amomi  (Sha Ren) | 30 g |
| Rhizoma Pinelliae  (Ban Xia) | 60 g |
| Radix Coptidis  (Huang Lian) | 6 g |
| Massa Fermentata Medicinalis  (Shen Qu) | 60 g |
| Radix Angelicae Sinensis  (Dang Gui) | 120 g |
| Radix Paeoniae Lactiflorae  (Bai Shao) | 60 g |
| Rhizoma Cyperi  (Xiang Fu) | 60 g |
| Radix Glycyrrhizae  (Gan Cao) | 30 g |
| Radix Platycodi  (Jie Geng) | 60 g |
| Rhizoma Zingiberis  (Gan Jiang) | 6 g |
| Fructus Ziziphi Jujubae  (Hong Zao) | 60 g |

The original records state that the Rhizoma Dio and Semen Coicis should be roasted, and the Radix Atractylodis Macrocephalae and Radix Paeoniae Lactiflorae be respectively roasted with earth and millet wine. The Semen Dolichoris, Rhizoma Pinelliae and Radix Coptidis should be roasted with ginger juice. The Rhizoma Cyperi should be prepared with infants' urine. The above ingredients were ground into powder and mixed with refined honey to make wax-coated pills of six grams each. One pill was taken each time with rice gruel.

### Comments

This prescription was formulated on the basis of Ginseng-Poria and Atracty-lodis Macrocephalae Pill (Shen Ling Bai Zhu Wan) as recorded in *Imperial Grace Formulary of the Tai Ping Era* (Tai Ping Hui Min He Ji Ju Fang), by adding certain ingredients, i.e. Radix Coptidis and Massa Fermentata Medicinalis, which incorporated the excellent therapeutic properties of both Coptidis Decoction for Regulating Middle Jiao (Lian Li Tang) and Peony-Licorice Decoction (Shao Yao Gan Cao Tang) into the prescription. The prescription was thus moderate, neither too hot nor too cold. It could be used either during or after diarrhea for regulating purposes, for it could help promote the anti-pathogenic *qi* and eliminate the pathogenic *qi*, thus achieving the effect of regulating the function of the spleen and nourishing the body.

## XIII.7. AUCHLANDIAE-AMOMUM PILL FOR NOURISHING THE STOMACH

One half of the conventional dose for Auchlandiae-Amomum Pill for Nourishing the Stomach (Xiang Sha Yang Wei Wan) was used, with no specific information as to when it was prepared.

### Ingredients

| | |
|---|---|
| Pericarpium Citri Reticulatae  (Chen Pi) | 60 g |
| Rhizoma Cyperi  (Xiang Fu) | 60 g |
| Massa Fermentata Medicinalis  (Shen Qu) | 60 g |
| Fructus Hordei Germinatus  (Mai Ya) | 60 g |
| Rhizoma Atractylodis Macrocephalae  (Bai Zhu) | 60 g |
| Fructus Aurantii  (Zhi Shi) | 45 g |
| Rhizoma Pinelliae  (Ban Xia) | 45 g |
| Rhizoma Atractylodis  (Cang Zhu) | 45 g |
| Poria  (Fu Ling) | 45 g |
| Cortex Magnoliae Officinalis  (Hou Po) | 45 g |
| Radix Platycodi  (Jie Geng) | 45 g |
| Rhizoma Coptidis  (Huang Lian) | 30 g |
| Fructus Amomi  (Sha Ren) | 30 g |
| Radix Auchlandiae  (Mu Xiang) | 30 g |
| Fructus Crataegi  (Shan Zha) | 30 g |
| Radix Glycyrrhizae  (Gan Cao) | 30 g |
| Fructus Gardeniae  (Zhi Zi) | 37.5 g |
| Herba Agastachis  (Huo Xiang) | 37.5 g |
| Rhizoma Ligustici Chuanxiong  (Chuan Xiong) | 37.5 g |

The original records state that the Rhizoma Cyperi, Fructus Aurantii, Cortex Magnoliae Officinalis and Rhizoma Pinelliae should be prepared before use. The Fructus Hordei Germinatus, Rhizoma Atractylodis and Fructus Crataegi should be roasted and the Rhizoma Atractylodis Macrocephalae be roasted with earth before use. The above ingredients were first ground into powder and made with water into pills the size of mung beans. Nine grams of the pills were taken each time with boiled water.

### Comments

Auchlandiae-Amomum Pill for Nourishing the Stomach contained more ingredients than recorded in *Sheng's Medical Experience* (Shen Shi Zun Yi Shu) by Sheng Jinao. Included here were Massa Fermentata Medicinalis, Fructus Crataegi, Fructus Hordei Germinatus, Rhizoma Atractylodis, Rhizoma Coptidis, Fructus Gardeniae and Rhizoma Ligustici Chuanxiong, while Fructus Amomi Kravanh was omitted. The pill was appropriate for poor appetite, irregular stools, and indigestion due to spleen and stomach deficiency.

## XIII.8. REINFORCED THREE ELIXIRS DECOCTION

Reinforced Three Elixirs Decoction (Jia Wei San Xian Yin) was carefully prepared by the imperial physician Yao Baosheng on the 16th day of the first month of the lunar calendar, with no mention of the year.

### *Ingredients*

| | |
|---|---|
| Fructus Crataegi  (Shan Zha) | 4.5 g |
| Massa Fermentata Medicinalis  (Shen Qu) | 4.5 g |
| Fructus Hordei Germinatus  (Mai Ya) | 4.5 g |
| Fructus Aurantii  (Zhi Ke) | 4.5 g |
| Pericarpium Citri Reticulatae  (Chen Pi) | 3 g |
| Radix Coptidis  (Huang Lian) | 2.4 g |
| Radix Rehmanniae  (Sheng Di) | 9 g |
| Rhizoma Phragmitis  (Lu Gen) | 2 |
| Flos Chrysanthemi  (Ju Hua) | 9 g |
| Folium Phyllostachys  (Zhu Ye) | 2.4 g |

The original records say that the Rhizoma Phragmitis (fresh) should be sliced. The Radix Coptidis should be ground and prepared with millet wine. The Fructus Aurantii should be roasted until it was yellow in colour. The above ingredients were decocted and taken orally while still warm.

### *Comments*

Three Elixirs Decoction (San Xian Yin), consisting of Fructus Crataegi, Massa Fermentata Medicinalis and Fructus Hordei Germinatus, as well as Reinforced Three Elixirs Decoction (Jia Wei San Xian Yin) were often prescribed for Empress Dowager Cixi for promoting digestion and strengthening gastric function. They apparently had good therapeutic effects. The large Crataegi Pill (Da Shan Zha Wan), popular in Beijing, Tianjin and Northeast China, actually produces a better therapeutic effect in the treatment of food retention, belching and acid regurgitation. Some of the large Crataegi Pills manufactured in these places also contained Pericarpium Citri Reticulatae and Fructus Aurantii. Here the formula included Radix Coptidis, Radix Rehmanniae, Flos Chrysanthemi, Rhizoma Phragmitis and Folium Phyllostachys. The role of these in the formula was to clear remaining heat from the stomach, produce fluid, relieve restlessness and quench thirst.

## XIII.9. REINFORCED THREE ELIXIRS DECOCTION II

The Reinforced Three Elixirs Decoction II (Jia Wei San Xian Yin Di Er Fang) was prepared on the 30th day of the first month of the lunar calendar. The year is not known.

*Ingredients*

| | |
|---|---|
| Fructus Crataegi  (Shan Zha) | 18 g |
| Massa Fermentata Medicinalis  (Shen Qu) | 18 g |
| Fructus Hordei Germinatus  (Mai Ya) | 18 g |
| Pericarpium Citri Reticulatae Rubra  (Ju Luo) | 2 |

*Comments*

Pericarpium Citri Reticulatae Rubra, pungent, warming and bitter, has the action of dispelling cold, regulating *qi*, dispelling dampness, resolving phlegm, and relieving food retention or a full sensation in the stomach. It can be applied for relieving food retention or symptoms due to over consumption of alcohol. It may also be applied to cough caused by invasion of wind-cold.

## XIII.10.  REINFORCED THREE ELIXIRS DECOCTION III

Empress Dowager Cixi's Reinforced Three Elixirs Decoction III (Jia Wei San Xian Yin Di San Fang) was prepared on the ninth day of the fourth month of the lunar calendar, with no mention of the year.

*Ingredients*

| | |
|---|---|
| Fructus Crataegi  (Shan Zha) | 9 g |
| Massa Fermentata Medicinalis  (Shen Qu) | 9 g |
| Fructus Hordei Germinatus  (Mai Ya) | 9 g |
| Semen Arecae  (Bing Lang) | 9 g |

The original records say that the Semen Arecae should be roasted before use. Then all the ingredients were decocted for oral administration, and taken while still warm.

On the ninth day of the fourth month of the lunar calendar six grams of ground Radix Curcumae were added to the above ingredients.

*Comments*

Radix Arecae acts to promote *qi* circulation and remove obstruction, while Semen Arecae promotes *qi*, clearing *qi* stagnation and food retention. These were combined with Fructus Crataegi, Massa Fermentata Medicinalis and Fructus Hordei Germinatus to enhance the effect in treating epigastric and abdominal pain, and loose stools following diarrhea.

## XIII.11.  REINFORCED THREE ELIXIRS DECOCTION IV

Empress Dowager Cixi's Reinforced Three Elixirs Decoction IV (Jia Wei San Xian Yin Di Si Fang) was prepared on the seventh day of the fifth month of the lunar calendar, with no mention of the year.

*Ingredients*

| | |
|---|---|
| Fructus Crataegi  (Shan Zha) | 3 g |
| Massa Fermentata Medicinalis  (Shen Qu) | 3 g |
| Fructus Hordei Germinatus  (Mai Ya) | 3 g |

| | |
|---|---|
| Pericarpium Citri Reticulatae Rubra (Ju Hong) | 2.4 g |
| Caulis Bambusae in Taeniam (Zhu Ru) | 9 g |
| Fructus Canarit (Qing Guo) | 7 |

According to the original records dry and ground Fructus Canarit should be used. The above ingredients were prepared in decoction for oral administration, and taken when still warm.

### Comments

Based on Fructus Crataegi, Massa Fermentata Medicinalis and Fructus Hordei Germinatus, this prescription included Caulis Bambusae in Taeniam and Fructus Canarit, in addition to Pericarpium Citri Reticulatae Rubra. It was recommended in the treatment of sore throat, swollen throat and cough with thick sputum due to heat retention in the lung and stomach. The mechanism is that Caulis Bambusae in Taeniam, sweet in flavour and slightly cold in property, acts to clear heat, resolve phlegm and stop vomiting, while Fructus Canarit, sweet and neutral, clears heat, relieves toxicity and resolves phlegm to improve the throat condition.

## XIII.12. REINFORCED THREE ELIXIRS DECOCTION V

Empress Dowager Cixi's Reinforced Three Elixirs Decoction V (Jia Wei San Xian Yin Di Wu Fang) was carefully prepared by the imperial physicians Zhang Zhongyuan and Yao Baosheng on the 24th day of the fifth month of the lunar calendar, with no information given as to the year.

### Ingredients

| | |
|---|---|
| Fructus Crataegi (Shan Zha) | 18 g |
| Massa Fermentata Medicinalis (Shen Qu) | 18 g |
| Fructus Hordei Germinatus (Mai Ya) | 18 g |
| Fructus Aurantii (Zhi Ke) | 6 g |
| Semen Arecae (Bing Lang) | 6 g |
| Pericarpium Arecae (Da Fu Pi) | 6 g |
| Cortex Magnoliae Officinalis (Hou Po) | 4.5 g |
| Radix Scutellariae (Huang Qin) | 6 g |
| Red Poria (Chi Fu Ling) | 12 g |
| Herba Agastachis (Huo Xiang) | 2.4 g |

The original records state that the Fructus Aurantii should be roasted and the Semen Arecae roasted until yellow. The Cortex Magnoliae Officinalis should be prepared before use. The Radix Scutellariae should be prepared with millet wine. The above ingredeints were decocted, and taken while still warm.

### Comments

This prescription contains more ingredients for promoting *qi* and therefore gave better effect in treating abdominal fullness and distention, and nausea caused by *qi* stagnation of the spleen and stomach.

## XIII.13. REINFORCED THREE ELIXIRS DECOCTION VI

Empress Dowager Cixi's Reinforced Three Elixirs Decoction VI (Jia Wei San

Xian Yin Di Liu Fang) was prepared on the 25th day of the sixth month of the lunar calendar with no information given as to the year.

### Ingredients

| | |
|---|---|
| Fructus Crataegi  (Shan Zha) | 9 g |
| Massa Fermentata Medicinalis  (Shen qu) | 9 g |
| Fructus Hordei Germinatus  (Mai Ya) | 9 g |
| Herba Dendrobii  (Shi Hu) | 9 g |
| Fructus Canarit  (Qing Guo) | 15 |

The original records stipulate that the Fructus Canarit (dried) should be pounded before use.

### Comments

Herba Dendrobii and Fructus Canarit were included in this prescription in addition to Fructus Crataegi, Massa Fermentata Medicinalis and Fructus Hordei Germinatus. Its actions therefore were to nourish lung and stomach Yin, clear heat, relieve toxicity and augment body fluid. The decoction was administered for treating dry vomiting, dry cough and poor appetite due to Yin deficiency of the lung and stomach.

## XIII.14.  REINFORCED THREE ELIXIRS DECOCTION VII

Empress Dowager Cixi's Reinforced Three Elixirs Decoction VII (Jia Wei San Xian Yin Di Qi Fang) was carefully prepared by the imperial physician Yao Baosheng on the 28th day of the eighth month of the lunar calendar, with no year given.

### Ingredients

| | |
|---|---|
| Fructus Crataegi  (Shan Zha) | 3 g |
| Massa Fermentata Medicinalis  (Shen Qu) | 3 g |
| Fructus Hordei Germinatus  (Mai Ya) | 3 g |
| Pericarpium Citri Reticulatae Rubra  (Ju Hong) | 4.5 g |
| Radix Scutellariae  (Huang Qin) | 6 g |
| Cortex Magnoliae Officinalis  (Hou Po) | 4.5 g |
| Flos Chrysanthemi  (Ju Hua) | 9 g |
| Cornu Antelopis  (Ling Yang Jiao) | 4.5 g |
| Caulis Bambusae in Taeniam  (Zhu Ru) | 9 g |
| Fructus Aurantii Immaturus  (Zhi Shi) | 4.5 g |

The original records state that the Fructus Crataegi, Massa Fermentata, Fructus Hordei Germinatus and Fructus Aurantii Immaturus should be roasted until burnt-yellow in colour, while the Cortex Magnoliae Officinalis should be prepared before use. The Radix Scutellariae should be prepared with millet wine. The above ingredients were decocted and taken while still warm.

### Comments

Cornu Antelopis and Flos Chrysanthemi were included in this prescription besides those ingredients for promoting digestion and invigorating Yin. Analysis of the prescription indicated that Empress Dowager Cixi had recurrence of an eye condition at that time, and the two additions were made for clearing heat and brightening vision.

## XIII.15. REINFORCED THREE ELIXIRS DECOCTION VIII

Reinforced Three Elixirs Decoction VIII (Jia Wei San Xian Yin Di Ba Fang) was worked out on the 24th day of the 10th month of the lunar calendar, with no year recorded.

*Ingredients*

| | |
|---|---|
| Fructus Crataegi (Shan Zha) | 9 g |
| Massa Fermentata Medicinalis (Shen Qu) | 9 g |
| Fructus Hordei Germinatus (Mai Ya) | 9 g |
| Cortex Mori Radicis (Sang Bai Pi) | 9 g |

According to the original records, the Fructus Crataegi, Massa Fermentata Medicinalis and Fructus Hordei Germinatus should be roasted till burnt-yellow in colour, while the Cortex Mori Radicis should be prepared before use.

*Comments*

It is apparent that Cortex Mori Radicis was added for helping disperse lung *qi*, stop cough and resolve phlegm. Comparison may be made with Pericarpium Citri Reticulatae Rubra appearing in the previous prescriptions.

## XIII.16. MIDDLE JIAO-REGULATING AND SPLEEN-HARMONIZING PASTE

Empress Dowager Cixi's Middle Jiao-Regulating and Spleen-Harmonizing Paste (Tiao Zhong Chang Pi Gao) was carefully worked out by imperial physician Zhang Zhongyuan on the 24th day of the second month of the lunar calendar, with no year given.

*Ingredients*

| | |
|---|---|
| Fructus Forsythiae (Lian Qiao) | 9 g |
| Flos Lonicerae (Jin Yin Hua) | 15 g |
| Poria (Fu Ling) | 18 g |
| Rhizoma Atractylodis Macrocephalae (Bai Zhu) | 15 g |
| Cortex Moudan Radicis (Mu Dan Pi) | 12 g |
| Cortex Magnoliae Officinalis (Hou Po) | 12 g |
| Fructus Crataegi (Shan Zha) | 18 g |
| Endothlium Corneum Geriae Galli (Ji Nei Jin) | 18 g |
| Radia Auchlandiae (Mu Xiang) | 6 g |
| Rhizoma Pinelliae (Ban Xia) | 12 g |
| Semen Arecae (Bing Lang) | 9 g |
| Massa Fermentata Medicinalis (Shen Qu) | 15 g |
| Fructus Hordei Germinatus (Mai Ya) | 15 g |
| Semen Pharbitidis (Hei Chou) | 9 g |
| Fructus Amomi Kravanh (Bai Kou Ren) | 6 g |
| Fructus Glycyrrhizae (Gan Cao) | 9 g |
| Flos Chrysanthemi (Jù Hua) | 9 g |
| Pericarpium Citri Reticulatae Viride (Qing Pi) | 15 g |
| Semen Raphani (Lai Fu Zi) | 12 g |

The above ingredients were well fried in 1.5 kg of sesame oil. After separating out the residue, the remaining oily liquid was mixed with one kilogram of red lead to make the paste.

### Comments

The prescription acts to regulate the function of the Middle Jiao, strengthen the stomach and harmonize the spleen by means of removing stagnation, regulating *qi* and promoting water metabolism. It is applicable for the treatment of indigestion manifested by poor appetite, gastric discomfort, nausea and vomiting, sour regurgitation, as well as abdominal fullness and distention due to disorder in the *qi* mechanism.

## XIII.17. SPLEEN-YANG INVIGORATION PASTE

Empress Dowager Cixi's Spleen-Yang Invigorating Paste (Yang He Qi Pi Gao) was prepared on the 23rd day of the third month of the lunar calendar, with no year given.

### Ingredients

Radix Codonopsis Pilosulae  (Dang Shen)
Rhizoma Atractylodis Macrocephalae  (Bai Zhu)
Radix Astragali seu Hedysari  (Huang Qi)
Cornu Cervi  (Lu Jiao)
Radix Angelicae Sinensis  (Dang Gui)
Rhizoma Cyperi  (Xiang Fu)
[The original records did not specify the dosages for the above five ingredients. —Tr.]

| | |
|---|---|
| Radix Paeoniae Lactiflorae  (Bai Shao) | 30 g |
| Rhizoma Ligustici Chuanxiong  (Chuan Xiong) | 30 g |
| Radix Angelicae Pubescentis  (Du Huo) | 30 g |
| Radix Aconiti Praeparata  (Fu Zi) | 30 g |
| Rhizoma Zingiberis Recens  (Sheng Jiang) | 30 g |
| Resina Ferulae  (A Wei) | 30 g |
| Exocarpium Citri Grandis  (Ju Pi) | 30 g |
| Rhizoma Sparganii  (San Leng) | 30 g |
| Pericarpium Zanthoxyli  (Chuan Jiao) | 30 g |

The original records call for dried Rhizoma Zingiberis Recens. Directions for the first six ingredients are not available from the original. The above ingredients were well fried in 1.5 kg of sesame oil and the residue separated out, leaving the remaining oily liquid to be further concentrated until its drops fell like morning dew or water in freezing cold. 560 grams of water-refined red lead were added into the liquid followed by nine grams each of the three ingredients, Cortex Cinnamomi (Rou Gui), Lignum Aquilariae Resinatum (Chen Xiang) and Flos Caryophylli (Ding Xiang).

The latter three ingredients, ground into fine powder, were added when the oily mixture had cooled down in order to make balls weighing 120-150 grams each. The balls were used in three days' time when they were completely cool. The red lead should be proper in amount and of good quality. Ten pastes were made first and the other herbal balls stored in porcelain containers.

## Comments

The prescription has the action of warming Yang, eliminating cold, nourishing and activating blood, and regulating the channels and collaterals. Empress Dowager Cixi suffered for a long time from spleen deficiency that inevitably affected her kidneys. The use of this Spleen Yang-Invigorating Paste eliminate cold, and regulate *qi* and blood circulation.

## XIII.18. SYRUP FOR PROMOTING ENERGY AND REINFORCING THE SPLEEN

Empress Dowager Cixi's Syrup for Promoting Energy and Reinforcing the Spleen (Zi Sheng Jian Pi Gao) was prepared on the 23rd day of the third month of the lunar calendar, with no information given as to the year.

### Ingredients

| | |
|---|---|
| Radix Codonopsis Pilosulae  (Dang Shen) | 60 g |
| Rhizoma Atractylodis Macrocephalae  (Bai Zhu) | 45 g |
| Fructus Amomi  (sha Ren) | 30 g |
| Radix Auchlandiae  (Mu xiang) | 30 g |
| Poria  (Fu Ling) | 60 g |
| Pericarpium Citri Reticulatae  (Chen Pi) | 36 g |
| Semen Biotae  (Bai Zi Ren) | 45 g |
| Fructus Crataegi  (Shan Zha) | 120 g |
| Massa Fermentata Medicinalis  (Shen Qu) | 120 g |
| Fructus Hordei Germinatus  (Mai Ya) | 120 g |
| Rhizoma Dio  (Shan Yao) | 30 g |
| Cortex Magnoliae Officinalis  (Hou Po) | 30 g |
| Fructus Aurantii Immaturus  (Zhi Shi) | 36 g |
| Radix Glycyrrhizae  (Gan Cao) | 15 g |

According to the original records, the Rhizoma Atractylodis Macrocephalae and Semen Biotae should be roasted. The Fructus Crataegi, Massa Fermentata Medicinalis and Fructus Hordei Germinatus should be roasted until yellow. The Fructus Amomi, Radix Auchlandiae, Poria and roasted Fructus Aurantii Immaturus should be powdered. The Radix Glycyrrhizae should be prepared and the Cortex Magnoliae Officinalis prepared with Rhizoma Zingiberis Recens and Folium Perillae. The above ingredients were well decocted, the residue was separated out and the remaining decoction further concentrated and mixed with refined honey to form the syrup which was stored in a porcelain vessel. Twelve grams of the syrup was taken orally with boiled water each time.

## Comments

This prescription was formulated by modifying the Life Benefiting Pill (Zi Sheng Wan) furmulated by Miao Zhongchun. The Radix Codonopsis Pilosulae, Rhizoma Atractylodis Macrocephalae, Radix Glycyrrhizae and Rhizoma Dio were sweet and neutral and tonified the spleen; Fructus Amomi, Pericarpium Citri Reticulatae, Cortex Magnoliae Officinalis, Fructus Crataegi, Massa Fermentata

Medicinalis, Fructus Hordei Germinatus and Fructus Aurantii Immaturus were pungent and fragrant, and regulated stomach *qi*, while Semen Biotae has moistening action for stool softening. All the ingredients in the prescription made it applicable for tonifying the body and promoting the spleen's role in transformation and transportation. It is therefore an excellent formula without the excessive dryness from Auchlandiae-Amomi Immaturus Orange and Atractylodis Macrocephalae Pill (Xiang Sha Zhi Zhu Wan) nor excessive greasiness from Ginseng-Poria Atractylodis Macrocephalae Powder (Shen Ling Bai Zhu Wan).

## XIII.19.  SYRUP FOR REGULATING *QI* AND RESOLVING FLUID

Syrup for Regulating *Qi* and Resolving Fluid (Li Qi Hua Yin Wan) was prepared on the 10th day of the fourth month of the lunar calendar, with no year given.

*Ingredients*

| | |
|---|---|
| Radix Adenonhorae Strictae  (Sha Shen) | 60 g |
| Rhizoma Atractylodis Macrocephalae  (Bai Zhu) | 45 g |
| Poria  (Fu Ling) | 60 g |
| Semen Arecae  (Bing Lang) | 60 g |
| Rhizoma Sparganii  (San Leng) | 60 g |
| Radix Auchlandiae  (Mu Xiang) | 30 g |
| Fructus Amomi  (Sha Ren) | 30 g |
| Rhizoma Atractylodis  (Cang Zhu) | 45 g |
| Cortex Magnoliae Officinalis  (Hou Po) | 45 g |
| Pericarpium Citri Reticulatae  (Chen Pi) | 45 g |
| Endothlium Corneum Gieriae Galli  (Ji Nei Jin) | 45 g |
| Fructus Aurantii Immaturus  (Zhi Shi) | 45 g |
| Radix Glycyrrhizae  (Gan Cao) | 24 g |

According to the original record, the Rhizoma Atractylodis Macrocephalae, Rhizoma Atractylodis and Fructus Aurantii Immaturus should be roasted. The Endothlium Corneum Gieriae Galli should be griddle-dried. The Cortex Magnoliae Officinalis should be prepared while raw Radix Glycyrrhizae should be used. The above ingredients were well decocted. After separating out the residue, the fluid decoction was further concentrated, then mixed with refined honey to make a syrup to be stored in a porcelain vessel.

*Comments*

The prescription was modified on the basis of Decoction of Auchlandiae-Amomum with Six Nobles Ingredients (Xiang Sha Liu Jun Tang) and Powder for Pacifying the Stomach (Ping Wei San). With the extra ingredients Fructus Aurantii Immaturus, Endothlium Corneum Gieriae Galli and Rhizoma Sparganii, it served to tonify the body and remove *qi* stagnation.

## XIII.20.  SYRUP FOR REGULATING THE SPLEEN AND RESOLVING DAMPNESS

Empress Dowager Cixi's Syrup for Regulating the Spleen and Resolving

Dampness (Li Pi Tiao Zhong Hua Shi Gao) was carefully prepared by the imperial physicians Zhang Zhongyuan and Yao Baosheng on the 10th day of the fourth month of the lunar calendar, with no year given.

### Ingredients

| | |
|---|---|
| Radix Codonopsis Pilosulae  (Dang Shen) | 18 g |
| Rhizoma Atractylodis Macrocephalae  (Bai Zhu) | 9 g |
| Cortex Moudan Radicis  (Mu Dan Pi) | 9 g |
| Gingered Radix Coptidis  (Jiang Huang Lian) | 6 g |
| Massa Fermentata Medicinalis  (Shen Qu) | 12 g |
| Fructus Oryzae Germinature  (Gu Ya) | 12 g |
| Fructus Amomi  (Sha Ren) | 12 g |
| Radix Ophiopogonis  (Mai Dong) | 18 g |
| Poria  (Fu Ling) | 18 g |
| Rhizoma Cyperi  (Xiang Fu) | 9 g |
| Herba Agastachis  (Hua Xiang) | 9 g |
| Radix Glycyrrhizae  (Gan Cao) | 12 g |

According to the original records, the Rhizoma Atractylodis Macrocephalae and Massa Fermentata Medicinalis were roasted while the Radix Coptidis was prepared with ginger. Roasted Fructus Oryzae Germinature and Fructus Amomi should be ground into powder and the Rhizoma Cyperi and Radix Glycyrrhizae prepared before use. The above ingredients were well decocted, the herbal residue separated out, the remaining decoction further concentrated and then mixed with refined honey. One spoonful of the syrup was taken with boiled water each time.

### Comments

The prescription was modified on the basis of Decoction of Auchlandiae-Amomi with Six Nobles Ingredients (Xiang Sha Liu Jun Tang). The addition of Herba Agastachis, Massa Fermentata Medicinalis, Fructus Oryzae Germinature and gingered Radix Coptidis give the syrup the action of invigorating the spleen, removing *qi* stagnation and resolving dampness.

## XIII.21. SPLEEN-YANG REINFORCING SYRUP

No information is available as to the time of the preparation of Empress Dowager Cixi's Spleen-Yang Reinforcing Syrup (Jian Pi Yang He Gao).

### Ingredients

| | |
|---|---|
| Radix Codonopsis Pilosulae  (Dang Shen) | 60 g |
| Rhizoma Atractylodis Macrocephalae  (Bai Zhu) | 30 g |
| Poria  (Fu Ling) | 60 g |
| Folium Eriobotrayae  (Pi Pa Ye) | 60 g |
| Fructus Aurantii  (Zhi Ke) | 45 g |
| Radix Platycodi  (Jie Geng) | 30 g |
| Radix Auchlandiae  (Mu Xiang) | 30 g |
| Alpiniae Katsumadai  (Cao Kou Ren) | 36 g |
| Fructus Crataegi  (Shan Zha) | 40 g |
| Massa Fermentata Medicinalis  (Shen Qu) | 40 g |
| Fructus Hordei Germinatus  (Mai Ya) | 40 g |

| | |
|---|---|
| Flos Magnoliae  (Xin Yi) | 30 g |
| Pericarpium Citri Reticulatae  (Chen Pi) | 45 g |
| Folium Perilliae  (Su Ye) | 45 g |
| Rhizoma seu Radix Notopterygii  (Qiang Huo) | 45 g |

According to the original records, the Rhizoma Atractylodis Macrocephalae and Fructus Aurantii should be roasted, while the Poria, Radix Auchlandiae and Alpiniae Katsumadai should be ground into powder. The Fructus Crataegi, Massa Fermentata Medicinalis and Fructus Hordei Germinatus should be roasted until yellow. The Folium Eriobotryae should be prepared before use. The above ingredients were well decocted, the herbal residue was separated out, and the remaining decoction further concentrated and mixed with refined honey. Twelve grams of the syrup was taken with boiled water each time.

### Comments

The prescription achieved its Yang-strengthening effect by means of invigorating the deficient spleen-Yang. It was therefore composed of herbs for warming the spleen and excluding those for tonifying kidney-Yang.

## XIII.22. MODIFIED SPLEEN-YANG REINFORCING SYRUP

Empress Dowager Cixi's Modified Spleen-Yang Reinforcing Syrup (Jia Jian Jian Pi Yang He Gao) was formulated on the 14th day of the fourth month of the lunar calendar, with no information given as to the year.

### Ingredients

| | |
|---|---|
| Radix Codonopsis Pilosulae  (Dang Shen) | 60 g |
| Rhizoma Atractylodis Macrocephalae  (Bai Zhu) | 45 g |
| Poria  (Fu Ling) | 60 g |
| Folium Eriobotryae  (Pi Pa Ye) | 60 g |
| Pericarpium Citri Reticulatae  (Chen Pi) | 45 g |
| Cortex Magnoliae Officinalis  (Hou Po) | 45 g |
| Radix Auchlandiae  (Mu Xiang) | 30 g |
| Alpiniae Katsumadai  (Cao Kou Ren) | 45 g |
| Fructus Crataegi  (Shan Zha) | 40 g |
| Massa Fermentata Medicinalis  (Shen Qu) | 40 g |
| Fructus Hordei Germinatus  (Mai Ya) | 40 g |
| Radix Platycodi  (Jie Geng) | 45 g |
| Rhizoma Atractylodis  (Cang Zhu) | 45 g |

The original records state that the Rhizoma Atractylodis Macrocephalae and Rhizoma Atractylodis were roasted, while the Poria, Radix Auchlandiae and Alpiniae Katsumadai should be ground into powder. The Fructus Crataegi, Massa Fermentata Medicinalis and Fructus Hordei Germinatus should be roasted until yellow. The Folium Eriobotryae should be prepared and the Cortex Magnoliae Officinalis prepared with ginger. The above ingredients were well decocted. After separating out the herbal residue, the remaining decoction was further concentrated, then mixed with refined honey. Twelve grams of the syrup were taken with boiled water each time.

*Comments*

In this prescription, Fructus Aurantii, Flos Magnoliae and Rhizoma seu Radix Notopterypii were omitted, while Rhizoma Atractylodis and Cortex Magnoliae Officinalis were added. There were apparently certain symptoms requiring the use of aromatic ingredients to resolve dampness.

## XIII.23. PILL FOR IMPROVING APPETITE AND BENEFITING THE DIAPHRAGM

Pill for Improving Appetite and Benefiting the Diaphragm (Kai Wei Li Ge Wan) was prepared by the imperial physician Li Deli on the 18th day of the 10th month of the lunar calendar, with no information given as to the year.

*Ingredients*

| | |
|---|---|
| Pericarpium Trichosnathis (Gua Lou Pi) | 18 g |
| Fructus Aurantii Immaturus (Zhi Shi) | 18 g |
| Lignum Aquilariae Resinatum (Luo Shui Chen) | 9 g |
| Fructus Amomi (Sha Ren) | 12 g |
| Rhizoma Cyperi (Xiang Fu) | 18 g |
| Radix Platycodi (Jie Geng) | 12 g |
| Fructus Amomi Kravanh (Bai Kou Ren) | 12 g |
| Rhizoma Atractylodis (Cang Zhu) | 12 g |
| Herba Agastachis (Huo Xiang) | 15 g |
| Cortex Moudan Radicis (Mu Dan Pi) | 18 g |
| Cortex Magnoliae Officinalis (Hou Po) | 15 g |
| Fructus Crataegi (Shan Zha) | 20 g |
| Massa Fermentata Medicinalis (Shen Qu) | 20 g |
| Fructus Hordei Germinatus (Mai Ya) | 20 g |

The original recipe calls for the Fructus Aurantii Immaturus and Rhizoma Atractylodis to be roasted, while the Fructus Crataegi, Massa Fermentata Medicinalis and Fructus Hordei Germinatus should also be roasted until yellow. The Rhizoma Cyperi and Cortex Magnoliae Officinalis should be prepared. The above ingredients were ground into fine powder and mixed with refined honey to make pills the size of sorghum seeds. Six grams of the pills were taken with boiled water each time.

*Comments*

The prescription acts to relieve *qi* stagnation, promote normal mechanism of the diaphragm and digestion. The pills were taken to relieve pain in the chest and epigastric region, and to eliminate food retention.

## XIII.24. HERBAL TEA FOR PRODUCING BODY FLUID

Empress Dowager Cixi's Herbal Tea for Producing Body Fluid (Sheng Jin Dai Cha Yin) was prepared on the 11th day of the third month of the lunar calendar, with no year given.

*Ingredients*

| | |
|---|---|
| Fructus Canarit (Qing Guo) | 5 |

| | |
|---|---|
| Herba Dendrobii  (Shi Hu) | 6 g |
| Flos Chrysanthemi  (Ju Hua) | 6 g |
| Bulbus Eleosharis Tuberosae  (Bi Qi) | 5 |
| Radix Ophiopogonis  (Mai Dong) | 9 g |
| Rhizoma Phragmitis  (Lu Gen) | 2 |
| Folium Mori  (Sang Ye) | 9 g |
| Caulis Bambusae in Taeniam  (Zhu Ru) | 6 g |
| Nodus Neclumbinis Rhizomatis  (Ou) | 10 |
| Pear  (Li) | 2 |

The original records say that the Bulbus Eleocharis Tuberosae and pear should be peeled; the Fructus Canarit should be ground into powder; the Rhizoma Phragmitis (fresh) should be chopped. The above ingredients were decocted as a beverage in place of the daily tea.

*Comments*

The prescription here was adapted from Five Juices Decoction (Wu Zhi Yin) as recorded in *Treatise on Differentiation and Treatment of Epidemic Febrile Diseases* (*Wen Bing Tiao Bian Lun*). The original ingredients included pear, Bulbus Eleocharis Tuberosae, fresh Rhizoma Phragmitis, Radix Ophiopogonis and Nodus Melumbinis Rhizomatis or sugar cane. A proper amount of the juice from each ingredient was mixed together and taken orally when the mixture was cold. It was used in treating febrile diseases with excessive heat injuring lung- and stomach-Yin manifested by thirst, cough, thin foamy sputum and sticky greasiness in the mouth. The mechanism of the treatment was to nourish body fluid and dispel dryness. Should the patient dislike the cold juice, a decoction of the above ingredients could be an option. As the prescription contains Fructus Canarit, Herba Dendrobii, Folium Mori, Caulis Bambusae in Taeniam and Flos Chrysanthemi, it produced remarkable therapeutic effects in promoting Yin and body fluid and dispelling dryness.

## XIII.25. PRESCRIPTION FOR PRODUCING FLUID AND NOURISHING THE STOMACH

Empress Dowager Cixi's Prescription for Producing Fluid and Nourishing the Stomach (Sheng Jin Zi Wei Fang) was carefully prepared by the imperial physicians Zhang Zhongyuan and Dai Jiayu on the 21st day of the 10th month of the lunar calendar in 1908.

*Ingredients*

| | |
|---|---|
| Semen Phaseoli Radiatus  (Lu Dou) | 15 g |
| Fructus Canarit  (Qing Guo) | 20 |
| Folium Phyllostachyos  (Zhu Ye) | 3 g |
| Fructus Citrus Junos  (Chen Zi) | 1 |

The original records say that the Semen Phaseoli Radiatus and fresh Fructus Canarit without tips should be ground into powder, while the Fructus Citrus Junos should be chopped. The above ingredients were decocted for oral administration.

*Comments*

Prescription for Producing Fluid and Nourishing the Stomach was formulated for Empress Dowager Cixi's incontinence due to renal failure caused heat retention in the liver and stomach the day before her death. Fructus Citrus Junos, acid and cool, has excellent actions in subduing the rebellious *qi*, harmonizing Middle Jiao, strengthening the stomach and easing the diaphragm.

## XIII.26. HERBAL TEA FOR NOURISHING THE STOMACH AND PACIFYING THE MIDDLE JIAO

Empress Dowager Cixi's Herbal Tea for Nourishing the Stomach and Pacifying the Middle Jiao (Zi Wei He Zhong Dai Cha Yin) was carefully prescribed by the imperial physicians Zhang Zhongyuan and Dai Jiayu during the hours 23:00 - 01:00 on the 22nd-23rd day of the 10th month of the lunar calendar in 1908.

### Ingredients
| | |
|---|---|
| Caulis Bambusae in Taeniam  (Zhu Ru) | 3 g |
| Fructus Canarit  (Qing Guo) | 10 |
| Flos Magnoliae Officinalis  (Hou Po Hua) | 1.5 g |
| Cornu Antelopis  (Ling Yang Jiao) | 1.5 g |

The original records state that the Caulis Bambusae in Taeniam should be mixed with Cinnabari and the Fructus Canarit (fresh and without tips) should be ground. The above ingredients were decocted for oral administration.

### Comments
Herbal Tea for Nourishing the Stomach and Pacifying the Middle Jiao was taken by Empress Dowager Cixi several hours before her death to ease her critical condition marked by excessive sputum blocking the throat due to *qi* deficiency, listlessness, shortened tongue, thirst and failure of the stomach to receive food. Shortly after this oral administration, another formula similar to Pulse-activating Powder (Sheng Mai San) was also tried as a rescue measure.

# XIV.  PRESCRIPTIONS FOR LIVER CONDITIONS

## XIV.1. LIVER-YIN REINFORCING PILL FOR CLEARING WIND AND SOOTHING LIVER-YANG

Liver-Yin Reinforcing Pill for Clearing Wind and Soothing Liver-Yang (Qing Feng Zhen Ni Yang Yin Wan) was worked out by the imperial physicians Xue Fuchen and Li Dechang on the seventh day of the seventh month of the lunar calendar in 1887.

### Ingredients
| | |
|---|---|
| Radix Rehmanniae  (Sheng Di Huang) | 60 g |
| Radix Angelicae Sinensis  (Dang Gui) | 45 g |
| Rhizoma Ligustici Chuanxiong  (Chuan Xiong) | 30 g |
| Radix Paeoniae Lactiflorae  (Bai Shao) | 45 g |
| Radix Bupleuri  (Chai Hu) | 24 g |

| | |
|---|---|
| Radix Scutellariae  (Huang Qin) | 30 g |
| Rhizoma Acori Graminei  (Shi Chang Pu) | 15 g |
| Rhizoma Pinelliae  (Ban Xia) | 45 g |
| Magnetitum  (Ci Shi) | 60 g |
| Radix Poria  (Fu Ling) | 45 g |
| Modified Massa Fermentata Medicinalis  (Jian Qu) | 45 g |
| Fructus Lycii  (Gou Qi Zi) | 24 g |
| Fructus Gardeniae  (Zhi Zi) | 24 g |

The original records require the Radix Angelicae Sinensis to be washed in millet wine. The Radix Scutelllariae should be roasted with millet wine. The Rhizoma Pinelliae should be prepared and the Radix Bupleuri prepared with vinegar. The Magnetitum (calcined) should be ground separately into extremely fine powder in water before use. The Modified Massa Fermentata Medicinalis should be roasted. The above ingredients were ground into extremely fine powder and mixed with refined honey to make cinnabar-coated pills the size of mung beans. Nine grams of the pills were taken orally with salty water before sleep.

### Comments

The prescription has actions in nourishing Yin, pacifying the liver and subduing liver-Yang. It was modified on the basis of Four Substances Decoction (Si Wu Tang), Carefree Powder (Xiao Yao San) and Magnetite-Cinnabar Pill (Ci Zhu Wan), recorded in *Prescriptions Worth a Thousand Gold* (Qian Jin Yao Fang), and indicated in dizziness and vertigo, blurred vision, tinnitus, deafness, irritability, insomnia and palpitation. Heavy dosage was prescribed for Magnetitum which is pungent, cold and heavy, to achieve the therapeutic effect of tranquilizing the mind, tonifying the kidney and soothing the liver by soothing the liver-Yang.

## XIV.2. *QI* CONDITIONING PILL

Qi Conditioning Pill (Jiao Gan Wan) was carefully worked out by the imperial physicians Zhang Zhouhe and Li Dechang on the 24th day of the fifth month of the lunar calendar in 1891.

### Ingredients

| | |
|---|---|
| Rhizoma Cyperi  (Xiang Fu) | 30 g |
| Poria  (Fu Ling) | 120 g |
| Succinum  (Hu Po) | 15 g |

The original records prescribe that the Rhizoma Cyperi be prepared before use. The above ingredients were ground into fine powder and mixed with refined honey to make pills of nine grams each to be taken with boiled water.

*Qi* Conditioning Pill was prescribed for treating all *qi* disorders caused by emotional disturbance such as depression or vexation resulting from unhappiness or disappointments in life. Clinical manifestations included poor appetite, sallow complexion, emaciation and stuffiness in the chest. One pill was chewed and swallowed with boiled water each morning and evening. It had an excellent effect in treating gynecological diseases as well. Emotional disturbance and rich foods should be avoided while using the pills.

*Comments*

The prescription, functioning in relieving *qi* stagnation and tranquilizing the mind, was formulated in imitation of *Qi* Conditioning Pill consisting of Rhizoma Cyperi and Radix Poria, as recorded in *Shen's Medical Experience* (Shen Shi Zun Sheng Shu), for *qi* stagnation, and another pill of the same name with Rhizoma Cyperi, Radix Poria, Rhizoma Coptidis, Cortex Cinnamomi and Flos Chrysanthemi for treating patients for sudden deafness due to anger as recorded in *Standards for Differentiation and Treatment* (Zheng Zhi Zhun Sheng) by Wang Kentang. Succinum was also included in this prescription, enhancing the therapeutic effect of pacifying the heart and mind. Empress Dowager Cixi's existing health records indicate that she often suffered from depression.

## XIV.3. REINFORCED CAREFREE POWDER

Reinforced Carefree Powder (Jia Wei Xiao Yao San) was presented for imperial use on the 22nd day of the fifth month of the lunar calendar, with no information given as to the year.

### Ingredients

| | |
|---|---|
| Radix Bupleuri  (Chai Hu) | 3 g |
| Radix Angelicae Sinensis  (Dang Gui) | 6 g |
| Radix Paeoniae Lactiflorae  (Bai Shao) | 6 g |
| Rhizoma Atractylodis Macrocephalae  (Bai Zhu) | 3 g |
| Poria  (Fu Ling) | 3 g |
| Rhizoma Glycyrrhizae  (Gan Cao) | 1.5 g |
| Rhizoma Zingiberis Recens  (Sheng Jiang) | 3 |
| Herba Menthae  (Bo He) | 0.3 g |
| Folium Mori  (Sang Ye) | 6 g |

The original records say that the Radix Glycyrrhizae should be prepared before use, and the Rhizoma Zingiberis Recens wrapped for char-baking. The above ingredients were ground into powder. Six grams of the powder were taken each time to make up a course of 10 doses. The soup made from half of a fresh lotus leaf was taken with the powder.

*Comments*

Carefree Powder (Xiao Yao San) acts to remove *qi* stagnation. Fresh lotus leaf and Folium Mori were added possibly to dispel wind and clear heat, or for clearing summer heat in early summer. They may cause the clear Yang of the spleen and stomach to rise, and clear liver heat to promote vision as well.

## XIV.4. REINFORCED ANCIENT ESCAPE RESTRAINT AND CAREFREE PILL

Reinforced Ancient Escape Restraint and Carefree Pill (Gu Fang Yun Ju Xiao

Yao Jia Wei Wan) was carefully prepared by the imperial physicians Zhuang Shouhe and Li Dechang on the 30th day of the eighth month of the lunar calendar in 1891.

### Ingredients

| | |
|---|---|
| Radix Angelicae Sinensis  (Dang Gui) | 12 g |
| Radix Paeoniae Lactiflorae  (Bai Shao) | 9 g |
| Rhizoma Ligustici Chuanxiong  (Chuan Xiong) | 4.5 g |
| Radix Bupleuri  (Chai Hu) | 4.5 g |
| Rhizoma Cyperi  (Xiang Fu) | 9 g |
| Rhizoma Atractylodis  (Cang Zhu) | 9 g |
| Fructus Gardeniae  (Zhi Zi) | 9 g |
| Massa Fermentata Medicinalis  (Shen Qu) | 9 g |
| Pericarpium Citri Reticulatae Rubra  (Ju Hong) | 6 g |
| Rhizoma Pinellae  (Ban Xia) | 9 g |
| Poria  (Fu Ling) | 12 g |
| Fructus Evodiae  (Wu Zhu Yu) | 4.5 g |
| Rhizoma Coptidis  (Huang Lian) | 4.5 g |
| Cortex Mori Radicis  (Sang Bai Pi) | 9 g |
| Cortex Lycci Radicis  (Di Gu Pi) | 9 g |
| Bulbus Fritillariae Cirhosae  (Chuan Bei) | 12 g |
| Radix Glycyrrhizae  (Gan Cao) | 4.5 g |

The original recipe calls for the Radix Paeoniae Lactiflorae, Rhizoma Atractylodis and Fructus Gardeniae to be roasted, the Rhizoma Cyperi, Rhizoma Pinellae and Cortex Mori Radicis to be prepared before use, and the Radix Bupleuri to be prepared with vinegar. The Massa Fermentata Medicinalis should be roasted until yellow. The above ingredients were ground into extremely fine powder and mixed with refined honey to make cinnabar-coated pills the size of mung beans. Nine grams of pills were taken each time with boiled water.

The combination of these ingredients served to relieve liver $qi$ stagnation, harmonize the liver, regulate the lung and spleen to ease the diaphragm and Middle Jiao, regulate the circulation of $qi$ to stop cough, resolve phlegm, tonify $qi$ and blood, and regulate the channels and collaterals. A TCM classic says, "All possible $qi$ stagnation involves the lung. Most $qi$ obstruction is related to the Middle Jiao. The lung, the metal, dominates $qi$ that distributes in both Yin and Yang of the body. Once its function is impaired, it will be difficult for the lung to perform its normal descending and ascending functions, leading to $qi$ stagnation. Clinical manifestations may include occasional stuffiness in the chest, borborygmus, belching, cough, or gastric discomfort. Regular use of the remedy will restore the $qi$ mechanism to normal so that the above symptoms disappear."

### Comments

By modifying Stagnancy Relieving Pill (Yue Ju Wan) and Carefree Pill (Xiao Yao Wan), the prescription showed much stronger action in removing $qi$ stagnation, easing Middle Jiao and tonifying the spleen and stomach. It was thus more appropriate for the treatment of liver and spleen disorders resulting from either emotional disturbance such as depression or anger, or from improper diet.

## XIV.5. SIX DEPRESSIONS RELIEVING PASTE

One dose of Six Depressions Relieving Paste (Kai Jie Liu Yu Gao) was prescribed for Empress Dowager Cixi, with no information given as to when it was prepared.

*Ingredients*

| | |
|---|---|
| Rhizoma Cyperi  (Xiang Fu) | 30 g |
| Radix Curcumae  (Yu Jin) | 30 g |
| Fructus Aurantii Immaturus  (Zhi Shi) | 24 g |
| Pericarpium Citri Reticulatae Viride  (Qing Pi) | 24 g |
| Shan Tian | 15 g |
| Rhizoma Curcumae Longae  (Jiang Huang) | 18 g |
| Radix Auchlandiae  (Mu Xiang) | 18 g |
| Pericarpium Citri Reticulatae Rubra  (Ju Hong) | 15 g |
| Flos Carthami  (Hong Hua) | 15 g |
| Radix Angelicae Sinensis  (Dang Gui) | 30 g |
| Canlis Perillae  (Su Geng) | 30 g |
| Lignum Aquilariae Resinatum  (Chen Xiang) | 15 g |
| Moschus  (She Xiang) | 6 g |
| Semen Raphani  (Lai Fu Zi) | 18 g |
| Semen Sinapis Albae  (Bai Jie Zi) | 18 g |
| Rhizoma Atractylodis  (Cang Zhu) | 15 g |

The original records note that the use of Moschus required special permission. The above ingredients were well fried in sesame oil. After separating out the herbal residue, red lead was added to make the paste for external application at Feishu (UB 13) and Shangwan (Ren 13).

*Comments*

Stagnancy Relieving Pill (Yue Ju Wan) has the action of relieving the five sorts of stagnations or depressions. This pill is called Six Depressions Relieving Pill (Liu Yu Wan) when Rhizoma Corydalis is included because this helps regulate *qi* and activate blood. As an external remedy it is applied locally at Feishu (UB 13) and Shangwan (Ren 13). The prescription consists mainly of ingredients that regulate *qi* and activate blood circulation, plus ingredients from the traditional formula known as Three Seeds Decoction for the Aged (San Zi Yang Qin Tang). Six Depressions Relieving Paste was intended to cope with the impairment of lung *qi*.

## XIV.6. SYRUP FOR CLEARING LIVER HEAT AND ACTIVATING COLLATERALS

Empress Dowager Cixi's Syrup for Clearing Liver Heat and Activating Collaterals (Qing Re Yang Gan Huo Luo Gao) was carefully prepared by the imperial physicians Zhuang Shouhe and Yao Baosheng on the 29th day of the third month of the lunar calendar in 1904.

*Ingredients*

| | |
|---|---|
| Radix Rehmanniae  (Sheng Di Huang) | 15 g |

| | |
|---|---|
| Radix Paeoniae Lactiflorae (Bai Shao) | 12 g |
| Radix Angelicae Sinensis (Dang Gui) | 12 g |
| Cornu Antelopis (Ling Yang Jiao) | 7.5 g |
| Rhizoma Gastrodiae (Tian Ma) | 6 g |
| Radix Gentianae Macrophyllae (Qin Jiao) | 6 g |
| Bombyx Batryticatus (Jiang Can) | 9 g |
| Pericarpium Citri Reticulatae Rubra (Ju Hong) | 6 g |
| Bulbus Fritellariae Cirhosae (Chuan Bei) | 9 g |
| Fructus Aurantii (Zhi Ke) | 6 g |
| Modified Massa Fermentata Medicinalis (Jian Qu) | 6 g |
| Radix Glycyrrhizae (Gan Cao) | 3 g |

The original records state that the Bombyx Batryticatus, Fructrus Aurantii and modified Massa Fermentata Medicinalis should be roasted. The Radix Angelicae Sinensis was to be prepared with millet wine. The Bulbus Fritillariae Cirhosae should be ground into fine powder before use. The above ingredients were well decocted. After separating out the herbal residue, the remaining decoction was further concentrated and then mixed with refined honey. Nine grams of syrup were taken with boiled water each time.

### Comments

The existing medical history of Empress Dowager Cixi in the third month of the lunar calendar in 1904 records "dizziness and vertigo with slight headache, and blurred vision." The prescription was appropriate in the treatment of symptoms due to retention of liver heat.

## XIV.7. SYRUP FOR CLEARING LIVER HEAT AND REGULATING COLLATERALS

Empress Dowager Cixi's Syrup for Clearing Liver Heat and Regulating Collaterals (Qing Re Yang Gan Huo Luo Gao) was carefully worked out by the imperial physicians Zhuang Shouhe and Yao Baosheng on the 18th day of the fourth month of the lunar calendar. No year is given.

### Ingredients

| | |
|---|---|
| Radix Curcumae (Yu Jin) | 9 g |
| Folium Mori (Sang Ye) | 12 g |
| Rhizoma Atractylodis Macrocephalae (Bai Zhu) | 9 g |
| Radix Rehmanniae (Sheng Di Huang) | 9 g |
| Radix Paeoniae Lactiflorae (Bai Shao) | 12 g |
| Radix Angelicae Sinensis (Dang Gui) | 9 g |
| Cornu Antelopis (Ling Yang Jiao) | 7.5 g |
| Rhizoma Gastrodiae (Tian Ma) | 6 g |
| Radix Gentianae Macrocephyllae (Qin Jiao) | 6 g |
| Bombyx Batryticatus (Jiang Cang) | 9 g |
| Pericarpium Citri Reticulatae Rubra (Ju Hong) | 6 g |
| Bulbus Fritillariae Cirhosae (Chuan Bei) | 9 g |
| Fructus Aurantii (Zhi Ke) | 6 g |
| Modified Massa Fermentata Medicinalis (Jian Qu) | 9 g |

Radix Glycyrrhizae  (Gan Cao)                                      3 g

The original records say that the Bombyx Batryticatus, Fructus Aurantii and modified Massa Fermentata Medicinalis should be roasted while the Radix Angelicae Sinensis should be prepared with millet wine. The above ingredients were well decocted. After separating out the herbal residue, the remaining decoction was further concentrated and then mixed with refined honey. Nine grams of the syrup were taken with boiled water each time.

*Comments*

The ingredients included in this prescription were not very different from the one above. The dosage for Cornu Antelopis remained the same in both, mainly because of its sweet flavour and neutral property without toxicity. Meng Shen said, "Cornu Antelopis, roasted with Fructus Schisandrae and soaked in millet wine overnight for internal use, is applicable for the treatment of rigid tendons and bones, and windstroke." Cornu Antelopis is characterized by its effect in nourishing the liver, clearing heat and calming liver wind.

## XIV.8. REINFORCED GENTIANA PILL FOR SOOTHING LIVER FIRE

Reinforced Gentiana Pill for Soothing Liver Fire (Jia Wei Long Dan Xie Gan Wan) was carefully prepared by the imperial physician Yang Jihe on the 12th day of the fourth month of the lunar calendar in 1900.

*Ingredients*

Radix Angelicae Sinensis  (Dang Gui)                              9 g
Radix Paeoniae Lactiflorae  (Bai Shao)                          15 g
Radix Rehmanniae  (Sheng Di Huang)                              15 g
Fructus Gardeniae  (Zhi Zi)                                      9 g
Radix Gentiana  (Long Dan Cao)                                   9 g
Radix Bupleuri  (Chai Hu)                                        9 g
Rhizoma Cyperi  (Xiang Fu)                                      12 g
Rhizoma Curmuae Longae  (Jiang Huang)                            9 g
Caulis Akebiae  (Mu Tong)                                      4.5 g
Rhizoma Alismatis  (Ze Xie)                                    4.5 g
Semen Plantaginis  (Che Qian Zi)                                 6 g
Radix Platycodis  (Jie Geng)                                     9 g
Ramulus Mori  (Sang Zhi)                                         9 g
Radix Glycyrrhizae  (Gan Cao)                                    3 g

The original prescription calls for the Radix Gentiana to be prepared with millet wine, while the Radix Bupleuri should be prepared with vinegar. The Rhizoma Cyperi should be stewed and the Rhizoma Curcumae Longae be sliced. The above ingredients were ground into extremely fine powder and mixed with refined honey to make pills the size of mung beans. 4.5 grams of the pills were taken with boiled water each time.

*Comments*

The prescription was formed on the basis of Decoction of Gentiana for

Purging Liver Fire (Long Dan Xie Gan Tang) as recorded in *Secret Records of the Orchid Chamber* (Lan Shi Mi Cang). The original prescription was formulated for treating excessive fire of the liver channel manifested by hypochondriac pain, bitter taste in the mouth, congested eyes and deafness, as well as downward flow of damp-heat from the liver channel as indicated by turbid urine, itching of the external genitalia or turbid leukorrhea in women. Modern research verifies its effect for various inflammatory diseases such as acute pelvic inflammation and herpes zoster. The prescription may also be applied for the treatment of hypertension due to flaring up of liver fire.

## XIV.9. MAJOR GENTIANA PILL FOR SOOTHING LIVER FIRE

Major Gentiana Pill for Soothing Liver Fire (Da Long Dan Xie Gan Wan) was prepared for Empress Dowager Cixi by the imperial physicians Yang Jihe and Zhong Xun on the 13th day of the fourth month of the lunar calendar, with no information concerning the year.

*Ingredients*

| | |
|---|---|
| Arissema cum Bile  (Dan Nan Xing) | 9 g |
| Retinervus Citri Fructus  (Ju Luo) | 4.5 g |
| Bombyx Batryticatus  (Jiang Cang) | 4.5 g |
| Radix Gentianae  (Long Dan Cao) | 9 g |
| Radix Angelicae Sinensis  (Dang Gui) | 9 g |
| Radix Paeoniae Lactiflorae  (Bai Shao) | 15 g |
| Radix Rehmanniae  (Sheng Di Huang) | 15 g |
| Fructus Gardeniae  (Zhi Zi) | 9 g |
| Radix Bupleuri  (Chai Hu) | 9 g |
| Rhizoma Curcumae Longae  (Jiang Huang) | 9 g |
| Caulis Akebiae  (Mu Tong) | 4.5 g |
| Rhizoma Alismatis  (Ze Xie) | 4.5 g |
| Semen Plantaginis  (Che Qian Zi) | 6 g |
| Radix Codonopsis Pilosulae  (Dang Shen) | 15 g |
| Radix Scutellariae  (Huang Qin) | 9 g |
| Ramulus Mori  (Sang Zhi) | 9 g |
| Radix Glycyrrhizae  (Gan Cao) | 3 g |

According to the original records, the Bombyx Batryticatus and Fructus Gardeniae should be roasted, while the Radix Gentianae and Radix Scutellariae should be prepared with millet wine. The Radix Bupleuri should be prepared with vinegar, while the Rhizoma Curcumae Longae should be sliced. The above ingredients were ground into fine powder and mixed with refined honey to make pills the size of mung beans. Six grams of the pills were taken with boiled water each time.

*Comments*

There is no great difference between Major Gentiana Pill for Soothing Liver Fire from the previous Reinforced Gentiana Pill for Soothing Liver Fire. In this prescription, Radix Scutellariae was kept as a conventional ingredient. In addition, Arissema cum Bile, Bombyx Batryticatus and Radix Codonopsis Pilosulae were added. And Retinervus Citri Fructus was used to replace Radix Platycodi. It therefore had stronger actions in reinforcing deficiency and resolving phlegm in comparison with Reinforced Gentiana Pill for Soothing Liver Fire.

## XIV.10. PILL FOR NOURISHING BLOOD AND HARMONIZING THE LIVER

Empress Dowager Cixi's Pill for Nourishing Blood and Harmonizing the Liver (Yang Xue Rou Gan Wan) was carefully prepared by the imperial physician Zhang Zhongyuan on the 13th day of the 11th month of the lunar calendar in 1905.

*Ingredients*

| | |
|---|---|
| Radix Angelicae Sinensis  (Dang Gui) | 6 g |
| Rhizoma Ligustici Chuanxiong  (Chuan Xiong) | 3 g |
| Radix Rehmanniae  (Sheng Di Huang) | 9 g |
| Radix Paeoniae Lactiflorae  (Bai Shao) | 6 g |

The original records state that the Radix Paeoniae Lactiflorae should be prepared with millet wine. The above ingredients were ground into fine powder and then mixed with refined honey to make pills the size of mung beans. Six grams of the pills were taken with boiled water each time.

*Comments*

The ingredients in this prescription were the same as those in Four Substances Decoction (Si Wu Tang) that first appeared in *The Imperial Grace Formulary of the Tai Ping Era* (*Tai Ping Hui Min He Ji Ju Fang*). Pill for Nourishing Blood and Harmonizing the Liver was indicated in conditions of blood deficiency or those complicated by blood stasis. It could be applied for nourishing blood, harmonizing the liver and regulating menstruation. The formula was not used for Empress Dowager Cixi for regulating her menstruation but for such symptoms as dizziness and dry eyes, because she was quite old in 1905. Modern research proved its effect in promoting the maturity of the reticulocytes.

## XIV.11. SYRUP FOR REGULATING THE LIVER AND STOMACH

Empress Dowager Cixi's Syrup for Regulating the Liver and Stomach (Tiao Gan He Wei Gao) was carefully prepared by the imperial physician Zhang Zhongyuan on the 19th day of the fifth month of the lunar calendar, with no year given.

*Ingredients*

| | |
|---|---|
| Radix Codonopsis Pilosulae  (Dang Shen) | 9 g |
| Radix Paeoniae Lactiflorae  (Bai Shao) | 12 g |
| Herba Dendrobii  (Shi Hu) | 12 g |
| Folium Mori  (Sang Ye) | 12 g |
| Caulis Bambusae in Taeniam  (Zhu Ru) | 9 g |
| Fructus Crataegi  (Shan Zha) | 27 g |
| Massa Fermentata Medicinalis  (Shen Qu) | 27 g |
| Fructus Hordei Germinatus  (Mai Ya) | 27 g |
| Radix Auchlandiae  (Mu Xiang) | 2.4 g |

| | |
|---|---|
| Fructus Aurantii  (Zhi Ke) | 6 g |
| Pericarpium Citri Reticulatae Rubra  (Ju Hong) | 4.5 g |
| Radix Glycyrrhizae  (Gan Cao) | 3 g |
| Rhizoma Atractylodis Macrocephalae  (Bai Zhu) | 6 g |

The original records state that the Fructus Crataegi, Massa Fermentata Medicinalis and Fructus Hordei Germinatus should be roasted until yellow. The Radix Auchlandiae should be ground, and the Fructus Aurantii roasted. The above ingredients were well decocted, and after separating out the herbal residue the remaining decoction was further concentrated and mixed with refined honey. Five grams of the syrup were taken with boiled water each time.

### Comments

This prescription acts to regulate the liver and stomach. The large proportion of the Radix Paeoniae Lactiflorae was to treat Empress Dowager Cixi's liver-Yin deficiency and disharmony between the spleen and stomach.

## XIV.12.  PILL FOR REGULATING THE LIVER AND HARMONIZING BLOOD

One dose of Pill for Regulating the Liver and Harmonizing Blood (Tiao Gan He Xue Wan) was prescribed on the 25th day of the eighth month of the lunar calendar. No year was given.

### Ingredients

| | |
|---|---|
| Radix Angelicae Sinensis  (Dang Gui) | 24 g |
| Radix Paeoniae Lactiflorae  (Bai Shao) | 15 g |
| Radix Bupleuri  (Chai Hu) | 9 g |
| Rhizoma Cyperi  (Xiang Fu) | 12 g |
| Herba Menthae  (Bo He) | 9 g |
| Cortex Moudan Radicis  (Mu Dan Pi) | 12 g |
| Fructus Gardeniae  (Zhi Zi) | 9 g |
| Radix et Rhizoma Rhei  (Da Huang) | 12 g |
| Cornu Rhinoceri Asiatici  (Xi Jiao) | 4.5 g |
| Radix Rehmanniae  (Sheng Di Huang) | 18 g |
| Pericarpium Citri Reticulatae Viride  (Qing Pi) | 6 g |

According to the original records, the Radix Bupleuri should be prepared with vinegar, while the Fructus Gardeniae should be roasted. The Radix et Rhizoma Rhei should be baked over charcoal fire. The above ingredients were ground into fine powder which was made into water-bound pills the size of mung beans.

### Comments

The prescription was formulated by modifying Carefree Powder of Moudan Bark and Cape Jasmine Fruit (Dan Zhi Xiao Yao San) and Decoction of Rhinoceri Horn and Rehmanniae (Xi Jiao Di Huang Tang). It nourishes blood, regulates the liver, and cools and harmonizes blood. Its extra herbal potency makes it appropriate for treating blood deficiency conditions due to liver-*qi* stagnation complicated by blood heat.

# XV. PRESCRIPTIONS FOR DIARRHEA DUE TO KIDNEY DEFICIENCY

## XV.1. MODIFIED FOUR GENTLEMEN AND FOUR MIRACLES PRESCRIPTION

One dose of Modified Four Gentlemen and Four Miracles Prescription (Si Jun He Si Shen Jia Jian Fang) was prescribed on the 13th day of the first month of the lunar calendar. The year was not given.

*Ingredients*

| | |
|---|---|
| Radix Codonopsis Pilosulae (Dang Shen) | 3 g |
| Rhizoma Atractylodis Macrocephalae (Bai Zhu) | 3 g |
| Fructus Psoraleae (Bu Gu Zhi) | 4.5 g |
| Poria (Fu Ling) | 3 g |
| Semen Myristicae (Rou Dou Kou) | 2.4 g |
| Fructus Evodiae (Wu Zhu Yu) | 1.2 g |
| Radix Bupleuri (Chai Hu) | 0.6 g |
| Fructus Schisandrae (Wu Wei Zi) | 1.8 g |

The original records state that the Rhizoma Atractylodis Macrocephalae should be roasted with powdered earth. The Fructus Psoraleae and Fructus Evodiae should also be roasted. The Semen Myristicae should be wrapped for baking over charcoal fire to rid it of the oily substance. The Fructus Schisandrae should be prepared, and the Radix Bupleuri be prepared with vinegar. The above ingredients were ground into fine powder and mixed with date paste to make pills 1.5 grams each. One pill was taken in the morning and one in the evening together with ginger tea.

*Comments*

This prescription, a combination of Four Gentlemen Decoction (Si Jun Zi Tang) and Four Miracles Pill (Si Shen Wan), suited Empress Dowager Cixi's condition of chronic diarrhea. Four Gentlemen Decoction acted specifically by strengthening the spleen and reinforcing *qi*. It was effective for loose stools resulting from digestive dysfunction, anorexia and general lassitude. However, it weakened Four Gentlemen Decoction and could deal only with chronic diarrhea or that caused by kidney deficiency. Four Miracles Pill (Si Shen Wan) was added here to tonify and warm the spleen and kidney while checking diarrhea. The double prescription introduced acts to treat chronic enteritis, intestinal tuberculosis and chronic dysentery, all manifested by deficient cold involving both the spleen and kidney. Four Miracles Pill (Si Shen Wan), a proved remedy, was recorded in *Standards for Syndrome Differentiation and Treatment (Zheng Zhi Zhun Shen)*. Contemporary studies show that Four Gentlemen Decoction (Si Jun Zi Tang) promotes the synthesis of hepatic glycogen. Its therapeutic effects are better when used together with other herbs.

## XV.2. TWO DAWN DIARRHEA PRESCRIPTIONS

Neither prescription introduced here has any clue as to the date of formulation or the names of the imperial physicians who prepared them for Empress Dowager Cixi.

*Ingredients (Dawn Diarrhea I)*

| | |
|---|---|
| Pericarpium Papaveris  (Ying Su Ke) | 12 g |
| Fructus Crataegi  (Shan Zha) | 3 g |
| Fructus Crataegi, burnt  (Jiao Shan Zha) | 3 g |

The above ingredients were taken with sugar water.

*Ingredients (Dawn Diarrhea II)*

| | |
|---|---|
| Radix Codonopsis Pilusolae  (Zheng Tai Shen) | 12 g |
| Fructus Lycii  (Gou Qi Zi) | 15 g |
| Arillus Longan  (Gui Yuan) | 12 g |
| Cortex Cinnamomi  (Zi You Gui) | 4.5 g |
| Millet wine  (Gan Jiu) | 1.5 g |

According to the original records, the Cortex Cinnamomi should be broken into pieces and steamed in millet wine before use.

*Comments*

The first prescription took the Pericarpium Papaveris as the main ingredient, with Fructus Crataegi added, for the treatment of chronic diarrhea. Also, ingredients for promoting digestion and checking diarrhea were combined in the same prescription. According to *Compendium of Enlargement of Materia Medica* (*Ben Cao Fa Hui*) by Xu Yanchun of the Ming Dynasty (1368-1644), Pericarpium Papaveris, astringent and neutral, enters the lung, large intestine and kidney channels. It acts to contract the lungs, stop cough, check diarrhea and ease pain, and is applicable for lingering cough, chronic dysentery or diarrhea, prolaspe of the rectum, epigastric pain and painful joints. *Compendium of Materia Medica* (*Ben Cao Gang Mu*) records: "Pericarpium Papaveris has a strong astringent effect and is therefore inappropriate to prescribe in the initial stage of a disease. Long-standing diarrhea or dysentery may lead to a weak *qi* concentration, giving rise to protracted loose stools and prolaspe of the rectum. Similarly, a chronic cough will cause poor concentration of pulmonary *qi* manifested by distending sensation in the chest and severe pain. At the same time, it would be appropriate to suggest the use of Pericarpium Papaveris for stopping diarrhea, lifting the prolapsed rectum and contracting the lungs." The chemical elements in Pericarpium Papaveris such as papaverine, narcotoline and erythritol are effective in stopping cough, relieving pain and relaxing smooth muscles of the internal organs and those of the blood vessels. The prescription was thus apparently appropriate for Empress Dowager Cixi at that time.

In the second prescription, Cortex Cinnamomi, pungent and sweet in flavour and hot in property, enters the kidney, spleen and liver channels. It can reinforce kidney Yang, warm up the spleen and stomach, and stop diarrhea due to cold retention. The cinnamic oil contained in Cortex Cinnamomi can promote digestion, remove *qi* stagnation and relieve spasm, while cinnamic aldehyde tranquilizes the patient and eliminates heat. It was used here together with Arillus Longan, Fructus Lycii and Radix Codonopsis Pilosulae for simultaneously reinforcing the spleen and kidney. It was rational also for millet wine to be used here to enhance the therapeutic effects of the other ingredients.

# XVI. PRESCRIPTIONS FOR CLEARING INTESTINES AND STOPPING INTESTINAL HEMORRHAGE

## XVI.1. Sophora Japonica Fruit Pill

Empress Dowager Cixi's Sophora Japonica Fruit Pill (Huai Jiao Wan) was carefully prepared on the ninth day of the fifth month of the lunar calendar in 1903.

### Ingredients

| | |
|---|---|
| Fructus Sophorae  (Huai Jiao) | 30 g |
| Fructus Aurantii  (Zhi Ke) | 15 g |
| Pericarpium Citri Reticulatae Rubra  (Ju Hong) | 9 g |
| Radix Glycyrrhizae  (Gan Cao) | 3 g |

According to the original records both the Fructus Sophorae Japonica and Fructus Aurantii should be roasted. The above ingredients were ground into fine powder and mixed with refined honey to make gold leaf-coated pills the size of mung beans. Six grams of pills were taken each time with pear or lotus soup.

### Comments

According to *Complete Works of Surgical Diseases* (*Yang Yi Da Quan*) by Gu Shicheng, Sophorae Japonica Fruit Pill consists of Fructus Sophorae, Flos Sophorae, Semen Arecae, Radix Scutellariae and Corium Erinacei for treating hemorrhoids. In this prescription, the Fructus Sophorae was heavily used. Having a strong action in clearing heat, cooling blood and stopping bleeding, it is applicable for defecation and hemorrhoids, and for stopping hemorrhage in dysentery. It is also indicated in bleeding involving the Upper and Lower Jiao, and epistaxis. Modern studies have shown that Fructus Sophoraecan can shorten the bleeding time, increase capillary resistance and prevent cerebral hemorrhage in hypertensive patients.

## XVI.2. ANTI-HEMORRHAGE PILL WITH COPTIDIS

Empress Dowager Cixi's Anti-hemorrhage Pill with Coptidis (Zang Lian Wan) was prescribed on the ninth day of the sixth month of the lunar calendar in 1903.

### Ingredients

Radix Ginseng  (Ren Shen)
Radix Angelicae Sinensis  (Dang Gui)
Fructus Sophorae  (Huai Jiao)
Rhizoma Coptidis  (Huang Lian)

Poria  (Fu Ling)
Radix Trichosanthis  (Tian Hua Fen)
Spina Gleditsiae  (Ya Zao)
Cortex Moudan Radicis  (Dan Pi)
Radix Rehmanniae  (Sheng Di Huang)
Rhizoma Alismatis  (Ze Xie)
Fructus Corni  (Shan Zhu Yu)
Rhizoma Dio  (Shan Yao)
Rhizoma Anemarrhenae  (Zhi Mu)
Cortex Phellodendri  (Huang Bai)

According to the original records, the ingredients of this prescription should be of equal amount and purchased only in Tianyitang Pharmacy in Haidian District of Beijing. All ingredients were ground into powder and stuffed into a length of raw clean pig intestine (colon) with the ends tied up. This was steamed on rice. When the pig colon was well done and purple in colour, it was removed from the rice and dried in the sun, after which it was ground into fine powder and mixed with refined honey to make pills the size of mung beans. Six grams of pills were taken each time with boiled water.

### Comments

Anti-hemorrhage Pill with Coptidis, recorded in *Standards of Syndrome Differentiation and Treatments* (*Zheng Zhi Zhun Shen*) by Wang Kentang, consisted only of Rhizoma Coptidis and male pig colon. The prepared pills were taken with warm liquor, millet wine or soup from Fructus Mume on an empty stomach. The remedy was applied to treat hemafecia with or without swelling and a sinking sensation in the anus. Empress Dowager Cixi's health records show that she suffered from occasional hemafecia, possibly due to hemorrhoids. The prescription for Anti-hemorrhage Pill with Coptidis, clearing heat from intestines and stopping bleeding as well as tonifying *qi* and nourishing Yin, was quite effective in treating both the symptoms (Biao) and root cause (Ben) at the same time.

## XVI.3. EXTERNAL WASH FOR CLEARING HEAT AND RESOLVING DAMPNESS

Empress Dowager Cixi's External Wash for Clearing Heat and Resolving Dampness (Qing Re Hua Shi Xi Yao Fang) was carefully prepared by the imperial physicians Zhuang Shouhe and Yao Baosheng on the 30th day of the ninth month of the lunar calendar in 1907.

### Ingredients

| | |
|---|---|
| Petiolus Sophorae  (Huai Tiao) | 60 g |
| Folium Artemisiae Argyi  (Ai Ye) | 30 g |
| Alumen  (Bai Fan) | 30 g |
| Herba Portulacae  (Ma Chi Xian) | 30 g |
| Radix Glycyrrhizae  (Gan Cao) | 30 g |

The above ingredients were decocted for local washing.

### Comments

This external wash for clearing heat from the intestines, eliminating dampness, relieving swelling and stopping pain was prescribed for Empress Dowager Cixi's hemorrhoids. According to *Folk Remedies* (*Chuan Xin Fang*), another method for treating hemorrhoids was to make a concentrated liquid from Petiolus Sophorae for local washing to be followed by igniting seven moxa cones on the local area to provide suitable heat for healing. This remedy depended greatly on the method of application for therapeutic effects.

## XVI.4.  ANUS COMPRESS

Anus Compress (Teng Xi Fang) was prepared for Empress Dowager Cixi's hemorrhoid condition, with no information given as to the date.

*Ingredients*

| | |
|---|---|
| Herba Plantaginis  (Ha Ma Cao) | 30 g |
| Radix Sophorae Flavescentis  (Ku Shen) | 30 g |
| Radix Ledebouriellae  (Fang Feng) | 21 g |
| Herba cum Radix Patrimiae  (Bai Jiang Cao) | 30 g |
| Mirabilite  (Po Xiao) | 9 g |
| Radix Glycyrrhizae  (Gan Cao) | 21 g |
| Fructus Aurantii  (Zhi Ke) | 21 g |
| Fructus Sophorae  (Huai Jiao) | 21 g |

The above ingredients were cooked in water for local application and washing.

*Comments*

Anus Compress has the action of clearing toxic heat and stopping hemorrhoid bleeding. Radix Sophorae Flavescentis was used for stopping bleeding due to hemorrhoids or dysentery, or to trichomonal vaginitis. According to *Comprehensive Summary of External Medicine* (*Wai Ke Da Chen*), Sophora Flavescentis and Rehmanniae Pill (Ku Shen Di Huang Wan) was applied for the treatment of hemorrhoid bleeding and enterorrhagia.

# XVII.  PRESCRIPTION FOR CLEARING HEAT AND PROMOTING URINATION

## XVII.1.  PILL FOR TREATING DARK YELLOW URINE

One dose of Pill for Treating Dark Yellow Urine (Dao Chi Dan) was prescribed for Empress Dowager Cixi without any information as to the date.

*Ingredients*

| | |
|---|---|
| Herba Menthae  (Bo He) | 3 g |
| Radix Ophiopogonis  (Mai Dong) | 3 g |
| Caulis Akebiae  (Mu Tong) | 3 g |
| Rhizoma Coptidis  (Huang Lian) | 3 g |
| Radix Rehmanniae  (Sheng Di Huang) | 3 g |
| Radix Platycodi  (Jie Geng) | 3 g |
| Radix Glycyrrhizae  (Gan Cao) | 3 g |

The above ingredients were ground into fine powder and mixed with refined honey to make cinnabar-coated pills of three grams each.

### Comments

Pill for Treating Dark Yellow Urine was modified by adding appropriate ingredients into the traditional Powder for Treating Dark Yellow Urine (Dao Chi San). This prescription, having the action of clearing and promoting urination, was applied to the treatment of dark, difficult or painful urination, ulcer in the mouth or on the tongue, and sore throat caused by excessive heat in the heart channel or from the heart channel transmitting to the small intestine channel. In terms of modern medicine, the above-mentioned conditions are encountered in acute urinary infections, ulcerative stomatitis and pharyngitis.

# XVIII. PRESCRIPTIONS FOR CONDITIONS OF THE FOUR LIMBS

## XVIII.1. HONG'S EXTERNAL WASH

Hong's External Wash (Hong Yi Xi Yao Fang) was prepared on the 28th day of the 11th month of the lunar calendar in 1882.

### Ingredients

| | |
|---|---:|
| Rhizoma seu Radix Notopterygii (Qiang Huo) | 9 g |
| Radix Ledebouriellae (Fang Feng) | 9 g |
| Radix Achyranthis Bidentatae (Niu Xi) | 6 g |
| Radix Angelicae Sinensis (Dang Gui) | 9 g |
| Flos Carthami (Hong Hua) | 6 g |
| Radix Stephaniae Tetrandrae (Fang Ji) | 6 g |
| Herba Speranskia Tuberculatae (Tou Gu Cao) | 6 g |
| Radix Glycyrrhizae (Gan Cao) | 6 g |
| Table salt (Shi Yan) | 12 g |
| Bulb Allii Fistulosi (Cong Bai) | 7 sticks |

The above ingredients were decocted and mixed with 45 grams of white spirit for local washing.

### Comments

This prescription, composed of ingredients for nourishing and activating blood, dispelling wind and regulating channels and collaterals, is effective for healing limb conditions by means of external washing so that the herbal effect penetrates into the affected areas. Its therapeutic effect in activating blood circulation is enhanced by combing with alcohol in clinical application.

## XVIII.2. BI-SYNDROME COMPRESS

One dose of Bi-syndrome Compress (Teng Xi Yao Fang) was recorded but with no information concerning the date.

### Ingredients

| | |
|---|---|
| Os Draconis  (Long Gu) | 12 g |
| Os Tigris  (Hu Gu) | 12 g |
| Radix Angelicae Dahuricae  (Bai Zhi) | 9 g |
| Radix Ledebouriellae  (Fang Feng) | 12 g |
| Rhizoma Ligustici Chuanxiong  (Chuan Xiong) | 12 g |
| Pericarpium Zanthoxyli  (Chuan Jiao) | 12 g |
| Fructus Chaenomelis  (Mu Gua) | 9 g |
| Radix Platycodi  (Jie Geng) | 12 g |
| Herba Schizonepetae  (Jing Jie) | 12 g |
| Radix Scutellariae  (Huang Qin) | 12 g |
| Herba Achillea Aplina  (Yi Zhi Hao) | 12 g |

### Comments

This prescription was made for external application in the treatment of painful joints, particularly for articular pain due to wind-dampness invasion. All the ingredients are common except for the Herba Achillea Alpina which was recorded in only a few herbal books such as *Compendium of Materia Medica* (*Ben Cao Gang Mu*), and *Supplement to Compendium of Materia Medica* (*Ben Cao Gan Mu Shi Yi*). Here, it was applied by the imperial physicians to treat Empress Dowager Cixi's painful joints. It showed that the imperial physicians were not only confined to the classical formulae of ancient times but also drew on useful folk remedies. Herba Achillea Alpina, possessing actions in activating blood circulation, eliminating wind, easing pain and relieving toxicity, was applied in Bi-syndrome and for healing traumatic injuries.

# XIX. PRESCRIPTION FOR WARMING UMBILICUS

## XIX.1. MIRACULOUS PASTE FOR WARMING UMBILICUS

The prescription for Miraculous Paste for Warming Umbilicus (Shen Xiao Nuan Qi Gao) was copied by imperial physicians from the Imperial Pharmacy on the 21st day of the third month of the lunar calendar in 1880.

### Ingredients

| | |
|---|---|
| Cortex Cinnamomi  (Rou Gui) | 45 g |
| Cortex Moudan Radicis  (Mu Dan Pi) | 24 g |
| Radix Astragali seu Hedyari  (Huang Qi) | 60 g |
| Radix Codonopsis Pilosulae  (Dang Shen) | 60 g |
| Radix Angelicae Sinensis  (Dang Gui) | 60 g |
| Radix Rehmanniae  (Sheng Di Huang) | 60 g |
| Radix Paeoniae Lactiflorae  (Bai Shao) | 30 g |
| Herba Cistanchis  (Rou Cong Rong) | 30 g |
| Radix Aconiti Praeparatae  (Fu Zi) | 30 g |
| Semen Momordica Cochinchinensis  (Mu Bie Zi) | 30 g |
| Herba Schizonepetae  (Jing Jie) | 15 g |
| Radix Ledebouriellae  (Fang Feng) | 15 g |

| | |
|---|---|
| Herba Ephedrae  (Ma Huang) | 15 g |
| Ramulus Cinnamomi  (Gui Zhi) | 15 g |
| Radix Bupleuri  (Chai Hu) | 15 g |
| Radix Peucedani  (Qian Hu) | 15 g |
| Rhizoma Cimicifugae  (Sheng Ma) | 15 g |
| Radix Puerariae  (Ge Gen) | 15 g |
| Folium Perillae  (Su Ye) | 15 g |
| Herba Menthae  (Bo He) | 15 g |
| Rhizoma seu Radix Notopertygii  (Qiang Huo) | 15 g |
| Radix Angelicae Pubescentis  (Du Huo) | 15 g |
| Radix Angelicae Dahuricae  (Bai Zhi) | 15 g |
| Rhizoma Ligustici  (Hao Ben) | 15 g |
| Rhizoma Ligustici Chuanxiong  (Chuan Xiong) | 15 g |
| Herba Asari  (Xi Xin) | 15 g |

The original records state that the Cortex Cinnamomi should be peeled and that the Semen Momordica Conchinchinensis should be used without the cortex, while the Radix Aconiti should be prepared. The above ingredients were mixed with 1.5 kg of sesame oil and 120 grams of chopped Fructus Allii Fistulosi and Rhizoma Zingiberis Recens. All the ingredients were simmered to a burnt yellow colour. After separating out the residue, the processed oil was weighed and mixed with red lead in the ratio of 2 to 1. The mixture was further concentrated to a paste which was kept in a porcelain vessel to be used after seven days.

A further dose of Miraculous Paste for Warming Umbilicus was made by adding 1.5 grams of Moschus.

### Comments

Paste for Warming Umbilicus (Nuan Qi Gao) contained different ingredients in different regions of China. Ten Fragrances Paste for Warming Umbilicus (Shi Xiang Nuan Qi Gao), e.g., varied in content according to the region of production, though both pastes used the same commercial name. The one made in Tianjin consisted of Bulbus Allii Fistulosi, Allium Tuberosum, raw Radix Aconiti, Pericarpium Zanthoxyli and Rhizoma Zingiberis. The one produced in Jinan contained Moschus, Cortex Cinnamomi, Fructus Cinnamomi and Lignum Aquillaricae Resinatum. And the one made in Hohhot, known as Paste for Sealing Umbilicus (Feng Qi Gao), contained Rhizoma Zingiberis, Radix Aconiti Praeparata and Fructus Evodiae. The actions were to relieve pain, stop diarrhea, dispel wind, eliminate dampness, strengthen the spleen and stomach, and warm the abdomen. It was indicated in abdominal pain and distention, vomiting and sour regurgitation caused by invasion of cold. In folk traditional practice it was also applied in the treatment of long-standing infertility and pain in the lumbosacral region.

# XX. PRESCRIPTIONS FOR DERMATOLOGICAL CONDITIONS

## XX.1. POWDER FOR ELIMINATING WIND AND DAMPNESS

Powder for Eliminating Wind and Dampness (Qu Feng Chu Shi San) was carefully prepared by the imperial physicians Zhuang Zhouhe and Yang Jihe on the 15th day of the second month of the lunar calendar, with no information as to the year.

### Ingredients

| | |
|---|---|
| Herba Schizonepetae (Jing Jie Sui) | 9 g |
| Radix Ledebouriellae (Fang Feng) | 9 g |
| Radix Angelicae Dahuricae (Bai Zhi) | 9 g |
| Bombyx Batryticatus (Jiang Can) | 6 g |
| Cortex Dictamni Dasyarpi Radicis (Bai Xian Pi) | 9 g |
| Fructus Kochiae (Di Fu Zi) | 9 g |
| Squama Manitis (Chuan Shan Jia) | 6 g |
| Talcum (Hua Shi) | 9 g |
| Alum, dried (Ku Fan) | 3 g |
| Cortex Moudan Radicis (Mu Dan Pi) | 6 g |
| Borneoleum Syntheticum (Bing Pian) | 1.5 g |

The original records say that the Bombyx Batryticatus should be roasted and that the Squama Manitis should be prepared before use. The above ingredients were ground into fine powder and sieved through silk before packing into a cloth bag for application.

### Comments

Functioning in dispelling wind-damp, stopping itching and clearing rashes, the powder was cool in nature for external use, and appropriate for skin conditions caused by heat retention in the blood.

## XX.2. EXTERNAL POWDER FOR DRYING DAMPNESS AND STOPPING ITCHING

External Powder for Drying Dampness and Stopping Itching (Li Shi Zhi Yang Pu Yao Fang) was worked out by the imperial physicians Li Dechang and Yang Jihe on the 17th day of the sixth month of the lunar calendar in 1886.

### Ingredients

| | |
|---|---|
| Fructus Kochiae (Du Fu Zi) | 30 g |
| Bombyx Batryticatus (Jiang Can) | 15 g |
| Cortex Dictami Dasycarpi Radicis (Bai Xian Pi) | 15 g |
| Radix Angelicae Dahuricae (Bai Zhi) | 9 g |
| Herba Schizonepetae (Jing Jie Sui) | 15 g |
| Herba Artemisiae Capillaris (Yin Chen) | 15 g |
| Herba cum Radice Patrimiae (Bai Jiang Cao) | 15 g |
| Alum (Bai Fan) | 9 g |
| Vital Energy Nourishing Powder (Yi Yuan San) | 15 g |

The original records require the Bombyx Batryticatus to be roasted and the alum calcined. The above ingredients were ground into fine powder and packed into a cloth bag for direct application to the affected areas.

### Comments

This prescription was formulated also for dispelling wind and dampness and for stopping itching in the treatment of skin conditions. It was prepared meticulously in the form of dusting powder. Among the ingredients the Fructus Kochiae, bitter and cold, was dominant. Fructus Kochiae has the effect of eliminating damp-heat and promoting urination. It is believed to inhibit the growth of certain dermatomyces. It is also effective in easing itching due to damp-heat. Adding Fructus Litseae Cubebae and Alum would enhance its effect in stopping itching. The use of Fructus Kochiae alone prepared for local bathing is applicable for scrotum eczema.

## XX.3.  EXTERNAL APPLICATION POWDER

Empress Dowager Cixi's External Application Powder (Fu Yao San) was prepared by the imperial physician Xu Benlin on the 26th day of the fourth month of the lunar calendar in 1902.

### Ingredients

| | |
|---|---|
| Semen Phaseoli Radiatus  (Lu Dou) | 30 g |
| Periostracum Cicadae  (Chan Tui) | 3 g |
| Herba Lycopi  (Ze Lan) | 9 g |
| Cortex Fraxini  (Qin Pi) | 6 g |
| Spica Prunellae  (Xia Ku Cao) | 6 g |
| Fructus Forsythiae  (Lian Qiao) | 9 g |
| Radix Angelicae Dahuricae  (Bai Zhi) | 9 g |
| Fructus Viticis  (Man Jing Zi) | 9 g |

The above ingredients were ground into fine powder, nine to 12 grams of which were mixed with dilute honey water for external application to the affected areas.

### Comments

Functioning in dispelling wind, clearing heat and relieving swelling, this powder is also applicable for treating skin conditions. Semen Phaseoli Radiatus is the main ingredient. Its external application eliminates toxic heat in the treatment of erysipelas and carbuncles. According to *Prescriptions for General Application* (*Pu Ji Fang*) Semen Phaseoli Radiatus was indicated in erysipelas and scattered furuncles: "Grind Semen Phaseoli Radiatus and Radix Rhei into powder and mix it with honey liquid prepared with Herba Menthae for external application." Another prescription containing Semen Phaseoli Radiatus for the treatment of carbuncles was also recorded in the same book. "Grind Semen Phaseoli Radiatus, Glycine Max and Rhizoma Curcumae Longae into extremely fine powder for external application." Ingredients for dispelling wind were added, making the remedy more effective. Reference to existing health histories of the Qing Dynasty on the 26th day of the fourth month of the lunar calendar in 1902 shows that a separate herbal wash was applied together with this prescription. It contained Fructus Viticis, Herba Schizonepetae, Fructus Tribuli, Folium Mori and Cortex Fraxini.

## XX.4. HERBAL WASH FOR CLEARING WIND-HEAT

Empress Dowager Cixi's Herbal Wash for Clearing Wind-Heat (Qu Feng Qing Re Xi Yao Feng) was carefully prepared by the imperial physicians Li Jun and Zhang Zhongyuan on the 26th day of the seventh month of the lunar calendar in 1906.

*Ingredients*

| | |
|---|---|
| Flos Carthami  (Hong Hua) | 6 g |
| Radix Ledebouriellae  (Fang Feng) | 9 g |
| Radix Angelicae Dahuricae  (Bai Zhi) | 6 g |
| Rhizoma seu Radix Notoptergyii  (Qiang Huo) | 6 g |
| Folium Mori  (Sang Ye) | 6 g |
| Flos Chrysanthemi  (Ju Hua) | 6 g |
| Herba Menthae  (Bo He) | 6 g |
| Bombyx Batryticatus  (Jiang Can) | 3 g |

The above ingredients were boiled in water and mixed with one spoonful of perfume for application.

*Comments*

Empress Dowager Cixi often complained of itching skin. This prescription, acting to elimminate wind, was reinforced by Flos Carthami for activating blood. Therapeutically, both blood and pathogenic wind were considered at the same time. The perfume was supposed to enhance the effect of stopping itching.

## XX.5. EXTERNAL POWDER FOR CLEARING WIND-DAMP AND STOPPING NUMBNESS AND ITCHING

External Powder for Clearing Wind-Damp and Stopping Numbness and Itching (Chu Shi Qu Feng Zhi Mu Yang Mian Yao) was carefully formulated by the imperial physician Li Dechang on the sixth day of the seventh month of the lunar calendar, with no year given.

*Ingredients*

| | |
|---|---|
| Radix Angelicae Dahuricae  (Bai Zhi) | 6 g |
| Radix Ledebouriellae  (Fang Feng) | 6 g |
| Fructus Kochiae  (Di Fu Zi) | 6 g |
| Plum Blossom Tongue Ulcer Pill  (Mei Hua Dian She Dan) | 4 pills |
| Bombyx Batryticatus  (Jiang Can) | 6 g |
| Vital Energy Nourishing Powder  (Yi Yuan San) | 6 g |
| Squama Manitis  (Chuan Shan Jia) | 6 g |
| Borneoleum syntheticum  (Bing Pian) | 0.6 g |

The original records call for the Bombyx Batryticatus and Squama Manitis to be roasted before use. The above ingredients were ground into extremely fine powder and placed in a cloth bag for external application to areas where numbness, itching or swelling were felt.

*Comments*

This prescription eliminates wind and dampness and relieves numbness in the elbow. Plum Blossom Tongue Ulcer Pill was added to the prepared powder, i.e., small portions of Resina Olibani, Resina Murrhae, Resina Draconis, Lignum Aquilariae Resinatum, Calculus Bovis, Venenum Bufonis, Moschus and pearl, ingredients that regulate *qi*, activate blood, and relieve both toxicity and swelling. External application of the reinforced powder to the local lesions helps alleviate swelling and ease itching.

## XX.6. EXTERNAL APPLICATION POWDER PLUS

One dose of External Application Powder Plus (Fu Yao You Fang) was prescribed for Empress Dowager Cixi on the 24th day of the eighth month of the lunar calendar, with no information given as to the year.

*Ingredients*

| | |
|---|---|
| Alum, dried  (Ku Fan) | 9 g |
| Realgar  (Xiong Huang) | 4.5 g |
| Radix Angelicae Dahuricae  (Bai Zhi) | 9 g |
| Cortex Phellodendri  (Huang Bai) | 6 g |
| Resina Murrhae  (Mu Yao) | 6 g |
| Rhizoma Atractylodis  (Cang Zhu) | 9 g |
| Herba Menthae  (Bo He) | 9 g |
| Radix Stemonae  (Bai Bu) | 9 g |

The above ingredients were ground into fine powder for external application. Four other doses were prescribed separately on the following four days.

*Comments*

This remedy in powder form for external application clears heat, dries dampness, eliminates wind and relieves toxicity. One application of 60 grams was given each day, though it is not certain what kind of skin condition Empress Dowager Cixi had at that time.

## XX.7. DERMATOLOGICAL OINTMENT

Four doses of Dermatological Ointment (Mian Yao Dao Gao Fang) were urgently prepared for Empress Dowager Cixi on the 12th day of the ninth month of the lunar calendar, with no information given as to the year.

*Ingredients*

| | |
|---|---|
| Semen Hydnocarpi  (Da Feng Zi) | 18 g |
| Alum, dried  (Ku Fan) | 9 g |
| Indigo Naturalis  (Qing Dai) | 9 g |
| Realgar  (Xiong Huang) | 6 g |
| Camphora  (Zhang Nao) | 6 g |
| Powdery Concha Meretricis seu Cyclinea  (Ge Fen) | 9 g |

The original records state that uncoated Semen Hydnocarpishould be used.

The above ingredients were ground into fine powder and mixed with 12 grams each of uncoated Semen Junlandis and salt, plus a proper amount of lard to make a paste.

### Comments

With Semen Hydnocarpi as the principal ingredient, the formula has the action of clearing heat, drying dampness and relieving toxicity. Experiments showed that water infusion made from Semen Hydnocarpi in the ratio of one portion of Semen Hydnocarpi to two portions of water has an inhibitory effect on sporular tinea fungi. The remedy apppeared effective in both tinea and neurodermatitis.

## XX.8. DERMATOLOGICAL OINTMENT PLUS

Four doses of Dermatological Ointment Plus (Mian Yao Dao Gao You Fang) were urgently prepared for Empress Dowager Cixi on the 12th day of the ninth month of the lunar calendar, with no year given.

### Ingredients

| | |
|---|---|
| Semen Hydnocarpi  (Da Feng Zi) | 18 g |
| Realgar  (Xiong Huang) | 6 g |
| Camphora  (Zhang Nao) | 6 g |
| Mirabilitum  (Feng Hua Xiao) | 6 g |
| Alum, dried  (Ku Fan) | 6 g |
| Powdery Concha Meretricis seu Cyclinea  (Ge Fen) | 9 g |
| Lithargyrum  (Mi Tuo Shen) | 9 g |
| Table salt  (Shi Yan) | 6 g |

According to the original records the Semen Hydnocarpi should be used without coating. The above ingredients were ground into fine powder and mixed with lard to make a paste for local application.

### Comments

What should be noted is that two more ingredients, Lithargyrum and salt, were added to the previous prescription. Experiments showed that Lithargyrum inhibited to various degrees such dermatophytes as metatarsal trichophyton, interphalangeal trichophyton and Epidermophyton floccosum. Its external application may relieve inflammation. However, the cause of the Empress Dowager's skin itching is still not understood.

# XXI. HERBAL BATH REMEDIES

## XXI.1. HERBAL BATH REMEDY I

Two portions of ingredients of Herbal Bath Remedy (Mu Yu Fang) were prescribed for Empress Dowager Cixi on the 18th day of the fourth month of the lunar calendar, with no year given.

### Ingredients

| | |
|---|---|
| Flos Eriocauli  (Gu Jing Cao) | 36 g |
| Herba Artemisiae  (Yin Chen) | 36 g |
| Concha Haliotidis  (Shi Jue Ming) | 36 g |
| Ramulus Mori  (Sang Zhi) | 36 g |
| Flos Chrysanthemi Morifolii  (Bai Ju Hua) | 36 g |
| Fructus Chaenomelis  (Mu Gua) | 45 g |
| Folium Mori  (Sang Ye) | 45 g |

### Comments

The prescription mainly consists of ingredients that have the action of clearing heat, dispelling wind, eliminating dampness, brightening the eyes and refreshing the mind. Among them, Flos Eriocauli has antibacterial effects on Bacillus pyocyaneus and inhibitory effects on dermatophytes. This bath remedy might prevent the onset of dermatological disorders and keep the skin healthy.

## XXI.2.  HERBAL BATH REMEDY II

Herbal Bath Remedy II (Mu Yu Er Fang) for Empress Dowager Cixi was formulated by the imperial physician Yao Baosheng on the fourth of the fifth month of the lunar calendar, with no year given.

### Ingredients

| | |
|---|---|
| Fructus Chaenomelis  (Mu Gua) | 30 g |
| Semen Coicis  (Yi Yi Ren) | 30 g |
| Ramulus Mori  (Sang Zhi) | 30 g |
| Folium Mori  (Sang Ye) | 30 g |
| Herba Artemisiae  (Yin Chen) | 18 g |
| Flos Chrysanthemi  (Ju Hua) | 30 g |
| Pericarpium Citri Reticulatae Viride  (Qing Pi) | 30 g |
| Periostracum Cicadae  (Chan Tui) | 30 g |
| Fructus Evodiae  (Wu Zhu Yu) | 6 g |
| Rhizoma Coptidis  (Huang Lian) | 6 g |

The original records say the above ingredients were ground into rough powder which was tied into a cloth bag to be boiled in water and used for bathing.

### Comments

This prescription was similar to the previous one in composition but with some additions: Periostracum Cicadae is used to clear wind-heat and help cure rashes and prevent skin eruptions; Rhizoma Coptidis helps clear heat and dry dampness; and Fructus Evodiae, despite its pungent bitter aroma and severe heat property, has antibacterial effects on Bacillus pyocyaneus and staphylococcus aureus. According to the principle that pungent ingredients dispel and bitter ones purge, Fructus Evodiae and Rhizoma Coptidis were used together in sedating the liver and pacifying the stomach. They were often used internally for treating nausea and vomiting, and for discomfort and pain in the epigastric region, while these two ingredients rendered for external application were rare in TCM literature. The reason for their being included in the bathing remedy was probably related to their actions in clearing heat, drying dampness and relieving toxicity.

# XXII. PRESCRIPTIONS FOR REGULATING MENSTRUATION

## XXII.1. PILL FOR REGULATING MENSTRUATION

Pill for Regulating Menstruation (Tiao Jing Wan) was prepared for young Cixi on the 30th day of the fourth month of the lunar calendar, with no year given.

*Ingredients*

| | |
|---|---|
| Rhzioma Cyperi  (Xiang Fu) | 30 g |
| Rhizoma Atractylodis  (Cang Zhu) | 30 g |
| Red Poria  (Chi Fu Ling) | 30 g |
| Rhizoma Ligustici Chuanxiong  (Chuan Xiong) | 9 g |
| Radix Linderae  (Wu Yao) | 30 g |
| Cortex Phellodendri  (Huang Bai) | 9 g |
| Herba Lycop  (Ze Lan) | 30 g |
| Cortex Moudan Radicis  (Mu Dan Pi) | 24 g |
| Radix Angelicae Sinensis  (Dang Gui) | 24 g |

The original records say the Rhizoma Cyperi should be prepared with urine from boys under 12 years of age and the Cortex Phellodendri should be roasted with millet wine. The above ingredients were ground into fine powder and made into water-bound pills the size of mung beans. Six grams of the pills were taken each time with boiled water on an empty stomach.

*Comments*

The prescription has the action of regulating menstruation, nourishing blood, stopping pain and relieving blood stasis. In addition to the use of ingredients for nourishing blood, activating blood and regulating *qi*, Rhizoma Atractylodis and Cortex Phellodendri were added for the purpose of clearing heat and eliminating dampness, resembling the therapeutic feature of Two Wonders Powder (Er Miao San). The use of Pill for Regulating Menstruation serves as a clear indication that Empress Dowager Cixi suffered from menstrual problems complicated by excessive leukorrhea in her youth.

## XXII.2. DAWN DEW PILL FOR PROMOTING MENSTRUATION

The use of Dawn Dew Pill for Promoting Menstruation (Tong Jing Gan Lu Yin) is recorded undated in imperial medical records.

*Ingredients*

| | |
|---|---|
| Radix Angelicae Sinensis  (Dang Gui) | 240 g |
| Cortex Moudan Radicis  (Mu Dan Pi) | 120 g |
| Fructus Aurantii  (Zhi Ke) | 60 g |
| Pericarpium Citri Reticulatae  (Chen Pi) | 60 g |
| Faeces Trogopterorum  (Wu Ling Zhi) | 90 g |
| Fructus Amomi  (Sha Ren) | 60 g |
| Radix Rehmanniae Praeparatae  (Shu Di Huang) | 120 g |
| Radix Rehamnniae  (Sheng Di Huang) | 120 g |
| Rhizoma Corydalis  (Yuan Hu Suo) | 120 g |

| Radix et Rhizoma Rhei  (Da Huang) | 240 g |
| Radix Paeoniae Rubra  (Chi Shao) | 90 g |
| Pericarpium Citri Reticulatae Viride  (Qing Pi) | 90 g |
| Rhizoma Cyperi  (Xiang Fu) | 750 g |
| Rhizoma Zingiberis Recens  (Sheng Jiang) | 60 g |
| Cortex Cinnamomi  (Rou Gui) | 60 g |
| Rhizoma Sparganii  (San Leng) | 240 g |
| Rhizoma Zedoaiae  (E Zhu) | 240 g |
| Radix Glycyrrhizae  (Gan Cao) | 60 g |
| Flos Carthami  (Hong Hua) | 60 g |

According to the original records, the Rhizoma Corydalis, Radix et Rhizoma Rhei and Rhizoma Cyperi should be prepared before use. The above ingredients were processed together with 1.5 kg of vinegar and 120 grams of Lignum Sappan decoction to make the pills.

### Comments

The prescription has the action of activating blood, removing blood stasis and promoting *qi* circulation to generate blood. It was indicated in obstructed menstruation, abdominal masses, distending pain in the lower lateral abdomen, and consumptive fever due to Yin deficiency. The pill made in different parts of China under the same patent name varied in constituents. Some included Moschus,while others contained fuligo. This prescription was probably made for Empress Dowager Cixi when she was middle-aged. It was recorded in *Original Prescription Records for Empress Dowager Cixi* (*Lao Fo Ye Yong Yao Di Bu*) during the era of Emperor Guangxu.

## XXII.3. BLACK GOLD PILL

Black Gold Pill (Wu Jin Wan) was copied from *A Collection of Recommended Prescriptions* (Liang Fang Ji Cheng) on the 20th day of the fifth month of the lunar calendar, with no information given as to the year.

### Ingredients

| Radix Lindera  (Tai Wu) | 90 g |
| Radix et Rhizoma Rhei  (Da Huang) | 90 g |
| Radix Ginseng  (Ren Shen) | 90 g |
| Rhizoma Zedoariae  (E Zhu) | 90 g |
| Rhizoma Sparganii  (San Leng) | 90 g |
| Radix Scutellariae  (Huang Qin) | 90 g |
| Rhizoma Corydalis  (Yuan Hu Suo) | 90 g |
| Cortex Moudan Radicis  (Mu Dan Pi) | 90 g |
| Colla Corii Asini  (E Jiao) | 30 g |
| Pollen Typhae  (Pu Huang) | 90 g |
| Rhizoma Cyperi  (Xiang Fu) | 90 g |
| Cortex Sojae Nignum  (Wu Dou Yi) | 90 g |
| Radix Rehmanniae  (Sheng Di Huang) | 90 g |
| Rhizoma Ligustici Chuanxiong  (Chuan Xiong) | 90 g |
| Herba Artemisia Anomalalliu  (Liu Ji Lu) | 60 g |
| Folium Artemisiae Argyi  (Qi Ai) | 60 g |

Semen Dolichoris (Bian Dou)        60 g

The original records say that the Radix et Rhizoma Rhei should be prepared before use. It was forbidden in this case to process the Radix Rehmanniae in an iron utensil. The above ingredients were first baked with the decoction made from Lignum Sappan and then ground into fine powder. The processed powder was then mixed with refined honey to make wax-coated pills of three grams each.

### Comments

Black Gold Pill, an empirical remedy, was indicated in women patients complaining of poor appetite, bitter taste in the mouth, dry throat, sallow complexion, emaciation, pricking pain in the chest and hypochondriac regions, massive uterine bleeding and turbid leukorrhea caused by the seven emotional disturbances, particularly depression. This prescription has a mild therapeutic effect in comparison with Dawn Dew Pill for Promoting Menstruation (Tong Jing Gan Lu Wan).

# XXIII. DELACTATION FORMULA AND RECIPE FOR PROMOTING APPETITE IN NEWBORNS

## XXIII.1. DELACTATION FORMULA AND PILL FOR HAPPINESS AND LONGEVITY

On the 25th day of the third month of the lunar calendar in 1856 the imperial physicians Luan Tai, Yang Chun and Li Dechang took the young Cixi's pulse and felt it slippery and deep. They believed that it was related to her lochia and gastrointestinal dryness. After consultation they prescribed one dose of Decoction for Delactation and Moistening the Stomach (Hui Ru Sheng Hua Tang) to be taken at noon.

On the 27th day of the third month of the lunar calendar in 1856, the imperial physicians Luan Tai, Yang Chun and Li Dechang felt the young Cixi's pulse moderately slippery. Although there was less stagnant blood, dryness in the stomach and intestines remained, which was marked by continued milk secretion and heat retention in the liver channel. One dose of Decoction for Clearing Liver Heat and Delactation (Qing Gan Hui Ru Yin) was prescribed for her to be taken at noon.

On the 29th day of the third month of the lunar calendar in 1856, the imperial physicians Luan Tai, Yang Chun and Li Dechang felt the young Cixi's pulse moderate. Lactation gradually stopped. Subcutaneous nodes were disappearing despite *qi* and blood disharmony and some remaining dormant heat. One dose of Decoction for Nourishing Body Fluid and Resolving Stasis (Tiao Ying Hua Chi Tang) was prescribed for her to be taken at noon.

On the 23rd day of the third month of the lunar calendar in 1856, the imperial physicians Luan Tai and Ying Wenxi observed the facial expression and pulse of the new-born boy, who later became Emperor Tongzhi, to be perfectly normal. Soy Powder for Happiness and Longevity (Fu Shou Dan) was prescribed for promoting his appetite.

*Ingredients*

| | |
|---|---|
| Cinnabari  (Zhu Sha) | 0.3 g |
| Rhizoma Coptidis  (Huang Lian) | 0.3 g |
| Radix Glycyrrhizae  (Gan Cao) | 0.15 g |

The above ingredients were processed in the form of powder to be taken with honey water.

*Comments*

The above records were abstracted from *Young Cixi's Happy Delivery of Baby Tongzhi* (Yi Fei Yi Xi Da A Ge). It was the imperial document that started on the 23rd day of the third month of the lunar calendar in 1856, providing the daily events concerning the delivery of the infant who later became Emperor Tongzhi.

The above-mentioned decoctions were only recorded by their names without listing the respective use of individual ingredients. However, their therapeutic effects were obvious, for the daily documents indicated the success of the treatment process.

# XXIV.  FEISHU PLASTER REMEDIES

## XXIV.1.  PLASTER FOR SOOTHING THE LIVER AND PROMOTING LUNG *QI*

Plaster for Soothing the Liver and Promoting Lung Qi (Li Gan Shu Fei He Mai Gao) was formulated for Empress Dowager Cixi by the imperial physicians Li Dechang and Zhang Zhongyuan on the 12th day of the third month of the lunar calendar, with no information given as to the year.

*Ingredients*

| | |
|---|---|
| Rhizoma Cyperi  (Xiang Fu) | 30 g |
| Radix Angelicae Pubescentis  (Du Huo) | 18 g |
| Herba Ephedrae  (Ma Huang) | 18 g |
| Bombyx Batryticatus  (Jiang Can) | 18 g |
| Pericarpium Citri Reticulatae Viride  (Qing Pi) | 24 g |
| Squama Manitis  (Chuan Shan Jia) | 18 g |
| Rhizoma Curcumae Longae  (Jiang Huang) | 15 g |
| Fructus Chaenomelis  (Mu Gua) | 30 g |
| Radix Angelicae Sinensis  (Dang Gui) | 30 g |
| Radix Paeoniae Lactiflorae  (Bai Shao) | 18 g |
| Rhizoma Ligustici Chuanxiong  (Chuan Xiong) | 15 g |
| Herba Sperankia Tuberculata  (Tou Gu Cao) | 24 g |
| Resina Olibani  (Ru Xiang) | 9 g |
| Resina Murrhae  (Mo Yao) | 9 g |
| Radix Dipsaci  (Xu Duan) | 24 g |
| Cortex Acanthopanacis Radicis  (Wu Jia Pi) | 18 g |

The original recipe calls for raw Rhizoma Cyperi, Squama Manitis and Radix Paeoniae Lactiflorae. The Rhizoma Curcumae Longae should be sliced. The above ingredients were well fried in two kilograms of sesame oil. After separating out the herbal residue, powdered red lead was added to make the paste for external application to Jianjing (GB 21) and Feishu (UB 13). 0.15 grams of Moschus was mixed with the paste during application.

### Comments

The prescription was prepared for external application. Analysis of the composition of the formula indicates that Empress Dowager Cixi was suffering from liver *qi* stagnation as manifested by distending pain in the chest and hypochondriac region, and tense tendons and muscles. Most of the ingredients were used to promote *qi* and activate blood. The large proportion of Rhizoma Cyperi was for soothing the liver and regulating *qi* circulation so as to stop pain. Herba Ephedrae was used to assist Rhizoma Cyperi in dispersing lung *qi* and regulating channels and collaterals. All were used only after deep consideration. The selection of ingredients and of acupuncture points was suited to treatment based on syndrome differentiation.

## XXIV.2. PLASTER FOR RELIEVING *QI* STAGNATION AND PROMOTING LUNG *QI*

Plaster for Relieving *Qi* Stagnation and Promoting Lung *Qi* (Jie Yu Shu Fei He Mai Gao) was carefully prepared by the imperial physicians Zhuang Shouhe, Li Dechang, Quan Shun and Nie Hongjun for Empress Dowager Cixi on the 16th day of the third month of the lunar calendar in 1895.

### Ingredients

| | |
|---|---|
| Rhizoma Cyperi  (Xiang Fu) | 18 g |
| Bombyx Batryticatus  (Jiang Can) | 15 g |
| Rhizoma Acori Graminei  (Shi Chang Pu) | 15 g |
| Canlis Perillae  (Su Geng) | 12 g |
| Semen Sinapis Albae  (Bai Jie Zi) | 12 g |
| Retinerus Citri Fructus  (Ju Luo) | 12 g |
| Radix Angelicae Sinensis  (Dang Gui) | 30 g |
| Pericarpium Citri Reticulatae Viride  (Qing Pi) | 15 g |
| Radix Paeoniae Lactiflorae  (Chi Shao) | 15 g |
| Radix Codonopsis Pilosulae  (Dang Shen) | 18 g |
| Rhizoma Curcumae Longae  (Jiang Can) | 15 g |
| Ramulus Mori  (Sang Zhi) | 30 g |
| Herba Speranskia Tuberculata  (Tou Gu Cao) | 24 g |
| Caulis Spatholobi Syrup  (Ji Xue Teng Gao) | 24 g |

According to the original records, raw Rhizoma Cyperi should be used. The Rhizoma Curcumae Longae should be sliced before use. The above ingredients were well fried in 1. 5 kilograms of sesame oil. After separating out the herbal residue, powdered red lead was added to make the paste for external application at Feishu (UB 13).

### Comments

The formulating principle of the prescription Plaster for Relieving *Qi* Stagnation and Promoting Lung *Qi* was similar to that above. It was intended to resolve phlegm and remove obstruction from channels and collaterals despite the variation of ingredients. Still, the underlying purpose of relieving *qi* stagnation was maintained. What is noteworthy is that plastering at acupuncture points coordinated with the philosophy of TCM. Such plasters are still in use today.

# XXV.  HERBAL TEA REMEDIES

## XXV.1.  HERBAL TEA FOR CLEARING HEAT AND REGULATING *QI*

Herbal Tea for Clearing Heat and Regulating *Qi* (Qing Re Li Qi Dai Cha Yin) was formulated with care for Empress Dowager Cixi by the imperial physician Yao Baosheng on the 16th day of the second month of the lunar calendar with no information given as to the year.

*Ingredients*

| | |
|---|---|
| Flos Chrysanthemi  (Ju Hua) | 9 g |
| Folium Mori  (Sang Ye) | 9 g |
| Pericarpium Citri Reticulatae Rubra  (Ju Hong) | 4.5 g |
| Rhizoma Phragmitis  (Lu Gen) | 2 |
| Massa Fermentata Medicinalis, modified  (Jian Qu) | 6 g |
| Fructus Aurantii  (Zhi Ke) | 4.5 g |
| Cornu Antelopis  (Ling Yang Jiao) | 1.5 g |
| Fructus Oryzae Germinature  (Gu Ya) | 9 g |

The original record stipulates that the Rhizoma Phragmitis (fresh) should be chopped before use, while the Fructus Aurantii, Massa Fermentata Medicinalis and Fructus Oryzae Germinature should be roasted. The above ingredients were prepared as a decoction to be taken while still warm.

*Comments*

Among the ingredients, the Flos Chrysanthemi and Folium Mori were applied to clear heat and promote vision; the Pericarpium Citri Reticulatae Rubra and Fructus Aurantii to regulate *qi* and harmonize the Middle Jiao; the Rhizoma Phragmitis to clear heat from the lung and stomach; and the Cornu Antelopis to clear heat from the liver and gallbladder. The prescription focused on clearing heat from the head, eyes and the Upper Jiao, and on regulating *qi* of the spleen and stomach. It was appropriate for Empress Dowager Cixi's conditions of recurrent eye disorders and disharmony between the spleen and stomach. The ingenious imperial physicians made the medicine in the form of herbal tea for the use of the imperial family. It was in fact widely applied for its purgative effect while avoiding the medicinal taste of a decoction. It could well be considered as an effective preventive beverage.

## XXV.2.  HERBAL TEA FOR CLEARING HEAT AND REGULATING *QI* PLUS

Empress Dowager Cixi's Herbal Tea for Clearing Heat and Regulating *Qi* Plus (Qing Re Li Qi Dai Cha Yin Fang You) was carefully prepared by the imperial physician Yao Baosheng on the 26th day of the second month of the lunar calendar, with no year given.

*Ingredients*

| | |
|---|---|
| Flos Chrysanthemi (Ju Hua) | 9 g |
| Folium Mori (Sang Ye) | 9 g |
| Cornu Antelopis (Ling Yang Jiao) | 1.5 g |
| Radix Ophiopogonis (Mai Men Dong) | 9 g |
| Poria (Fu Ling) | 12 g |
| Fructus Aurantii (Zhi Ke) | 4.5 g |
| Rhizoma Alismatis (Ze Xie) | 4.5 g |
| Fructus Oryzae Germinature (Gu Ya) | 9 g |

The original records say that the Fructus Aurantii and Fructus Oryzae Germinature should be roasted. The above ingredients were prepared in decoction form to be taken while still warm.

*Comments*

Compared with the previous prescription, this has fewer ingredients for strengthening the spleen and easing the stomach while those for clearing heart heat and eliminating dampness were more. Radix Ophiopogonis with its cores enters into the heart channel. It was used here not only to clear heart heat and produce fluid; it was also used to disperse turbid *qi* from the heart channel. Further, its sweet flavour and bland taste made it suitable for combination with other ingredients for preparation in the form of tea.

## XXV.3. HERBAL TEA I FOR CLEARING DAMP-HEAT

Empress Dowager Cixi's Herbal Tea I for Clearing Damp-Heat (Qing Re Hua Shi Dai Cha Yin Fang Yi) was carefully prepared by the imperial physicians Zhang Zhongyuan and Yao Baosheng on the 12th day of the first month of the lunar calendar with no year given.

*Ingredients*

| | |
|---|---|
| Rhizoma Phragmitis (Lu Gen) | 2 |
| Caulis Bambusae in Taeniam (Zhu Ru) | 4.5 g |
| Fructus Crataegi (Shan Zha) | 9 g |
| Fructus Oryzae Germinature (Gu Ya) | 9 g |
| Pericarpium Citri Reticulatae Rubra (Ju Hong) | 2.4 g |
| Folium Mori (Sang Ye) | 6 g |

According to the original manuscript the Rhizoma Phragmitis should be chopped while the Fruotus Oryzae Germinature (fresh) roasted, and the Fruotus Crataegi also roasted until yellow. The above ingredients were prepared in decoction form to be used as tea.

*Comments*

Herbal tea remedies accepted in the imperial palaces were those that would help eliminate pathogenic factors, without weakening the antipathogenic *qi*. This remedy has the action of clearing the ascending heat in the head and eyes, while harmonizing the spleen and stomach. Dampness was eliminated when the spleen and stomach were strengthened, and the head and eyes were cleared when the heat was dispelled. This prescription used less and smaller amounts of the ingredients which the Empress Dowager Cixi appreciated.

## XXV.4. HERBAL TEA II FOR CLEARING DAMP-HEAT

Empress Dowager Cixi's Herbal Tea II for Clearing Damp-Heat (Qing Re Yang Yin Dai Cha Yin Fang Er) was prepared with care by the imperial physician Yao Baosheng on the 20th day of the second month of the lunar calendar, with no year given.

### Ingredients

| | |
|---|---|
| Flos Chrysanthemi  (Ju Hua) | 9 g |
| Cortex Mori Radicis  (Sang Bai Pi) | 3 g |
| Folium Mori  (Sang Ye) | 3 g |
| Radix Scutellariae  (Huang Qin) | 4.5 g |
| Poria  (Fu Ling) | 9 g |
| Cornu Antelopis  (Ling Yang Jiao) | 1.5 g |
| Massa Fermentata Medicinalis, modified  (Jian Qu) | 6 g |
| Rhizoma Alismatis  (Ze Xie) | 4.5 g |
| Fructus Aurantii  (Zhi Ke) | 4.5 g |

The original records state that the Radix Scutellariae should be prepared with millet wine while the Massa Fermentata Medicinalis (modified) and Fructus Aurantii should be roasted. The above ingredients were prepared in decoction form to be taken while still warm.

### Comments

In this prescription, in addition to the use of Radix Scutellariae and Cornu Antelopis for clearing heat, and Poria for eliminating dampness from the urinary system, Rhizoma Alismatis was added, apparently for enhancing the effect of eliminating dampness through the urine. However, too strong an effect in eliminating dampness would impair the body's Yin. Light dosage of such ingredients was therefore to be considered if the herbal tea was to be taken regularly.

## XXV.5. HERBAL TEA III FOR CLEARING DAMP-HEAT

Empress Dowager Cixi's Herbal Tea III for Clearing Damp-Heat (Qing Re Hua Shi Dai Cha Yin Fang San) was carefully formulated by the imperial physician Yao Baosheng on the 22nd day of the second month of the lunar calendar with no year given.

### Ingredients

| | |
|---|---|
| Flos Chrysanthemi  (Ju Hua) | 9 g |
| Folium Mori  (Sang Ye) | 9 g |
| Radix Scutellariae  (Huang Qin) | 4.5 g |
| Poria  (Fu Ling) | 12 g |
| Cornu Antelopis  (Ling Yang Jiao) | 1.2 g |
| Massa Fermentata Medicinalis, modified  (Jian Qu) | 9 g |
| Pericarpium Citri Reticulatae  (Chen Pi) | 4.5 g |

Rhizoma Phragmitis (Lu Gen) 2

The original records require the Radix Scutellariae to be prepared with millet wine, while the Massa Fermentata Medicinalis (modified) was roasted. Fresh Rhizoma Phragmitis should be chopped before use. The above ingredients were prepared in decoction form to be taken while still warm.

### Comments

This prescription contained Radix Scutellariae, bitter and cold for clearing heat from the Upper Jiao, and Poria, sweet and bland, for eliminating dampness via the urinary system. The selection of ingredients, indications, formulation of the prescription and therapeutic principle coincided with the name of the remedy, i.e. clearing heat and eliminating dampness.

## XXV.6. HERBAL TEA FOR CLEARING HEAT AND NOURISHING YIN

Empress Dowager Cixi's Herbal Tea for Clearing Heat and Nourishing Yin (Qing Re Yang Yin Dai Cha Yin) was carefully formulated by the imperial physician Yao Baosheng on the 24th day of the second month of the lunar calendar without information concerning the year.

### Ingredients

| | |
|---|---|
| Flos Chrysanthemi (Ju Hua) | 9 g |
| Folium Mori (Sang Ye) | 9 g |
| Cornu Antelopis (Ling Yang Jiao) | 1.5 g |
| Radix Ophiopogonis (Mai Men Dong) | 9 g |
| Poria (Fu Ling) | 12 g |
| Pericarpium Citri Reticulatae (Chen Pi) | 4.5 g |
| Fructus Aurantii (Zhi Ke) | 4.5 g |
| Rhizoma Phragmitis (Lu Gen) | 2 |

According to the original records, the Radix Ophiopogonis together with its cores should be used. The Fructus Aurantii should be roasted and the Phragmitis (fresh) chopped before use.

### Comments

Regular use of herbs for eliminating dampness through urination would damage the body's Yin. Since the 20th day of the second month of the lunar calendar, Empress Dowager Cixi had been taking herbal tea containing Poria and Rhizoma Alismatis. Even though it was not a very long time, the body fluid and Yin were probably injured. Therefore, Radix Ophiopogonis was added for the purpose of "appeasing the undiseased part first," demonstrating how careful the imperial physicians were in applying herbal ingredients.

## XXV.7. HERBAL TEA FOR CLEARING HEAT

Empress Dowager Cixi's Herbal Tea for Clearing Heat (Qing Re Dai Cha Yin) was carefully formulated by the imperial physician Yao Baosheng between 5:00 and 7:00 p.m. on the second day of the second month of the lunar calendar, with no year given.

*Ingredients*

| | |
|---|---|
| Fructus Canarit  (Qing Guo) | 20 |
| Rhizoma Phragmitis  (Lu Gen) | 4 |

The original records say that the Fructus Canarit should be used without cores and the Phragmitis (fresh) chopped. The above ingredients were prepared in decoction form to be drunk as tea.

*Comments*

Fresh Fructus Canarit has the action of clearing the lungs and promoting the throat, clearing fire and resolving phlegm. It was applied for treating conditions of excessive heat in the lungs and stomach as manifested by pain and swelling of the throat and profuse sputum. Fructus Canarit was often included in prescriptions suggested for Empress Dowager Cixi. Rhizoma Phragmitis not only helped clear lung heat and eliminate sputum and abscess, it cleared stomach heat, promoted body fluid and stopped vomiting. The two in combination had a strong and concentrated effect in clearing lung and stomach heat. Empress Dowager Cixi was believed to have complained of throat unease at that time.

## XXV.8. HERBAL TEA FOR CLEARING HEAT AND STOPPING COUGH

Empress Dowager Cixi's Herbal Tea for Clearing Heat and Stopping Cough (Qing Re Zhi Ke Dai Cha Yin) was carefully and promptly prepared by the imperial physician Yao Baosheng in late afternoon on the sixth day of the second month of the lunar calendar, with no year given.

*Ingredients*

| | |
|---|---|
| Flos Chrysanthemi  (Ju Hua) | 6 g |
| Folium Mori  (Sang Ye) | 6 g |
| Pericarpium Citri Reticulatae  (Chen Pi) | 3 g |
| Folium Eriobotryae  (Pi Pa Ye) | 6 g |
| Radix Rehmanniae  (Sheng Di Huang) | 4.5 g |
| Fructus Aurantii  (Zhi Ke) | 4.5 g |
| Radix Scutellariae  (Huang Qin) | 3 g |
| Rhizoma Phragmitis  (Lu Gen) | 2 |

The original records state that the Folium Eriobotryae should be prepared and wrapped before use, while the Fructus Aurantii should be roasted until yellow. The Radix Scutellariae should be prepared with millet wine, and the Rhizoma Phragmitis (fresh) chopped. The above ingredients were prepared as a decoction to be taken while still warm.

*Comments*

In this prescription, Folium Eriobotryae and Pericarpium Citri Reticulatae were added in addition to those herbs for clearing heat and those aiming at assisting Radix Scutellariae and Rhizoma Phragmitis in clearing lung heat. The formula therefore has actions in clearing heat for resolving exterior syndrome as well as in stopping cough. This example indicated that the ingredients used in preparing herbal tea could be quite flexible. It was believed to be applicable only in chronic conditions, or for the treatment of local disorders of the throat and stomach. Its effect was too mild and slow for use in severe or critical cases, and other measures should be considered.

# XXVI. MEDICATED WINE

## XXVI.1. PRESCRIPTION FOR MEDICATED WINE

Prescription for Medicated Wine (Pao Jiu Fang) was formulated for Empress Dowager Cixi on the 10th day of the ninth month of the lunar calendar in 1906.

*Ingredients*

| | |
|---|---|
| Rhizoma Acori Graminei (Shi Chang Pu) | 18 g |
| Fructus Chaenomelis (Mu Gua) | 18 g |
| Ramulus Loranthi (Sang Ji Sheng) | 30 g |
| Fructus Foeniculi (Xiao Hui Xiang) | 6 g |
| Flos Chrysanthemi (Ju Hua) | 18 g |

The original records say fresh Rhizoma Acori Graminei and Flos Chrysanthemi should be used. On the same day, 10 doses of the formula were prescribed without the use of Radix Achyranthis Bidentatae, which should be added in a dosage of six grams in case of leg pain. It was not used on that day. The above ingredients were immersed in 1.5 kilograms of liquor for use after seven days. One small cup of the medicated wine was taken every morning.

*Comments*

Referring to the health archives of Empress Dowager Cixi in the ninth month of the lunar calendar in 1906, she "had a deep wiry and thready pulse on the left, while it was deep and slippery on the right." Constitutional deficiency of kidney essence and poor function of the spleen in transforming water and dampness blocked the normal dispersing of Yang *qi*. Hence such clinical manifestations as "dizziness and vertigo, aversion to cold due to Yang deficiency, poor digestion, tinnitus and weakness in walking." Imperial physicians, including Zhang Zhongyuan, also prepared a prescription for promoting Empress Dowager Cixi's spleen function of removing dampness. Prescription for Medicated Wine was prepared as a secondary approach in helping improve Empress Dowager Cixi's condition.

## XXVI.2. RAMULUS ALBIZIAE WINE

Ramulus Albiziae Wine (Ye He Zhi Jiu) was prepared on the second day of the sixth month of the lunar calendar in 1908.

*Ingredients*

| | |
|---|---|
| Ramulus Albiziae (Ye He Zhi) | 150 g |

| | |
|---|---|
| Ramulus Phellodendri  (Huang Bai Zhi) | 150 g |
| Ramulus Sophorae  (Huai Zhi) | 150 g |
| Ramulus Mori  (Sang Zhi) | 150 g |
| Ramulus Granati  (Shi Liu Pi) | 150 g |
| Semen Oryzae Glutinosae  (Nuo Mi) | 5,175 ml |
| Glycine Max  (Hei Dou) | 51,754 ml |
| unidentified | |
| unidentified | |
| Massa Fermentata Medicinalis  (Shen Qu) | 3.75 kg |

According to the original records, fresh Ramulus Albiziae, Ramulus Phellodendri, Ramulus Sophorae, Ramulus Mori and Ramulus Granati should be taken for processing. Either the Ramulus Phellodendri, or Ramulus Sophorae or Ramulus Mori was first decocted in 51.75 litres of water, as the exact Chinese character forming part of the ingredient in the prescription was illegible. Then, 26 litres of the decoction were to be mixed with the Semen Oryzae Glutinosae and Glycine Max for further steaming. This done, the Massa Fermentata Medicinalis and the two other unidentified ingredients were added. After the mixture had been sealed hermetically for 21 days it was squeezed to obtain the fluid only. One small cup only of the wine was prescribed each time for oral administration, since overdose would make Empress Dowager Cixi drunk and vomit. It was applied for muscular atrophy resulting from windstroke.

### Comments

According to *Illustrated Materia Medica* (*Ben Cao Tu Jing*), Ramulus Albiziae bore two Chinese names, i.e. Ye He Zhi (branch with leaves closed at night) and He Huan Zhi (branch with leaves open in daytime). Its leaves, very fine and dense, look like those of Gleditsiae that close at night, thus the name. Regarding the action of Ramulus Albiziae, *Supplement to Amplification of Materia Medica* (*Ben Cao Yan Yi Shi Yi*) contains the following record, "Ramulus Albiziae produces immediate effect for nourishing Yin, and for the growth of muscles and recovery of tendons and bones." However, its therapeutic effect for traumatic injuries was often neglected. According to *Secret Records of Mother and Son* (*Zi Mu Mi Lu*), powdered Flos Albiziae was mixed with two spoonfuls of millet wine for treating pain due to traumatic injuries. *Peaceful Holy Benevolent Prescription* (*Tai Ping Shen Hui Fang*) also recorded the use of Ramulus Albiziae Pill (*Ye He Hua Wan*) for the treatment of chronic pain in the lumbar region and foot. The above use of Ramulus Albiziae is based on its functions in promoting the growth of muscles and bones and helping the recovery of tendons. The use of different ramuluses prescribed for the preparation of medicated wine was in consideration of their actions in activating blood vessels and removing obstruction from channels and collaterals. The medicated wine was therefore also applicable for the treatment of muscular spasm encountered in windstroke.

# XXVII.  COSMETIC SOAP

## XXVII.1.  REINFORCED COSMETIC SOAP

The prescription for Reinforced Cosmetic Soap (Jia Wei Xiang Fei Zao Fang) was formulated on the 11th day of the second month of the lunar calendar in 1904.

### Ingredients

Lignum Santali  (Tan Xiang)
Radix Auchlandiae  (Mu Xiang)
Flos Caryophylli  (Ding Xiang)
Herba Lysimachia  (Ling Ling Cao)
Spina Gledistiae  (Zao Jiao Ci)
Rhizoma Nardostachyos  (Gan Song)
Plumula Nelumbinis  (Lian Zi Xin)
Rhizoma Kaempferiae  (Shan Nai)
Bombyx Batryticatus  (Jiang Can)
Moschus  (She Xiang)
Borneolum Syntheticum  (Bing Pian)

The original records give no dosages for any of the above ingredients, all of which were ground into extremely fine powder and mixed with water prepared with brown sugar to make soap cakes of six grams each.

### Comments

Facial cosmetic ways and means drew much attention in the imperial palace. Reinforced Cosmetic Soap was formulated by using different fragrant herbs plus Flos Rosae, Plumula Nelumbinis and Spina Gledistiae. Among them, Lignum Santali, Herba Lysimachia Capillipes and Herba Lysimachia all had rich fragrant aromas. Using them for bathing helped clear turbidity and refresh the mind. Soap made from Lignum Santali was considered top quality in those days. *Compendium of Materia Medica* (*Ben Cao Gang Mu*) says to "apply Lignum Santali onto the body" for its delicate and lasting scent. This soap, formulated by the imperial physicians, was applied to maintain facial skin in good condition, cleanse the body and give it a fragrant scent.

# XXVIII.  PRESCRIPTIONS FOR RELIEVING SUMMER HEAT

## XXVIII.1.  ELSHOLTZIA PILL

The prescription for Elsholtzia Pill (Xiang Ru Wan) was copied on the 28th day of the fifth month of the lunar calendar in 1881.

### Ingredients

| | |
|---|---:|
| Herba Elsholtzia  (Xiang Ru) | 150 g |
| Herba Agastachis  (Huo Xiang) | 300 g |
| Folium Perillae  (Su Ye) | 240 g |
| Radix Glycyrrhizae  (Gan Cao) | 210 g |

| Fructus Chaenomilis (Mu Gua) | 105 g |
| Lignum Santali (Tan Xiang) | 45 g |
| Flos Caryophylli (Ding Xiang) | 45 g |
| Poria (Fu Ling) | 450 g |

The above ingredients were processed into extremely fine powder and made into honey pills of 4.5 grams each.

*Comments*

The prescription mainly consists of fragrant ingredients for refreshing the mind and sour-sweet ones for nourishing Yin. To enhance its action, a few ingredients of bland flavour for eliminating dampness from the urine were added to the prescription. Lignum Santali, pungent and warm, was heavily used to relieve exterior cold syndrome, clear summer heat and resolve dampness. It was applicable for conditions caused by summer heat manifested by nausea, vomiting, dry mouth with bitter taste, general lassitude, poor appetite, and spasm. Study of the origin of the prescription reveals that it was actually the Elsholtzia Pill (Xiang Ru Wan) from *Imperial Grace Formulary of the Tai Ping Era* (*Tai Ping Hui Min He Ji Ju Fang*), plus Folium Perillae. It should have been most appropriate for summer heat conditions complicated by cold symptoms and signs. In the imperial palace, it was applied to harmonize the stomach and intestines with fragrant ingredients functioning in eliminating dampness. It was different from Elsholtzia Decoction (Xiang Ru Yin) recorded in *Imperial Grace Formulary of the Tai Ping Era* and Newly Reinforced Elsholtzia Decoction (Xin Jia Xiang Ru Yin) recorded in *Treatise on Differentiation and Treatments of Epidemic Febrile Diseases* (*Wen Bing Tiao Bian*) since both were characterized by greater use of bitter and warming ingredients to help dry the dampness.

## XXVIII.2. ELSHOLTZIA DECOCTION FORMULA

One dose of Elsholtzia Decoction Formula (Xiang Ru Tang Fang) was recorded with no information concerning the date.

*Ingredients*

| Herba Elsholtzia (Xiang Ru) | 45 g |
| Radix Glycyrrhizae (Gan Cao) | 45 g |
| Semen Dolichoris (Bian Dou) | 45 g |
| Red Poria (Chi Pian Dou) | 35 g |
| Radix Astragali seu Hedysaria (Huang Qi) | 6 g |
| Cortex Magnoliae Officinalis (Hou Po) | 6 g |
| Pericarpium Citri Reticulatae (Chen Pi) | 6 g |
| Flos Chrysanthemi (Ju Hua) | 3 g |

The above ingredients were prepared in decoction form for oral administration.

*Comments*

According to the tradition in the imperial palace, every summer from May to July, decoction for preventing summer heat was distributed to princes, dukes, ministers and others serving in the imperial palace. The decoction was sent to the

Palace of Heavenly Purity, Palace of Longevity and Peace, Mind Cultivation Hall, and the Summer Palace. This decoction was prepared specifically for preventing summer heat. It was a reinforced prescription on the basis of Elsholtzia Decoction (Xiang Ru Yin) as recorded in *Imperial Grace Formulary of the Tai Ping Era* (*Tai Ping Hui Min He Ji Ju Fang*). Since "summer heat could injure *qi* and bring dampness together to attack the body," Radix Astragali seu Hedysari, Red Poria, Pericarpium and Radix Glycyrrhizae were added with the intention of tonifying the *qi* and regulating the Middle Jiao. Summer heat could thus be cleared without injuring *qi* while the dampness could be eliminated without consuming Yin. It was an ideal remedy for the summer season.

## XXVIII.3. SUMMER HEAT DECOCTION

One dose of Summer Heat Decoction (Shu Tang Fang) was prescribed with no information concerning the date.

*Ingredients*

| | |
|---|---|
| Herba Elsholtzia (Xiang Ru) | 9 g |
| Herba Agastrachis (Huo Xiang) | 15 g |
| Poria (Fu Ling) | 45 g |
| Pericarpium Citri Reticulatae (Chen Pi) | 15 g |
| Semen Dolichoris (Bian Dou) | 45 g |
| Rhizoma Atractylodis (Cang Zhu) | 24 g |
| Cortex Magnoliae Officinalis (Hou Po) | 12 g |
| Fructus Chaenomelis (Mu Gua) | 15 g |
| Talcum (Hua Shi) | 30 g |
| Radix Glycyrrhizae (Gan Cao) | 15 g |
| Lignum Santali (Tan Xiang) | 15 g |
| Fructus Mume (Wu Mei) | 10 |
| Ignited Yellow Earth (Fu Long Gan) | 90 g |
| Radix Astragali seu Hedysari (Huang Qi) | 9 g |
| Radix Ophiopogonis (Mai Dong) | 30 g |
| Rhizoma Atractylodis Macrocephalae (Bai Zhu) | 18 g |

The original records state that the Semen Dolichoris, Rhizoma Atractylodis and Rhizoma Atractylodis Macrocephalae should be prepared. All the above ingredients should then be decocted for oral administration.

*Comments*

This prescription was specially prepared for distribution in the imperial palace for preventing summer heat. It was formed by mixing Elsholtzia Pill (Xiang Ru Wan) and Elsholzia Decoction (Xiang Ru Yin) as described in *Imperial Grace Formulary of the Tai Ping Era* (*Tai Ping Hui Min He Ji Ju Fang*). Adding Radix Astragali seu Hedysari, Rhizoma Atractylodis Macrocephalae, Radix Ophiopogonis and Fructus Mume, with astringent and sour-flavoured ingredients, enhanced the therapeutic effect of promoting *qi* and body fluid. This coincided with the idea of ancient medical practitioners that "the treatment of summer heat condition should be characterized by first using pungent ingredients of cooling property, second using sweet ingredients of cold property, and finally using astringent ingredients for clearing heat with no consideration of purgatives." It also agreed with the principle in *Compendium on Seasonal Febrile Diseases* (*Wen Re Jing Wei*): "Summer heat consumes Yin. Treatment focusing on clearing summer heat while tonifying primary *qi* is sure to be successful." This prescription may be considered as one way to clear summer heat and reinforce *qi*.

## XXVIII.4.  REINFORCED NOONDAY TEA

Reinforced Noonday Tea (Jia Wei Wu Shi Cha) was prepared on the sixth day of the fourth month of the lunar calendar, without the year given.

*Ingredients*

| | |
|---|---|
| Noonday Tea  (Wu Shi Cha) | 1 portion |
| Fructus Crataegi  (Shan Zha) | 6 g |
| Massa Fermentata Medicinalis  (Shen Qu) | 6 g |
| Fructus Hordei Germinatus  (Mai Ya) | 6 g |
| Unidentified | 9 g |
| Pericarpium Citri Reticulatae Rubra  (Ju Hong) | 3 g |
| Pericarpium Citri Reticulatae Viride  (Qing Pi) | 2.4 g |

The original records say the Fructus Crataegi, Massa Fermentata Medicinalis and Fructus Hordei Germinatus should be roasted until yellow, and the Pericarpium Citri Reticulatae Viride should also be roasted. The above ingredients were decocted for oral use while still warm.

*Comments*

Noonday Tea (Wu Shi Cha) was originally a modification of Midday Tea (Tian Zhong Cha) from *A Collection of Outstanding Prescriptions* (*Ba Cui Liang Fang*). Its indications included common cold caused by wind-cold invasion, vomiting or diarrhea due to food retention and diarrhea accompanied by abdominal pain. Pungent drugs of warming property, aromatic drugs for resolving dampness, and ingredients for appeasing the stomach and clearing dampness were all included in the prescription. It had good therapeutic effects in treating common cold caused by cold invasion in summer, headache and diarrhea, and so gained great popularity. Empress Dowager Cixi used a modified prescription for what was believed to be *qi* stagnation resulting from food retention related to her preference for sweet and greasy food and over-use of imperial authority. The introduction of Noonday Tea (Wu Shi Cha) into the imperial palace offered a glimpse of the wide application of Chinese medicinal ingredients in the Qing Dynasty.

## XXVIII.5.  GOLDEN SUMMER HEAT PILL

Golden Summer Heat Pill (Jin Yi Qu Shu Wan) was copied by imperial physicians serving in the Imperial Pharmacy on the 28th day of the fifth month of the lunar calendar in 1881.

*Ingredients*

| | |
|---|---|
| Herba Agastachis  (Huo Xiang) | 120 g |
| Herba Elsholtzia  (Xiang Ru) | 120 g |
| Ramulus seu Folium Canlis Perillae  (Su Geng Ye) | 120 g |

| | |
|---|---|
| Rhizoma Atractylodis  (Cang Zhu) | 60 g |
| Rhizoma Atractylodis Macrocephalae  (Bai Zhu) | 60 g |
| Cortex Magnoliae Officinalis  (Hou Po) | 75 g |
| Radix Platycodi  (Jie Geng) | 30 g |
| Semen Dolichoris  (Bian Dou) | 75 g |
| Pericarpium Citri Reticulatae  (Chen Pi) | 75 g |
| Poria  (Fu Ling) | 120 g |
| Radix Angelicae Dahuricae  (Bai Zhi) | 30 g |
| Pericarpium Arecae  (Da Fu Pi) | 30 g |
| Rhizoma seu Radix Notopterygii  (Qiang Huo) | 45 g |
| Rhizoma Pinelliae  (Ban Xia) | 30 g |
| Fructus Chaenomelis  (Mu Gua) | 45 g |
| Polyporus Umbellatus  (Zhu Ling) | 90 g |
| Rhizoma Alismatis  (Ze Xie) | 30 g |
| Radix Glycyrrhizae  (Gan Cao) | 30 g |

The original records call for the Rhizoma Atractylodis Macrocephalae to be roasted with powdered earth. The Rhizoma Atractylodis and Semen Dolichoris should be plain roasted and the Cortex Magnoliae Officinalis and Rhizoma Pinelliae should be roasted with ginger juice. The above ingredients were processed to an extremely fine powder and mixed with refined honey to make patent pills coated with Cinnabari and Aurum of 4.5 grams each.

### Comments

Most important in treating summer heat is to clear heat and resolve dampness. To this end, the prescription for Golden Summer Heat Pill was prepared on the basis of Peptic Powder (Ping Wei San), Powder of Five Drugs with Poria (Wu Ling San) and Elsholtzia Powder (Xiang Ru San). The application of Cinnabari and Aurum to coat that pill was to help clear heart fire and tranquilize the mind. For treating summer heat conditions the pill could be either taken alone or together with a decoction in summer. In comparison with the conventional Golden Summer Heat Pill, ingredients for strengthening the spleen and resolving dampness were added in this recipe, e.g. Rhizoma Atractylodis Macrocephalae, Rhizoma Atractylodis, Radix Platycodi, Cortex Magnoliae Officinalis, Semen Dolichoris, Pericarpium Citri Reticulatae, Radix Angelicae Dahuricae, Pericarpium Arecae, Rhizoma seu Radix Notopterygii, Polyporus Umbellatus and Rhizoma Alismatis.

## XXVIII.6.  SIX ACTIONS PILL FOR EASING SUNSTROKE

Six Actions Pill for Easing Sunstroke (Liu He Ding Zhong Wan) was also copied by the imperial physicians serving in the Imperial Pharmacy on the 28th day of the fifth month of the lunar calendar in 1881.

### Ingredients

| | |
|---|---|
| Herba Elsholtzia  (Xiang Ru) | 120 g |
| Folium Perillae  (Su Ye) | 120 g |
| Cortex Magnoliae Officinalis  (Hou Po) | 45 g |
| Fructus Aurantii  (Zhi Ke) | 75 g |
| Fructus Amomi  (Suo Sha Ren) | 30 g |

| | |
|---|---|
| Radix Glycyrrhizae  (Gan Cao) | 15 g |
| Semen Dolichoris  (Bian Dou) | 75 g |
| Red Poria  (Chi Fu Ling) | 60 g |
| Flos Caryophylli  (Ding Xiang) | 30 g |
| Rhizoma Pinelliae  (Ban Xia) | 60 g |
| Herba Agastachis  (Huo Xiang) | 120 g |

According to the original records, the Cortex Magnoliae Officinalis and Rhizoma Pinelliae should be prepared before use. The Fructus Aurantii and Semen Dolichoris should be roasted. The above ingredients were processed into extremely fine powder and then mixed with some refined honey to make pills of 7.5 grams each.

*Comments*

The prescription for Six Actions Pill for Easing Sunstroke originated from *New Revision of Concise Formulas (Yi Fang Yi Jian Xin Bian)* by Gong Zizhang of the Qing Dynasty. It has the action of clearing summer heat, eliminating dampness, harmonizing the Middle Jiao and stopping diarrhea. It was indicated in conditions of sunstroke or summer heat and dampness seen in malaria, dysentery or cholera manifested by stuffiness in the chest, nausea, headache, abdominal pain, and vomiting or diarrhea. It was also recognized as a reinforced formula of Elsholtzia Pill (Xiang Ru Wan). In addition to clearing summer heat, it had the action of easing the stomach as well. As for prescriptions for treating summer heat conditions, those recorded in *Imperial Grace Formulary of the Tai Ping Era (Tai Ping Hui Min He Ji Ju Fang)* were most preferred for reference of imperial physicians, possibly because the book was officially compiled.

## XXVIII.7. MUME-PERILLA PILL

Mume-Perilla Pill (Mei Su Wan) was prescribed on the 12th day of the ninth month of the lunar calendar in 1887.

*Ingredients*

| | |
|---|---|
| Sacharum Granorum  (Yi Tang) | 740 g |
| Fructus Mume  (Wu Mei Rou) | 30 g |
| Radix Puerariae  (Ge Gen) | 3 g |
| Folium Perillae  (Su Ye) | 1.5 g |
| Lignum Santali  (Tan Xiang) | 3 g |
| Herba Menthae  (Bo He) | 1.5 g |

The above ingredients were processed into fine powder and made into water-bound pills the size of eurylae seeds. Imperial physicians Quan Shun and Yang Jihe worked out this prescription. Rock sugar, 120 grams, was added to each dose. The formula was the same as that of Tong Ren Tang Pharmacy.

*Comments*

Mume-perilla Pill was similar to Mume-desiring Pill (Wang Mei Wan) as recorded in *Prescriptions in Rhyme (Tang Tou Ge Jue)*. With sour- and sweet-flavoured drugs nourishing Yin and those pungent-tasting of cold property for relieving summer heat, the prescription cleared summer heat, nourished body fluid and quenched thirst. It was applicable in such summer heat conditions as vertigo, thirst, dryness in the throat and fullness in the chest. Fructus Mume and Radix Puerariae in combination produced good therapeutic effects in nourishing stomach Yin and elevating stomach *qi*. They were often applied for extreme thirst occurring in summer heat conditions. Perilla Pill (Wei Su Wan) is best kept in the mouth for gradual dissolving.

# XXIX. ONE-INGREDIENT PRESCRIPTIONS

## XXIX.1. FRUCTUS SCHISANDRAE SYRUP

Fructus Schisandrae Syrup (Wu Wei Zi Gao) was prepared on the eighth day of the sixth month of the lunar calendar with no information concerning the year.

### Ingredient

Fructus Schisandrae (Wu Wei Zi)                                          240 g

The above amount of the Fructus Schisandrae was immersed in water after being washed clean. It was then well decocted. After separating out the residue, the remaining decoction was further concentrated until it became as thick as maltose. Refined honey was then added to make the syrup.

### Comments

Fructus Schisandrae, sour and sweet in taste and warm in property, enters the lung and kidney channels, promoting the lung in dispersing, nourishing the kidney, producing body fluid, arresting sweating, checking seminal emission and stopping diarrhea. The use of Schisandrae alone has both astringent and tonifying effects. It is listed as one of the best herbs in *Original Classics* (*Ben Jing*), claiming that it could "tonify *qi*, treat cough with dyspnea and weakness and emaciation due to internal injuries caused by overstrain, reinforce the deficiency, nourish Yin and replenish vital essence in men." Among 30 miscellaneous tonifying prescriptions recorded in *Prescriptions Worth a Thousand Gold* (*Qian Jin Yao Fang*), 16 contained Fructus Schisandrae. The famous Tang Dynasty medical scientist Sun Simiao (581-682) once wrote, "Frequent use of Fructus Schisandrae in May may help tonify *qi* of the five Zang organs." "Frequent use of Schisandrae in June may help tonify *qi*. It can reinforce the lung in the Upper Jiao and the kidney in the Lower Jiao." The above-mentioned medical classics all confirm its nourishing value.

According to modern pharmaceutical research, Fructus Schisandrae was believed to regulate the functions of the central nervous system. Fructus Schisandrae grown or produced in northeast or north China offered similar effect to that of ginseng in promoting cardiac function. In case of circulatory failure, it could be used together with ginseng and Radix Ophiopogonis to adjust or raise the blood pressure. Today, Fructus Schisandrae tincture and Fructus Schisandrae syrup are used for treating insomnia due to neurasthenia. The prescription here was prepared for Empress Dowager Cixi in lunar June as a tonifying and tranquilizing agent.

## XXIX.2. PROCESSED ARECAE SLICES I

The prescription for Processed Arecae Slices I (Fa Zhi Bing Lang Pian) was carefully prepared by the imperial physicians Dong Wenbin and Quan Shun on the 11th day of the seventh month of the lunar calendar in 1885.

### Ingredients

| | |
|---|---|
| Radix Codonopsis Pilosulae  (Dang Shen) | 60 g |
| Rhizoma Atractylodis Macrocephalae  (Bai Zhu) | 30 g |
| Radix Astragali seu Hedysari  (Huang Qi) | 30 g |
| Cortex Magnoliae Officinalis  (Hou Po) | 15 g |
| Caulis Bambusae in Taeniam  (Zhu Ru) | 30 g |
| Fructus Amomi  (Sha Ren) | 18 g |
| Flos Caryohpylli  (Ding Xiang) | 6 g |
| Radix Auchlandiae  (Mu Xiang) | 6 g |
| Medullae Junci Effusi  (Deng Xin Cao) | 9 g |

The original recipe requires the Cortex Magnoliae Officinalis to be prepared, while the Fructus Amomi should be ground for use. The above ingredients were well boiled in water to produce a decoction without any herbal residue. Then 120 grams of Arecae slices were added and boiled in the decoction until the mixture was dry. The Arecae slices processed in this way were further dried under the sun and roasted with salty water until they turned yellow. The proportion of table salt was 1.5 grams per slice.

### Comments

Semen Arecae promotes *qi*, corrects food retention and kills parasites. It is most beneficial in promoting digestion and increasing the appetite after it has been processed with herbs for tonifying *qi*, harmonizing the Middle Jiao and invigorating the spleen and was thus suitable for Empress Dowager Cixi's condition of weak function of the spleen and stomach. Such a method of preparing herbal slices instead of herbal decoctions deserves further study.

## XXIX.3. PROCESSED ARECAE SLICES II

Processed Arecae Slices II (Fa Zhi Bing Lang Pian) was carefully prescribed by the imperial physicians Li Dechang and Li Deli on the 24th day of the ninth month of the lunar calendar with no information as to the year.

### Ingredients

| | |
|---|---|
| Pericarpium Citri Grandis  (Ju Pi) | 60 g |
| Cortex Magnoliae Officinalis  (Hou Po) | 60 g |
| Rhizoma Atractylodis  (Cang Zhu) | 60 g |
| Radix Curcumae  (Yu Jin) | 60 g |
| Fructus Amomi  (Sha Ren) | 60 g |
| Caulis Bambusae in Taeniam  (Zhu Ru) | 45 g |
| Rhizoma Acori Graminei  (Shi Chang Pu) | 15 g |

The original recipe calls for the Cortex Magnoliae Officinalis to be prepared and the Rhizoma Atractylodis dried. All ingredients were well decocted so that no residue remained; 120 grams of sliced Semen Arecae were added and boiled into the decoction. After drying the processed Semen Arecae slices under the sun, they were roasted with salty water. (See above for salt proportion.)

*Comments*

Radix Codonopsis Pilosulae, Radix Astragali seu Hedysari, Flos Caryophylli and Radix Auchlandiae were omitted from the above prescription, while Pericarpium Citri Grandis, Radix Curcumae and Rhizoma Acori Graminei were added. It was assumed that Empress Dowager Cixi was troubled by excessive sputum or stagnant *qi*. Drugs were therefore added to resolve phlegm, clear the mind, promote *qi* and remove stagnation in addition to ingredients for promoting the stomach in digestion and invigorating the spleen. The therapeutic effect of Semen Arecae processed with different drugs in different ways varied accordingly. The imperial physicians at the time were apparently of high professional level in TCM.

# XXX. MISCELLANEOUS PROVED PRESCRIPTIONS

## XXX.1. REINFORCED YELLOW JADE CREAM

The prescription for Reinforced Yellow Jade Cream (Jia Wei Huang Yu Gao) was carefully worked out by the imperial physician Li Dechang on the 15th day of the 11th month of the lunar calendar in 1874.

*Ingredients*

| | |
|---|---|
| Rhizoma Coptidis  (Huang Lian) | 3 g |
| Cortex Phellodendri  (Huang Bai) | 9 g |
| Bombyx Batryticatus  (Jiang Can) | 9 g |
| Resina Olibani  (Ru Xiang) | 6 g |
| Radix Angelicae Dahuricae  (Bai Zhi) | 9 g |
| Ramulus Sophorae  (Huai Zhi) | 9 g |
| Cortex Dictamni Dasycarpi Radicis  (Bai Xian Pi) | 9 g |
| Radix Glycyrrhizae  (Gan Cao) | 4.5 g |

The above ingredients were well fried in 90 grams of sesame oil and 120 grams of lard. After removing the herbal residue, nine grams of the lard and 15 grams of an unrecognized ingredient were added to the remaining oily substance for further processing. 2.4 grams of Borneoleum Syntheticum was finally added to make the proper cream.

*Comments*

Yellow Jade Cream (Huang Yu Gao), a secret palace formula, was seldom seen in other formulary books. The prescription was made on the 15th day of the 11th month of the lunar calendar in 1874 when Emperor Tongzhi had just recovered from variola and was likely prepared specifically for the disease, composed as it was of herbs acting to clear heat and toxicity, dry dampness and stop itching. It may also have been effective in treating Empress Dowager Cixi's boils.

## XXX.2. COSMETIC CREAM

This prescription for Cosmetic Cream (Ou Zi Fang) was carefully worked out by the imperial physician Zhuang Shouhe on the 21st day of the ninth month of the lunar calendar in 1878.

*Ingredients*

Radix Ledebouriellae  (Fang Feng)
Radix Angelicae Dahuricae  (Bai Zhi)
Unidentified
Rhizoma Kaepmferiae  (Shan Nai)
Poria  (Fu Ling)
Rhizoma Bletillae Striatae  (Bai Ji)
Rhizoma Typhonii Gigantei  (Bai Fu Zi)
Unidentified

The amount of each ingredient is not specified in the original records. All were processed into large granules and then well boiled down to one kilogram of liquor. After separating out the residue, the remaining decoction was mixed with rock sugar and honey. When it was cool, Borneoleum Syntheticum and powdered Cinnabari were added. The mixture was then well stirred and stored in a porcelain container.

*Comments*

The Chinese phrase *ou zi*, meaning literally to immerse substances in water to become foamy, is another name for cosmetic creams in general. All types of cosmetics were generally prepared in the form of oily cream, moist and foamy. The description that "foamy and soapy with strong fragrant aromas for lifting up one's spirit," in *Deep Forest Verse* (*Shang Ling Fu*) by the famous Western Han Dynasty poet Sima Xiangru (179-117 B.C.) helps classify prescriptions under the name "Ou Zi" as cosmetic creams to make the skin appear more attractive and tender. This prescription, containing such fragrant herbs as Rhizoma Kaempferiae, made it unique among cosmetic formulae recorded in *Prescriptions Worth a Thousand Gold* (*Qian Jin Yao Fang*) and *The Medical Secrets of an Official* (*Wai Tai Mi Yao*).

## XXX.3. NINE-PORTION POWDER

Nine-portion Powder (Jiu Fen San Fang) was prescribed on the 30th day of the second month of the lunar calendar in 1879.

*Ingredients*

| | |
|---|---|
| Resina Olibani  (Ru Xiang) | 120 g |
| Resina Murrhae  (Mo Yao) | 120 g |
| Semen Strychni  (Ma Qian Zi) | 120 g |
| Herba Ephedrae  (Ma Huang) | 120 g |
| Eupolyphaga seu Steleopnaga  (Tu Bie Cong) | 12 g |
| Pryitum  (Zi Ran Tong) | 12 g |

The above ingredients were processed into extremely fine powder.

*Comments*

This prescription was for activating blood and removing stagnation. With fewer ingredients but in larger amounts, the powder had a strong and concentrated action. Known as an effective remedy for traumatic injuries, its actions included removing blood stasis and stopping pain. It was thus applicable for injured tendons and bones causing pain, redness and swelling. It was also applied for healing imperial punishments. Its name came from the powder being prescribed each time in packages of portions of nine to one. Believed to have been copied from the Palace of Heavenly Purity, the prescription was used frequently in the imperial palace with proved therapeutic effect. Nine-portion Powder made in Nanjing today is based on the same prescription and referred to as the one used in the Qing imperial palace and so enjoyed a high reputation in China.

## XXX.4. FOLIUM PERILLA AND CORTEX MAGNOLIAE OFFICINALIS PILL

The prescription for Folium Perilla and Cortex Magnoliae Officinalis Pill (Zi Po Wan) was merely copied by an imperial physician from *A Collection of Recommended Prescriptions* (*Liang Fang Ji Cheng*) and presented on the 17th day of the seventh month of the lunar calendar in 1881.

*Ingredients*

| | |
|---|---|
| Folium Perilla processed with Cortex Magnoliae Officinalis  (Zi Po) | 45 g |
| Fructus Crataegi  (Zhan Zha) | 60 g |
| Semen Raphani  (Lai Fu Zi) | 60 g |
| Rhizoma Sparganii  (San Leng) | 30 g |
| Rhizoma Zedoariae  (E Zhu) | 30 g |
| Fructus Aurantii Immaturus  (Zhi Shi) | 45 g |
| Fructus Forsythiae  (Lian Qiao) | 45 g |
| Pericarpium Citri Reticulatae Viride  (Qing Pi) | 45 g |
| Pericarpium Citri Reticulatae  (Chen Pi) | 45 g |
| Herba Asari  (Xi Xin) | 30 g |

The original records prescribe that the Folium Perilla should be processed with Cortex Magnoliae Officinalis, while the Fructus Aurantii Immaturus and Pericarpium Citri Reticulatae Viride should be roasted. The above ingredients were processed into extremely fine powder and made into pills of 4.5 grams each. Two pills were to be taken with boiled water.

The powder was especially effective in treating cholera, epidemic infections, febrile diseases due to summer heat invasion, and conditions characterized by food retention or phlegmatic attack into the Zang-Fu organs in summer. Manifestations of the above could include umbilical pain, vomiting, irritability, fullness in the chest, and constipation.

*Comments*

The prescription, having the action of relieving chest stuffiness, descending *qi* and removing food retention, was formulated for treating epidemic infectious diseases. The main ingredient, pronounced as *zi po* in Chinese, was prepared by mixing Cortex Magnoliae Officinalis with Folium Perilla and Rhizoma Zingiberis Recens by means of steaming. Its action was to strengthen the functions of the spleen in transforming and transporting, drying dampness from the spleen with fragrant aroma and relieving abdominal distention by promoting *qi* and removing *qi* stagnation with its warm and dry properties. Modern pharmaceutical studies have shown it applicable in various diseases. It showed antibacterial effects on bacillus typhi. Cortex Magnoliae Officinalis processed in this way had little side-effect on the throat, but stronger actions in promoting *qi* and easing the stomach.

## XXX.5. TREASURE FLOWER PILL FOR EPIDEMIC INVASIONS

The prescription for Treasure Flower Pill for Epidemic Invasions (Hua Sha Bao Hua Wan) was copied from *A Collection of Recommended Prescriptions* (*Liang Fang Ji Cheng*) and presented on the 17th day of the seventh month of the lunar calendar in 1881.

*Ingredients*

| | |
|---|---|
| Radix Curcumae  (Yu Jin) | 60 g |
| Herba Asari  (Xi Xin) | 60 g |
| Lignum Dalbergiae Odorriferae  (Jiang Xiang) | 150 g |
| Herba Schizonepetae  (Jing Jie) | 180 g |

The above ingredients were processed into extremely fine powder and made into honey pills of six grams each. One pill was taken each time together with Chinese tea.

The pills are specially effective for food retention and that of body fluid due to cold or heat accumulation caused by invasion of summer heat and dampness, as well as invasion of cold, or unconciousness caused by pathogenic factors of the summer that block the channels and collaterals. One pill was taken each time with slightly cool tea.

*Comments*

The four ingredients are mainly fragrant and pungent, of warm properties to prompt *qi* and resolve stagnation so as to relieve exterior syndrome. It was a quite unique approach in treating acute seasonal unhygienic diseases. As reviewed by medical experts of the past generations, the conventional treatment for acute seasonal unhygienic diseases was achieved through sweating. The 180 grams of Herba Schizonepetae may have been prescribed for the purpose of causing perspiration.

## XXX.6. RELIEVING SUFFERING PILL

Relieving Suffering Pill (Jiu Ku Dan) from *A Collection of Recommended Prescriptions* (*Liang Fang Ji Cheng*) was presented on the 17th day of the seventh month of the lunar calendar in 1881.

*Ingredients*

| | |
|---|---|
| Fructus Aurantii Immaturus  (Zhi Zhi) | 60 g |
| Semen Raphani  (Lai Fu Zi) | 60 g |
| Radix Curcumae  (Yu Jin) | 18 g |
| Radix Linderae  (Wu Yao) | 45 g |
| Frcutus Forsythiae  (Lian Qiao) | 45 g |

The original records prescribe that the Fructus Aurantii Immaturus should be roasted. The above ingredients were ground into extremely fine powder to make honey pills of one gram each. Two pills were taken each time with tea.

### Comments

This Relieving Suffering Pill was different from the other two patent remedies bearing the same name in two separate history books. First, it was different from the Relieving Suffering Pill (Jiu Ku Dan) recorded in *Standards for Syndrome Differentiation and Treatments* (*Zheng Zhi Zhun Shen*) written by Wang Kentang. Wang's remedy was intended to eliminate wind and activate blood in an attempt to treat patients for eye conditions. Second, it was different from the Relieving Suffering Pill recorded in *Compendium of Fine Prescriptions for Women* (*Fu Ren Liang Fang Da Quan*) written by Chen Ziming. Chen's remedy was intended to treat women patients for warming up the channels and collaterals and dizziness from excessive loss of blood from induced abortion. The three showed different therapeutic effects despite their common Chinese name. The prescription here was composed of ordinary ingredients but focused on promoting *qi* and removing stagnation. The normal circulation of *qi* would ensure that of blood. Only when both appeared normal could there be a thorough alleviation of the abovementioned conditions. It was more than just relieving the patient from the suffering from cholera and summer unhygienic diseases. It also served as an example of treating a severe condition by using fewer ingredients in the remedy.

## XXX.7. GOLDEN LOZENGE

Golden Lozenge (Chi Jin Ding) from *A Collection of Recommended Prescriptions* (*Liang Fang Ji Cheng*) was presented by the director of the Department of the Imperial Household Li Lianying on the 11th day of the fifth month of the lunar calendar in 1885.

### Ingredients

| | |
|---|---|
| Niter (Huo Xiao) | 240 g |
| Red lead (Zhang Dan) | 30 g |
| Melanterite (Hei Fan) | 30 g |
| Cinnabari (Zhu Sha) | 1.5 g |
| Mercury with Sulphur (Ying Zhu) | 1.5 g |

The above ingredients were melted in an iron utensil and poured over a stone slab. The thin chips were collected when they were cold.

### Comments

Golden Lozenge was used externally for subduing toxic boils. Red lead, also known as Qian Dan or Zhang Dan in Chinese, is pungent, slightly cold in property and toxic. Its external application helps expel toxins, remove necrotic tissue and regenerate new muscle. Mercury with Sulphur, also known as Xin Hong, is a chemical mixture with processed sulphur. It has similar actions to those of calomel. The prescription may have been called Golden because of its colour and remarkable effect in healing boils.

## XXX.8. OX GALLSTONE PILL FOR AGILE WALKING

Ox Gallstone Pill for Agile Walking (Niu Huang Jian Bu Wan) from *A Collection of Recommended Prescriptions* (*Liang Fang Ji Cheng*) was presented by the director of the Department of the Imperial Household Li Lianying on the 12th day of the ninth month of the lunar calendar in 1883.

### Ingredients

| | |
|---|---|
| Calculus Bovis  (Niu Huang) | 9 g |
| Radix Codonopsis Piosulae  (Dang Shen) | 75 g |
| Arisaema cum Bile  (Dan Nan Xing) | 30 g |
| Rhizoma Gastrodiae  (Tian Ma) | 30 g |
| Cornu Cervi Pantotrichum  (Lu Rong) | 30 g |
| Herba Menthae  (Bo He) | 9 g |
| Radix Poria  (Fu Shen) | 30 g |
| Radix Polygalae  (Yuan Zhi) | 30 g |
| Rhizoma Acori Graminei  (Shi Chang Pu) | 30 g |
| Semen Ziziphi Spinosae  (Suan Zao Ren) | 30 g |
| Fructus Chaenomelis  (Mu Gua) | 30 g |
| Semen Coicis  (Yi Yi Ren) | 30 g |
| Rhizoma seu Radix Notopterygii  (Qiang Huo) | 30 g |
| Radix Angelicae Pubescentis  (Du Huo) | 30 g |
| Radix Ledebouriellae  (Fang Feng) | 30 g |
| Pericarpium Citri Reticulatae Rubra  (Ju Hong) | 45 g |
| Radix Astragali seu Hedysari  (Huang Qi) | 45 g |
| Radix Angelicae Sinensis  (Dang Gui) | 45 g |
| Fructus Lycii  (Gou Qi Zi) | 45 g |
| Plastrum Testudinis  (Gui Ban) | 45 g |
| Fructus Psoraleae  (Po Gu Zhi) | 45 g |
| Rhizoma Atractylodis Macrocephalae  (Bai Zhu) | 60 g |
| Radix Paeoniae Lactiflorae  (Bai Zhao) | 60 g |
| Radix Rehmanniae  (Sheng Di Huang) | 60 g |
| Os Tigris  (Hu Gu) | 60 g |
| Radix Achyranthis Bidentatae  (Niu Xi) | 60 g |
| Cortex Eucommiae  (Du Zhong) | 60 g |
| Cortex Phellodendri  (Huang Bai) | 60 g |
| Rhizoma Anemarrhenae  (Zhu Mu) | 60 g |
| Radix Ophiopogonis  (Mai Men Dong) | 60 g |
| Lignum Aquilariae Resinatum  (Chen Xiang) | 15 g |
| Fructus Schisandrae  (Wu Wei Zi) | 15 g |

The original recipe calls for the Arisaema to be roasted with ginger juice. The Radix Polygalae with no cores should be infused in water and prepared with Radix Glycyrrhizae. The Cornu Cervi Pantotrichum, Plastrum Testudinis, and Os Tigris should be prepared until crisp. The Semen Ziziphi Spinosae and Semen Coicis should be roasted, while the Rhizoma seu Radix Notopterygii, Radix Angelicae Pubescentis, Radix Ledebouriellae, Radix Angelicae Sinensis, Radix Rehmanniae and Radix Achyranthis Bidentatae should be washed in millet wine. The Radix Astragali seu Hedysari should be roasted with salt water. The Rhizoma Atractylodis Macrocephalae containing no cores should be roasted with powdered earth, while the Radix Paeoniae Lactiflorae and Fructus Psoraleae should be roasted with salt and millet wine. The Cortex Eucommiae should be roasted with ginger-prepared millet wine. The Cortex Phellodendri and Rhizoma Anemarrhenae should be roasted with millet wine and mixed with salt and human milk. The Radix Ophiopogonis without cores should be used. The above ingredients were processed into fine powder and made into pills of 4.5 grams mixed with refined honey and pig spinal cord. The pills were coated with gold leaf and wrapped in wax.

Ox Gallstone Pill for Agile Walking was made specially for treating wind-stroke and syncope manifested by unconsciousness, sudden fainting, deviation of the mouth and eyes, hemiplegia or difficult walking, aphasia, profuse salivation and sputum, poor concentration, and Bi-syndrome caused by pathogenic wind and characterized by contracture of limbs, muscular spasm and joint pain. One pill was taken each time with either salt water or warm millet wine. In severe cases it was taken regularly.

*Comments*

According to traditional Chinese medicine, the liver dominates tendons and the kidney dominates bones. Liver and kidney deficiency consequently leads to Wei-syndrome marked by difficulty in walking. *On Wei-syndrome in Plain Questions* (*Su Wen*: "Wei Lun") states, "Liver heat forces the excretion of bile with such symptoms as bitter taste in the mouth and rigidity of tendons, and finally Wei-syndrome involving the tendons occurs. Heat in the kidney makes it difficult for patients to stretch the back, which is followed by malnutrition of bones and marrow. Thus, Wei-syndrome involving bones takes place."

The prescription focused on reinforcing the liver and kidney. At the same time, attention was paid to eliminating wind and phlegm. It therefore was applicable for the various types of Wei- and Bi-syndrome caused by wind-phlegm. Compared with Hidden Tiger Pill for Agile Walking (Jian Bu Hu Qian Wan), Ox Gallstone Pill for Agile Walking contained more ingredients for eliminating wind and phlegm. Calculus Bovis, the main ingredient, was shown to enter the heart and liver channels. It was to clear the heart and calm the mind, and calm the mind by resolving phlegm and clearing heat. One of the features of the pill was that it not only helped activate blood circulation in channels and collaterals for agile walking; it also treats heart and mental conditions. Empress Dowager Cixi had it prepared to treat her facial paralysis as well as for her general health.

## XXX.9.  EPIDEMIC HEAT DETOXICATING PILL

The prescription for Epidemic Heat Detoxicating Pill (Qing Wen Jie Du Wan) was prepared on the 11th day of the fourth month of the lunar calendar in 1884.

*Ingredients*

| | |
|---|---|
| Radix Scutellariae  (Huang Qin) | 60 g |
| Radix Scrophulariae  (Xuan Shen) | 90 g |
| Radix Platycodi  (Jie Geng) | 60 g |
| Pericarpium Citri Reticulatae  (Chen Pi) | 60 g |

| | |
|---|---|
| Rhizoma Coptidis  (Huang Lian) | 45 g |
| Rhizoma Cimicifugae  (Sheng Ma) | 15 g |
| Lasiphaera seu Calvatia  (Ma Bo) | 45 g |
| Fructus Arctii  (Niu Bang Zi) | 45 g |
| Radix Bupleuri  (Chai Hu) | 30 g |
| Fructus Forsythiae  (Lian Qiao) | 60 g |
| Radix Isatidis  (Ban Lan Gen) | 45 g |
| Bombyx Batryticatus  (Jiang Can) | 60 g |
| Radix Glycyrrhizae prepared in urine | 45 g |
| Ren Zhong Huang  (human feces extract prepared in bamboo) [its dosage not specified in the original records—tr.] | |
| Fructus Gardeniae  (Zhi Zi) | 60 g |
| Semen Sojae Praeparatum  (Dan Dou Chi) | 60 g |
| Cornu Rhinoceri Asiatici  (Xi Jiao) | 30 g |
| Herba Menthae  (Bo He) | 30 g |

The above ingredients were processed into fine powder and made into pills of nine grams each.

### Comments

On the basis of reinforcing Universal Benefit Decoction to Eliminate Toxin (Pu Ji Xiao Du Yin), the prescription has the action of dispelling wind, eliminating other pathogenic factors and clearing heat toxins. By adding Radix Glycyrrhizae prepared in human urine, Cornu Rhinoceri Asiatici, Fructus Gardeniae and Semen Sojae Praeparatum meant a stronger therapeutic effect in clearing heat and toxins. Thus, it was also appropriate for resolving epidemic heat and toxins.

## XXX.10.  EIGHT TREASURES AND RED MIRACLE POWDER

An imperial edict was passed by the eunuch Chang Tai to present the prescription for Eight Treasures and Red Miracle Powder (Ba Bao Hong Ling San) on the fourth day of the fifth month of the lunar calendar in 1884.

### Ingredients

| | |
|---|---|
| Aurum  (Chi Jin) | 20 |
| Borneoleum syntheticum  (Bing Pian) | 3 g |
| Moschus  (She Xiang) | 3 g |
| Cinnabari  (Zhu Sha) | 15 g |
| Mirabilitum  (Ya Xiao) | 15 g |
| Borax  (Peng Sha) | 3 g |
| Chlorite  (Meng Shi) | 3 g |
| Realgar  (Xiong Huang) | 9 g |

The original script calls for the Cinnabari to be ground into pieces, washed in water and dried in the sun. Raw Chlorite should be used. The above ingredients were ground into extremely fine powder and stored in a porcelain utensil at noon on the fifth day of the fifth month of the lunar calendar.

Eight Treasures and Red Miracle Powder was applicable to a number of conditions. For unspecific pyogenic infections, it was mixed with vinegar for external application. For abdominal pain due to cold or heat, 0.15 gram of powder was prescribed for oral administration with boiled water. For conditions manifested by vomiting, diarrhea, abdominal pain and tenesmus in adults or children, 0.15 gram of the powder was prescribed for oral administration with boiled water. For dizziness and tinnitus due to over exposure to summer sun, 0.15 gram of the powder was prescribed for oral administration with Chinese tea. For symptoms of regurgitation of clear fluid, lumbar pain, greenish complexion, cold hands and cold sweat, 0.15 gram of the powder was prescribed for oral administration with Chinese tea. For dry cholera, 0.15 gram of the powder was prescribed for oral administration with tea. For epidemic infectious diseases, the powder could be applied externally on the canthi of the right eye in women and on the left eye in men. Covering the patient with blankets to force perspiration could bring the cure. It was contraindicated in pregnant women. For all kinds of diseases caused by pathogenic fire, 0.15 gram of the powder was prescribed for oral administration with boiled water. For vomiting and diarrhea resulting from cholera or climate sickness, 0.15 gram of the powder was prescribed for oral administration. For difficult swallowing due to tonsillitis, 0.15 gram of the powder was sprayed on the throat through a length of bamboo tube so as to bring an immediate cure. Stimulating food should be avoided during the treatment. For eczema on external genitalia, it could be applied directly to the lesion to bring an immediate cure. For linking herpes of white colour appearing in the lumbar region in children, 0.06-0.09 gram of the powder mixed with vinegar should be applied externally to the local area as soon as possible for a quick cure. For acute conjunctivitis, symptoms would disappear soon after the powder was applied to the eye canthi. For lumbodorsal cellulitis or other carbuncles with substantial abscess, the powder could be applied externally at any stage to remove sloughed tissue and generate new. For irregular menstruation marked by either advanced or delayed flow with abdominal pain, 0.09-0.12 gram of the powder could be taken with millet wine. In this case, covering the body with a heavy blanket to force sweating could improve the patient's condition. For furuncles on fingers, 0.15 gram of the powder was inserted into an egg through a small orifice and the affected finger placed in the broken egg. One egg was generally sufficient, while another egg would be needed in severe cases. The powder was helpful in preventing epidemic infectious diseases. Even in epidemic infectious conditions in animals, external application of the powder was made to the canthi of the affected animals, while they should be kept away from water during the treatment. For traumatic injuries, insect bites, or tetanus, the powder was used externally with satisfactory results. Intake of stimulating food was contraindicated during treatment.

### Comments

This recipe, originally from *Jade Calendar Collection of Fine Prescriptions* (*Yu Li Hui Lu Liang Fang*), has the action of clearing heat and toxins, tranquilizing the mind and resuscitating the patient. It was believed to be a proper remedy in the imperial palace for sunstroke, fulminant dysentery, cholera and other epidemic infections. The original recipe bears a footnote: "The imperial edict passed by Changtai on the fifth day of the fifth month of the lunar calender ordered the omission of the ingredient Mirabilitum."

## XXX.11. PEACE PILL

Peace Pill (Ping An Wan) was worked out by the imperial physician Li Dechang on the ninth day of the fifth month of the lunar calendar in 1884.

### Ingredients

| | |
|---|---|
| Lignum Santali  (Tan Xiang) | 60 g |
| Lignum Aquilariae Resinatum  (Luo Shui Chen) | 60 g |
| Radix Auchlandiae  (Mu Xiang) | 60 g |
| Flos Caryophylli  (Ding Xiang) | 60 g |
| Fructus Amomi Kravanh  (Bai Kou Ren) | 60 g |
| Semen Myristicae  (Rou Kou Ren) | 60 g |
| Fructus Galangae  (Hong Kou) | 60 g |
| Alpiniae Katsumadai  (Cao Dou Kou) | 60 g |
| Pericarpium Citri Reticulatae  (Chen Pi) | 60 g |
| Cortex Magnoliae Officinalis  (Hou Po) | 60 g |
| Rhizoma Atractylodis  (Cang Zhu) | 60 g |
| Massa Fermentata Medicinalis  (Shen Qu) | 60 g |
| Radix Glycyrrhizae  (Gan Cao) | 60 g |
| Fructus Hordei Germinatus  (Mai Ya) | 60 g |
| Fructus Crataegi  (Shan Zha) | 60 g |

The original records prescribe that the Cortex Magnoliae Officinalis should be prepared before use. The Fructus Hordei Germinatus should be roasted and the Fructus Crataegi roasted until burnt yellow. The above ingredients were processed into extremely fine powder and made into honey pills of 6 grams each.

### Comments

All of the ingredients were therapeutically good for the spleen and stomach. The four fragrant ingredients could help promote the circulation of *qi* and invigorate the spleen. Fructus Amomi Kravanh, Semen Myristicae, Fructus Galangae and Alpiniae Katsumadai helped eliminate dampness from the spleen. The ingredients from the traditional formula for Stomach Easing Powder (Ping Wei San) strengthened the spleen in transforming and transporting, and pacified the stomach. The prepared "three elixirs," i.e. Fructus Hordei Germinatus, Massa Fermentata Medicinalis and Fructus Crataegi, helped increase the appetite. In TCM most of the formulary books traced their basic philosophy to the ideas in the *Yellow Emperor's Internal Medicine* (*Huang Di Nei Jing*) that "the stomach provides the essence for human beings." Ancient TCM doctors maintained that the spleen and stomach formed the root for the acquired essence. A healthy condition of these two ograns would ensure that a person would live rather peacefully and healthily. It was possible that Peace Pill was named according to this reasoning. The prescription was prepared for Empress Dowager Cixi for her chronic spleen and stomach conditions. Peace Pill was useful to healthy persons for its help to the spleen.

# XXX.12.  RENEWAL PILL

Renewal Pill (Zai Zhao Wan) was prepared by the imperial physician Li Dechang on the 26th day of the first month of the lunar calendar in 1885.

### *Ingredients*

| | |
|---|---|
| Agkistrodon Halys  (Qi She) | 30 g |
| Lignum Santali  (Tan Xiang) | 7.5 g |
| Herba Asari  (Xi Xin) | 15 g |
| Calculus Bovis  (Niu Huang) | 4.5 g |
| Lumbricus  (Di Long) | 7.5 g |
| Rhizoma Cyperi  (Xiang Fu) | 15 g |
| Radix Notoginseng  (Han San Qi) | 7.5 g |
| Pericarpium Citri Reticulatae Viride  (Qing Pi) | 15g |
| Monascus Purpureus  (Hong Qu) | 7.5 g |
| Radix Ledebouriellae  (Fang Feng) | 30 g |
| Cornu Rhinoceri Asiatici  (Xi Jiao) | 10.8 g |
| Goat blood  (Shan Yang Xue) | 15 g |
| Radix Rehmanniae Praeparatae  (Shu Di) | 30 g |
| Flos Caryophylli  (Ding Xiang) | 15 g |
| Concretio Silicea Bambusae  (Tian Zhu Huang) | 15 g |
| Radix Scrophylariae  (Xuan Shen) | 30 g |
| Rhizoma Curcumae Longae  (Jiang Huang) | 4.5 g |
| Resina Olibani  (Ru Xiang) | 15 g |
| Fructus Amomi Kravanh  (Bai Kou Ren) | 15 g |
| Radix Polugomi Multifori  (He Shou Wu) | 30 g |
| Rhizoma Ligustici Chuanxiong  (Chuan Xiong) | 30 g |
| Radix Anemone Raddeana  (Liang Tou Jian) | 30 g |
| Ramulus Loranthi  (Sang Ji Sheng) | 30 g |
| Radix Puerariae  (Ge Gen) | 22.5 g |
| Rhizoma Drynariae  (Gu Sui Bu) | 15 g |
| Cinnabari  (Zhu Sha) | 15 g |
| Os Tigris  (Hu Gu) | 15 g |
| Rhizoma Dioscoreae Septemlobae  (Bi Xie) | 30 g |
| Plastrum Testudinis  (Gui Ban) | 15 g |
| Borneoleum Syntheticum  (Bing Pian) | 3.6 g |
| Radix Astragali seu Hedysari  (Huang Qi) | 30 g |
| Poria  (Fu Ling) | 15 g |
| Rhizoma Coptidis  (Huang Lian) | 30 g |
| Radix et Rhizoma Rhei  (Da Huang) | 30 g |
| Herba Agastachis  (Huo Xiang) | 30 g |
| Herba Ephedrae  (Ma Huang) | 30 g |
| Scorpio  (Quan Xie) | 22.5 g |
| Radix Aconiti Praeparatae  (Zhi Fu Zi) | 15 g |
| Bombyx Batryticatus  (Jiang Can) | 15 g |
| Squama Manitis  (Chuan Shan Jia) | 15 g |
| Lignum Aquilariae Resinatum  (Chen Xiang) | 15 g |
| Rhizoma Gastrodiae  (Tian Ma) | 30 g |
| Radix Angelicae Sinensis  (Dang Gui) | 15 g |
| Rhizoma Atractylodis Macrocephalae  (Bai Zhu) | 15 g |

| | |
|---|---|
| Alpiniae Katsumadai  (Cao Dou Kou) | 30 g |
| Cortex Cinnamomi  (Rou Gui) | 30 g |
| Moschus  (She Xiang) | 7.5 g |
| Radix Ginseng  (Ren Shen) | 30 g |
| Resina Murrhae  (Mo Yao) | 30 g |
| Radix Clematis  (Wei Ling Xian) | 22.5 g |
| Rhizoma seu Radix Notopterygii  (Qiang Huo) | 30 g |
| Radix Angelicae Dahuricae  (Bai Zhi) | 30 g |
| Resina Draconis  (Xue Jie) | 10 g |
| Radix Paeoniae Lactiflorae  (Bai Shao) | 30 g |
| Radix Linderae  (Wu Yao) | 30 g |

The original recipe calls for the kernel of the Agkistrodon Halys to be used. The Radix Glycyrrhizae, Radix Polugomi Multifori, Plastrum Testudinis, Radix Astragali seu Hedysari, Squama Manitis, Resina Murrhae and Radix Clematis should be prepared before use. The hooks of the Scorpio should be removed and the Bombyx Batryticatus roasted. The above ingredients were processed into fine powder and made in the form of honey pills of 6 grams each, double-wrapped with both rice paper and wax.

### Comments

Having the action of relaxing tendons and collaterals, eliminating wind and resolving phlegm, this prescription was indicated in pain involving tendons and bones caused by dampness invasion into the channels and collaterals, numbness of the limbs, hemiplegia, deviation of the mouth and eye, contracture of the hand or foot, and aphasia. Its name, Renewal Pill, meaning "to bring life or to rebuild life," basically applied to its numerous indications. It was given to Empress Dowager Cixi to activate blood, regulate channels and collaterals and dispel wind.

There were also special remarks concerning the administration of the pill. It was traditionally given together with different guiding decoctions for the affected sides whether left or right; e.g. a disease on the left side of the body would likely be related to the blood. Four Substances Decoction (Si Wu Tang) was provided as the guiding decoction. On the other hand, a disease on the right side would likely be related to qi. Four Gentlemen Decoction (Si Jun Zi Tang) was provided as the guiding decoction. As far as other conditions were concerned, either ginger juice or millet wine would be recommended to assist the administration of the pill.

## XXX.13.  REINFORCED MINOR-COLLATERAL INVIGORATING PILL

Reinforced Minor-collateral Invigorating Pill (Xiao Huo Luo Dan Jia Wei) was carefully formulated by the imperial physicians Li Dechang, Zhuang Shouhe and Dong Wenbin on the 17th day of the second month of the lunar calendar in 1886.

### Ingredients

| | |
|---|---|
| Radix Aconiti  (Chuan Wu) | 15 g |
| Radix Aconiti Kusneziffii  (Cao Wu) | 15 g |
| Arisaema cum Bile  (Dan Nan Xing) | 12 g |

| | |
|---|---|
| Lumbricus  (Di Long) | 15 g |
| Resina Olibani  (Ru Xiang) | 12 g |
| Resina Murrhae  (Mo Yao) | 12 g |
| Rhizoma Gastrodiae  (Tian Ma) | 12 g |
| Herba Siegesbeckiae  (Xi Qian Cao) | 18 g |
| Rhizoma Atractylodis Macrocephalae  (Bai Zhu) | 24 g |
| Radix Angelicae Sinensis  (Dang Gui) | 30 g |
| Radix Paeoniae Lactiflorae  (Bai Shao) | 24 g |
| Ramulus Loranthi  (Sang Ji Sheng) | 24 g |
| Rhizoma Ligustici Chuanxiong  (Chuan Xiong) | 12 g |
| Radix Rehmanniae  (Sheng Di Huang) | 30 g |
| Pericarpium Citri Reticulatae Rubra  (Ju Hong) | 15 g |

The original records prescribe that the cortices from the Radix Aconiti and Radix Aconiti Kusneziffii should be removed through processing. The Lumbricus should be washed clean and roasted and the Resina Olibani oil extracted before use. The raw Rhizoma Atractylodis Macrocephalae should be used, while the Radix Paeoniae Lactiflorae should be roasted. The above ingredients were ground into extremely fine powder and made into wax-coated pills of 4.5 grams each. An equal amount of millet wine and refined honey were used for binding the pills. One pill was prescribed for oral administration each time with millet wine.

### Comments

This prescription was formulated on the basis of Minor-collateral Invigorating Pill (Xiao Huo Luo Dan) plus Rhizoma Gastrodiae, Herba Siegesbeckiae, Ramulus Loranthi, Rhizoma Atractylodis Macrocephalae and Pericarpium Citri Reticulatae Rubra in combination with Four Substances Decoction (Si Wu Tang). Minor-collateral Invigorating Pill was originally intended for treating windstroke manifested by chronic numbness of limbs due to phlegm-damp and blood stasis in the channels and collaterals, occasional mild pain in the body, muscular contraction and motor impairment. Composed of herbal ingredients drastic in action, it was applicable for patients whose constitutions were normally strong. For Empress Dowager Cixi, whose body was considered to be "the most precious of the era," it was therefore modified. The ingredients from Four Substances Decoction (Si Wu Tang) were added for nourishing blood. It was also intended to build up the antipathogenic *qi* and calm the internal wind in addition to nourishing blood. Ingredients for eliminating wind-damp, nourishing the liver and reinforcing the kidney were also added. The thoroughness of the imperial physicians who formulated the prescription was undeniable. The imperial physician Li Dechang claimed that "Reinforced Minor-collateral Invigorating Pill (Xiao Huo Luo Dan Jia Wei) was good for clearing heart fire, improving eyesight, removing stuffiness in the chest, regulating channels and collaterals, reinforcing both the nutrient and defensive systems, regulating the function of the spleen and resolving dampness and was thus applicable in coping with general Bi-syndromes resulting from the invasion of wind and dampness. The clinical manifestations included painful shoulders, pain in the upper back, lumbar regions and knees, various types of headache, deviation of the mouth and eye, hemiplegia, muscular contracture, numbness, aching and heaviness of muscles and skin itching." Moreover, regular use of the pill by the middle-aged who remained in good physical condition could help greatly in preventing possible windstroke attack.

## XXX.14. TEN FRAGRANCES RESUSCITATING PILL

Ten Fragrances Resuscitating Pill (Shi Xiang Fan Hun Dan) was copied from *A Collection of Recommended Prescriptions* (Liang Fang Ji Cheng) on the 20th day of the fifth month of the lunar calendar in 1886.

*Ingredients*

| | |
|---|---|
| Lignum Aguilariae Resinatum (Jia Nan Xiang) | 60 g |
| Flos Syzygii Aromatis (Gong Ding Xiang) | 60 g |
| Resina Liquidambar Orientalis (Su He You) | 60 g |
| Lignum Santali (Tan Xiang) | 60 g |
| Lignum Dalbergiae Odoriferae (Jiang Xiang) | 60 g |
| Resina Olibani (Ru Xiang) | 60 g |
| Herba Agastachis (Huo Xiang) | 60 g |
| Bombyx Batryticatus (Jiang Can) | 60 g |
| Rhizoma Gastrodiae (Tian Ma) | 60 g |
| Rhizoma Cyperi (Xiang Fu) | 60 g |
| Cinnabari (Zhu Sha) | 60 g |
| Amber (Xue Po) | 30 g |
| Benzoinum (An Xi Xiang) | 30 g |
| Calculus Bovis (Niu Huang) | 30 g |
| Moschus (She Xiang) | 30 g |
| Borneolum Syntheticum (Bing Pian) | 15 g |
| Fructus Chebulae (He Zi) | 60 g |
| Semen Trichosanthis (Gua Lou Ren) | 60 g |
| Semen Nelumbinis (Lian Zi) | 60 g |
| Radix Curcumae (Yu Jin) | 60 g |
| Chlorite (Meng Shi) | 60 g |

The original recipe calls for the oil from the Resina Olibani and Semen Trichosanthis to be extracted before use. The Bombyx Batryticatus without the head should be roasted, while the Rhizoma Gastrodiae should be used slightly warm. The Cinnabari should be ground in water into extremely fine powder. The Rhizoma Cyperi should be processed four times in succession respectively with urine of a boy under the age of 12, salt water, millet wine and vinegar. Lotion prepared from Benzoinum should be used. The plumule and radicle of Semen Nelumbinis should be taken. The chlorite should be calcined with vinegar nine times.

The above ingredients were processed into extremely fine powder in their exact doses, followed by decocting the powder with 120 grams of Radix Glycyrrhizae for further concentration to make the goldleaf-coated honey pills of three grams each.

*Comments*

Ten Fragrances Resuscitating Pill (Shi Xiang Fan Hun Dan) was formed on the basis of Liquid Amber Orientalis Pill (Su He Xiang Wan) from *Imperial Grace Formulary of the Tai Ping Era* (*Tai Ping Hui Min He Ji Ju Fang*) plus other ingredients having the action in eliminating pathogenic wind and dampness. Rich in fragrant ingredients, the pill possessed the action of clearing the mind and resolving phlegm in order to resuscitate patients. Its indications included phlegmatic syncope, windstroke attacking the Zang or Fu organs or *qi* manifested by deviation of the mouth and eye, clenched teeth and fainting or loss of consciousness. It was indicated in such conditions as talking to oneself due to wind invasion, and mental confusion with abnormal laughing and crying. Pungent fragrant ingredients of a wandering nature were applied to clear the mind and eliminate the turbid dampness. Specifically, Chlorite, Semen Trichosanthis and Radix Curcumae were used to eliminate phlegm. Bombyx Batryticatus and Rhizoma Gastrodiae were used to dispel wind. Cinnabari and Amber helped calm the mind. The rational combination of all the above ingredients jointly achieved the therapeutic effect of eliminating wind-dampness clearing the mind and bringing resuscitation from syncope. The pill was named Ten Fragrances Resuscitating Pill because it contained ten fragrant ingredients. TCM literature records it in both *A Collection of Recommended Prescriptions* (*Liang Fang Ji Cheng*) and *Spring Walking Collection* (*Chun Jiao Ji*). Here, it was prepared by the imperial physicians in the fifth month of the lunar calendar in 1886 for Empress Dowager Cixi. At that time the Empress Dowager had chronic facial spasm, and the prescription was introduced into the imperial palace to treat her and also to be prepared for palace emergency use. Various instructions for administrations were written to cope with various conditions. One pill was prescribed for oral administration in adults and half a pill for children.

Appendix: Instructions for Specific Applications

In case of windstroke attacking the Zang organs manifested by deviation of the mouth and eye, clenched teeth and syncope, or wind syndromes with corybantism as if being chased by ghosts, talking to onesalf, involuntary crying or laughing, reckless climbing on trees or buildings, and fearfulness due to phlegm obstruction, the pill was taken with boiled water and ginger juice.

In case of syncope due to sunstroke in summer, the pill was taken orally together with Elsholtziae Decoction (Xiang Ru Tang).

In case of sudden unconsciousness in the seventh, eighth or ninth month of pregnancy, known as pregnancy dizziness, the pill was taken together with a decoction made from packed ginseng and Cinnabari floating on water in order to guide the medicine to work quickly in the body.

In case of acute or chronic infantile convulsions accompanied by eyes staring upward, vomiting of foamy phlegm and spasmodic limbs, the pill was taken with decoction made from Herba Menthae or with Medulla Junci Effusi and Ramulus Uncariae cum Uncis.

## XXX.15. PRESCRIPTION FOR INFECTIOUS EPIDEMIC DISEASES

An imperial edict was conveyed by the eunuch Xiangfu for working out

Prescription for Infectious Epidemic Diseases (Zhi Wen Bing Fang) on the fifth day of the third month of the lunar calendar in 1889.

### Ingredients

| | |
|---|---:|
| Borneolum Syntheticum (Bing Pian) | 9 g |
| Moschus (She Xiang) | 9 g |
| Borax (Peng Sha) | 18 g |
| Cinnabari (Zhu Sha) | 30 g |
| Realgar (Xiong Huang) | 18 g |
| Mirabilitum (Ya Xiao) | 3 g |
| Chlorite (Meng Shi) | 18 g |
| Goldleaves (Jin Bo) | 50 |

The above ingredients were processed into extremely fine powder of 0.3 gram to be taken each time with rain or snow water, or simply for smelling. The powder should be carried on the person for convenient use in case of sickness.

### Comments

The prescription was composed of aromatic herbs to drive away turbid pathogenic factors and resolve toxins to protect the heart. Among those ingredients, Borneoleum Syntheticum and Moschus, pungent, fragrant and wandering, removed obstruction so as to resuscitate the patient. It was used with Cinnabari according to TCM convention to treat infectious epidemic diseases. Chlorite was used to resolve phlegm and goldleaf to calm the heart. The remedy prepared in this way was believed to be effective in preventing and treating infectious epidemic diseases.

## XXX.16. THREE SAGES PILL

An imperial edict was delivered to prepare three doses of Three Sages Pill (San Shen Wan) on the 25th day of the sixth month of the lunar calendar in 1891.

### Ingredients

| | |
|---|---:|
| Rhizoma Atractylodis Macrocephalae (Bai Zhu) | 120 g |
| Rhizoma Coptidis (Huang Lian) | 15 g |
| Pericarpium Citri Reticulatae (Ju Hong) | 30 g |

According to the original recipe, the Rhizoma Coptidis should be roasted, and the Rhioma Atractylodis Macrocephalae also roasted until yellow. The above ingredients were processed into fine powder and made into pills the size of Chinese mung beans, together with decoction from Massa Fermentata Medicinalis. Fifty pills were taken each time with ginger soup on an empty stomach.

### Comments

Three Sages Pill (San Shen Wan) was taken from *Standards of Syndrome Differentiation and Treatments* (*Zheng Zhi Zhun Sheng*) by Wan Kentang. Acting to relieve food retention, it was applied in treating discomfort in the epigastric region. As Empress Dowager Cixi liked rich food, remedies for promoting digestion were often prepared for her in the imperial palace. In this prescription Rhizoma Atractylodis Macrocephalae was used to strengthen the spleen; Rhizoma Coptidis and Pericarpium Citri Reticulatae Rubra, one bitter with descending action and the other pungent with opening action, to relieve abdominal distention and fullness. A small amount of Rhizoma Coptidis strengthened gastric function. It was claimed to have the effect of "regulating the stomach and intestines" in the book entitled *Transactions of Famous Physicians* (*Ming Yi Bie Lu*). Pericarpium Citri Reticulatae Rubra was used to harmonize the stomach. The combination of the three was believed to strengthen the spleen and pacify the stomach.

Attention should also be paid to distinguishing three other pills of the same name as recorded in other sources. Specifically, the Three Sages Pill for treating malaria as recorded in *Therapeutic Standards for the Six Medical Departments* (*Liu Ke Zhun Shen*) consisted of the following: Squama Manitis, Radix Dichroae and Semen Arecae. The one recorded in *Formulas for the Living* (*Ji Sheng Fang*) was composed of Flos Caryphylli, Mylabris and Moschus, and was for treating scrofula. The third Three Sages Pill in the book *Complete Works on External Therapeutics* (*Yang Yi Da Quan*), composed of Hydrargyrum, Camphora and Semen Hynocarpi, was formulated for treating scabies.

## XXX.17. REINFORCED THREE SAGES PILL

Reinforced Three Sages Pill (Jia Wei San Shen Wan) was carefully worked out by the imperial physicians Li Dechang and Yang Jihe on the 29th day of the sixth month of the lunar calendar in 1891.

*Ingredients*

| | |
|---|---|
| Rhizoma Atractylodis Macrocephalae  (Bai Zhu) | 60 g |
| Rhizoma Coptidis  (Huang Lian) | 7.5 g |
| Pericarpium Citri Reticulatae Rubra  (Ju Hong) | 15 g |
| Cornu Antelopis  (Ling Yang Jiao) | 9 g |
| Arisaema cum Bile  (Dan Nan Xing) | 6 g |
| Fructus Aurantii Immaturus  (Zhi Shi) | 15 g |
| Folium Perillae  (Su Ye) | 9 g |
| Pericarpium Trichosanthis  (Gua Lou Pi) | 12 g |
| Semen Trichosanthis  (Gua Lou Zi) | 12 g |

According to the original records, the Rhizoma Atractylodis Macrocephalae, Rhizoma Coptidis and Fructus Aurantii Immaturus were roasted. The above ingredients were processed into fine powder and mixed with Massa Fermentata Medicinalis paste to make pills the size of Chinese mung beans. One hundred and fifty grams of the pills were taken each time with boiled water.

*Comments*

Reinforced Three Sages Pill (Jia Wei San Shen Wan) was formulated by modifying the ingredients of the original Three Sages Pill (San Shen Wan). Cornu Antelopis and Arisaema cum Bile were added in order to clear liver fire and resolve phlegm. Folium Perillae and Pericarpium Citri Reticulatae Rubra were added in case of possible symptoms and signs of an exterior syndrome.

## XXX.18. HEART-SPLEEN REINFORCING PILL FOR SOOTHING THE LIVER AND CLEARING THE LUNG

Heart-Spleen Reinforcing Pill for Soothing the Liver and Clearing the Lung (Yang Xin Li Pi Jie Yu Qing Fei Huan Gan Wan) was carefully formulated by the imperial physicians Zhuang Shouhe, Li Dechang, Quan Shun and Nie Hongjun on the 19th day of the third month of the lunar calendar in 1895.

### Ingredients

| | |
|---|---:|
| Radix Poria  (Fu Shen) | 18 g |
| Semen Ziziphi Spinosae  (Suan Zao Ren) | 15 g |
| Radix Polygalae  (Yuan Zhi) | 12 g |
| Pericarpium Citri Reticulatae Rubra  (Ju Hong) | 12 g |
| Rhizoma Polygonati Odorati  (Yu Zhu) | 15 g |
| Radix Angelicae Sinensis  (Dang Gui) | 18 g |
| Radix Rehmanniae  (Sheng Di Huang) | 24 g |
| Radix Paeoniae Lactiflorae  (Bai Shao) | 15 g |
| Rhizoma Cyperi  (Xiang Fu) | 18 g |
| Radix Platycodi  (Jie Geng) | 12 g |
| Flos Magnoliae Officinalis  (Hou Po Hua) | 12 g |
| Radix Curcumae  (Yu Jin) | 12 g |
| Bulbus Fritillariae Cirhosae  (Chuan Bei) | 12 g |
| Caulis Spatholobi syrup  (Ji Xue Teng Gao) | 15 g |
| Semen Coicis  (Yi Yi Ren) | 15 g |

The original recipe calls for the Semen Ziziphi Spinosae to be roasted until yellow. The Radix Paeoniae Lactiflorae and Semen Coicis should be simply roasted, while the Rhizoma Cyperi should be prepared. The above ingredients were processed into extremely fine powder and mixed with refined honey to make Cinnabari-coated pills the size of mung beans. Nine grams of the pills were taken each time with boiled water.

### Comments

This prescription characterized by a balanced effort between soothing and regulating could be prescribed regularly. Although the heart, spleen, lung and liver were treated at the same time, the focus lay in the first two organs. Therefore, the formula was modified on the basis of Decoction for Invigorating the Spleen and Nourishing the Heart (Gui Pi Tang), replacing those ingredients for nourishing qi with those for nourishing blood for the purpose of strengthening the spleen and nourishing the heart. Among the various ingredients, those for nourishing the heart were dominant. As in military strategy, "Following the orders from the central commander, field forces could fight against the enemy troops with a clear sense though the enemies attacked from different routes on the front line." In 1895 Empress Dowager Cixi was past 60, and besides remedies for her chronic cough and disharmony between heart and stomach, others were prescribed for nourishing the heart and soothing the liver, thought to be a way to achieve longevity.

# XXX.19. MOISTENING COPTIDIS PASTE FOR CLEARING WIND-HEAT

Moistening Coptidis Paste for Clearing Wind-Heat (Qing Run Huang Lian Gao) was prepared by the imperial physician Zhuang Shouhe on the 12th day of the fourth month of the lunar calendar in 1900.

*Ingredients*

| | |
|---|---|
| Rhizoma Coptidis  (Huang Lian) | 4.5 g |
| Radix Angelicae Sinensis  (Dang Gui) | 9 g |
| Radix Rehmanniae  (Sheng Di Huang) | 9 g |
| Cortex Phellodendri  (Huang Bai) | 9 g |
| Rhizoma Curcumae Longae  (Jiang Huang) | 6 g |
| Gypsum Fribrosum  (Shi Gao) | 9 g |
| Herba Menthae  (Bo He) | 3 g |

The above ingredients were prepared in concentrated decoction. After separating out the residue, 0.6 gram of Borneoleum Syntheticum and a suitable amount of refined honey were added to make a paste.

*Comments*

Moistening Coptidis Paste for Clearing Wind-Heat was made by enriching the Coptidis Paste (Huang Lian Gao) from *Golden Mirror of Medical Tradition* (*Yi Zong Jin Jian*). With a satisfactory therapeutic effect, the original Coptidis Paste was applied in treating nasal boils, pain, dryness, itching and skin eruptions due to wind invasion. By adding Gypsum Fribrosum for clearing heat from the lung and stomach, and Herba Menthae for dispelling head wind, the reinforced paste for external application had stronger action in clearing toxic heat, curing boils and dispelling pathogenic wind.

# XXX.20. TAIYI PURPLE LOZENGE

An imperial edict was carried out by the Longevity Pharmacy for preparing three doses of Taiyi Purple Lozenge (Tai Yi Zi Jin Ding) on the fourth day of the fifth month of the lunar calendar in 1903.

*Ingredients*

| | |
|---|---|
| Meretrix  (Wen Ge) | 3 kg |
| Radix Euphorbiae Pekinensis  (Da Ji) | 1.5 kg |
| Rhizoma Pleionis  (Shan Ci Gu) | 2.06 kg |
| Semen Euphorbiae Lathyridis  (Qian Jin Zi) | 920 g |
| Realgar  (Xiong Huang) | 515 g |
| Moschus  (She Xiang) | 270 g |
| Cinnabari  (Zhu Sha) | 650 g |

According to the original recipe the oil should be removed from the Semen Euphorbiae Lathyridis. The Moschus could be used only with special permission. The above ingredients were first ground into fine powder, then 2.24 kg of Semen Oryzae Glutinosae were steamed into paste. The powder from the ingredients was next mixed with the paste and pounded with a stick until the paste became moist and sticky.

### Comments

Taiyi Purple Lozenge, also known as Tai Yi Jade Pivot Pill (Tai Yi Yu Shu Dan), was recorded in the book entitled *Synopsis of Cholera* (*Huo Luan Lun*). Its actions are to clear turbid dampness and epidemic toxins. Conventionally, it was applied for treating mental confusion, nausea and vomiting, diarrhea, infantile syncope and boils due to invasion of turbid dampness or seasonal epidemics. It was also applicable to amenorrhea if taken internally with Flos Carthami decoction. In windstroke with deviation of the mouth and eye, the lozenge was ground into powder and taken with millet wine. In Empress Dowager Cixi's later years she was susceptible to chronic facial spasm. Three doses were ordered at once, indicating how urgent the lozenge was needed in order to relieve her chronic facial disorder. Internal application of the remedy helped clear toxic heat while external application helped relieve swelling and boils. It also acted in clearing epidemic heat and promoting the motor functions of joints.

## XXX.21.  VINEGAR CAKE PRESCRIPTION

Vinegar Cake Prescription (Cu Bing Fang) was prepared on the 16th day of the ninth month of the lunar calendar in 1903.

### Ingredients

| | |
|---|---:|
| Wheat flour paste  (Jiao Ni Mian) | 1,000 g |
| Folium Artemisiae Argyi  (Ai Rong) | 60 g |
| Table salt  (Shi Yan) | 60 g |

The above ingredients were mixed with vinegar and made into cakes with holes in the centre to be impaled on a bamboo stick.

### Comments

Many a herbal book states that vinegar could help relieve toxicity, disperse stasis and promote the stomach in digestion. Mixing vinegar with wheat flour paste could help disperse the stagnant blood caused by traumatic injuries and relieve swelling due to boils. Folium Artemisiae Argyi was applied here to eliminate cold, ease pain, warm the channels and stop bleeding. The cake prepared with vinegar might also help prevent miscarriage and stop abdominal pain. By 1903, Empress Dowager Cixi had already undergone menopause, and perhaps the cake was applied for the purpose of relieving toxicity, subduing carbuncles or regulating both *qi* and blood. Preparing powdered ingredients and vinegar together with flour into herbal cakes for healing was a new thing at the time.

## XXX.22.  PILL FOR CLEARING DAMP-HEAT

One dose of Pill for Clearing Damp-Heat (Qing Re Hua Shi Wan) was prescribed for Empress Dowager Cixi by the imperial physicians Zhang Zhongyuan and Yao Baosheng on the 25th day of the fourth month of the lunar calendar in 1906.

*Ingredients*

| | |
|---|---|
| Radix Codonopsis  (Dang Shen) | 18 g |
| Poria  (Fu Ling) | 24 g |
| Rhizoma Alismatis  (Ze Xie) | 18 g |
| Rhizoma Dioscoreae Septemlobae  (Bi Xie) | 18 g |
| Caulis Akebiae  (Mu Tong) | 12 g |
| Radix Achyranthis Bidentatae  (Niu Xi) | 24 g |
| Rhizoma Cyperi  (Xiang Fu) | 24 g |
| Glycyrrhizae Uralensis Fish  (Gan Cao Shao) | 18 g |

The original recipe says the Rhizoma Cyperi should be prepared before use. The above ingredients were mixed with herbal residue left from the previous three days. They were then processed into fine powder and made into honey pills of 6 grams each for oral administration with boiled water.

*Comments*

Empress Dowager Cixi's health records in the fourth month of the lunar calendar in 1906, says she had "a wiry, slippery and rapid pulse in the liver region, but a deep slippery one in the lung and spleen regions." The composition of this prescription shows similarity to Eight Health-restoring Powder (Ba Zheng San) and that it was based on its recipe. Bland ingredients for eliminating dampness were assisted by those having the action of clearing heat from urine. Glycyrrhizae Uralensis Fish was used for dealing with painful urination. It was thought that Empress Dowager Cixi suffered from urinary tract infections as well as leukorrhea, leading the imperial physicians Zhang Zhongyuan and Yao Baosheng to diagnose "downward flowing of damp-heat due to dysfunction of the spleen." The prescription had no unfavourable side-effects in her situation and therefore should be effective in her case.

For readers' reference, prescriptions presented on the previous three days are listed as follows:

The prescription of the 22nd day of the fourth month of the lunar calendar in 1906 includes:

| | |
|---|---|
| Red Poria  (Chi Fu Ling) | 12 g |
| Rhizoma Atractylodis Macrocephalae  (Bai Zhu) | 6 g |
| Rhizoma Alismatis  (Ze Xie) | 4.5 g |
| Rhizoma Dioscoreae Septemlobae  (Bi Xie) | 9 g |
| Herba Dianthi  (Qu Mai) | 9 g |
| Semen Plantaginis  (Che Qian Zi) | 9 g |
| Herba Polygoni Avicularis  (Bian Xu) | 9 g |
| Radix Angelicae Sinensis  (Dang Gui) | 9 g |
| Semen Caesalpiniae  (Ku Shi Lian) | 6 g |
| Glycyrrhizae Uralendis Fish  (Gan Cao Shao) | 6 g |

Among the ingredients the Semen Plantaginis should be wrapped and the Rhizoma Cyperi prepared before use. Two pieces of Medulla Junci Effusi and 3 pieces of Herba Lophatheri were used as dominant drugs.

The prescription on the 23rd day was otherwise the same as that of the 22nd except for the omission of the two dominant drugs.

The prescription of the 24th day had Radix Ginseng, Radix Ophiopogonis and Cortex Moudan Radicis to replace the Rhizoma Dioscoreae Septemlobae, Semen Plantaginis and Rhizoma Cyperi in that used on the 22nd. The rest remained the same.

## XXX.23.  LIQUID STYRAX PILL

One dose of Liquid Styrax Pill (Su He Xiang Wan) was prescribed for Empress Dowager Cixi on the 23rd day of the 11th month of the lunar calendar in 1906.

*Ingredients*

| | |
|---|---|
| Lignum Aquilariae Resinatum  (Chen Xiang) | 30 g |
| Radix Auchalandiae  (Mu Xiang) | 30 g |
| Flos Caryophylli  (Ding Xiang) | 30 g |
| Lignum Santali  (Tan Xiang) | 30 g |
| Benzoinum  (An Xi Xiang) | 30 g |
| Rhizoma Cyperi  (Xiang Fu) | 30 g |
| Rhizoma Atractylodis Macrocephalae  (Bai Zhu) | 30 g |
| Fructus Chebulae  (He Zi) | 30 g |
| Fructus Piperis Longi  (Bi Bo) | 30 g |
| Cinnabari  (Zhu Sha) | 30 g |
| Borneolum Syntheticum  (Bing Pian) | 15 g |
| Resina Liquidambar Orientalis  (Su He You) | 15 g |

The above ingredients were processed into extremely fine powder and made into wax-coated honey pills of 4.5 grams each.

*Comments*

The prescription for Liquid Styrax Pill was originally from *Imperial Grace Formulary of the Tai Ping Era* (*Tai Ping Hui Min He Ji Ju Fang*). It was a fragrant, warming resuscitating remedy largely consisting of pungent and fragrant ingredients of warming property. In terms of actions, it was different from the pungent cooling resuscitations such as Bezoar Pill for Resurrection (Niu Huang Qing Xin Wan), Treasured Pill (Zhi Bao Dan) and Purple Snow Pill (Zi Xue Dan). According to the existing health records of Empress Dowager Cixi, she suffered from facial paralysis, diabetes, depressed liver *qi*, and amenorrhea. The prescription should be on the principle of promoting the circulation of *qi* and blood in the channels and collaterals since it largely consisted of fragrant, pungent ingredients of a wandering nature. It was good for the treatment of *qi* stagnation, blood stasis and obstruction of the channels and collaterals.

## XXX.24.  IMPERIAL PEACE PILL

An imperial edict was presented by the eunuch Xishou to Longevity Pharmacy to prepare seven doses of Imperial Peace Pill (Yu Zhi Ping An Wan) on the 27th day of the fifth month of the lunar calendar, with no information given as to the year.

*Ingredients*

| | |
|---|---|
| Moschus  (She Xiang) | 840 g |

| | |
|---|---:|
| Ash of Medulla Junci Effusi  (Deng Xin Cao Hui) | 504 g |
| Spina Gleditsiae  (Zhu Ya Zao) | 2.52 kg |
| Unidentified | 1.58 kg |
| Borneolum Syntheticum  (Bing Pian) | 840 g |
| Unidentified | 840 g |
| Realgar  (Xiong Huang) | 840 g |
| Cinnabari  (Zhu Sha) | 840 g |
| Fuligo Plantae  (Bai Cao Shuang) | 840 g |
| Semen Arecae  (Bing Lang) | 2.1 kg |
| Rhizoma Atractylodis  (Cang Zhu) | 2.1 kg |
| Poria  (Fu Ling) | 3.26 kg |
| Pericarpium Citri Reticulatae  (Chen Pi) | 1.68 kg |
| Cortex Acanthopanacis Radicis  (Wu Jia Pi) | 1.68 kg |
| Herba Agastachis  (Huo Xiang) | 2.52 kg |

The original recipe requires that the Rhizoma Atractylodis should be roasted and Cortex Magnoliae Officinalis prepared before use. The above ingredients were processed into extremely fine powder.

### Comments

The ancient Peace Pill (Ping An Wan) was indicated in nine sorts of pain in the chest and epigastric regions, pulling pain from time to time, distention and fullness in the chest and diaphragm, nausea, discomfort in the epigastrium, belching and sour regurgitation. Modified on the basis of Peace Pill, the Imperial Peace Pill acquired the action of relieving turbid dampness and epidemics, clearing summer heat, and strengthening spleen and stomach functions. Regular use of the pill should free a person from the bother of illness, and in the imperial palace the pill was often made and used by emperors, empresses, ladies-in-waiting and ministers.

## XXX.25.  PANACEA LOZENGE

An imperial edict was presented to Longevity Pharmacy for preparing four doses of Panacea Lozenge (Wan Ying Ding) on the 14th day of the fourth month of the lunar calendar, with no year given.

### Ingredients

| | |
|---|---:|
| Rhizoma Picrorhizae  (Hu Huang Lian) | 2 kg |
| Rhizoma Coptidis  (Huang Lian) | 2 kg |
| Acacia Cateche  (Er Cha) | 2 kg |
| Cinnabari  (Zhu Sha) | 120 g |
| Ful Ursi  (Xiong Dan) | 60 g |
| Borneolum Syntheticum  (Bing Pian) | 60 g |
| Moschus  (She Xiang) | 60 g |
| Old pine-oil ink  (Gu Mo) | 3.12 kg |

The original records state that Moschus and old pine-oil ink should be used only with special permission. The above ingredients were processed into fine powder and made into bile-bound pills the size of rice grains and coated with goldleaf.

*Comments*

Nowadays, Panacea Lozenges manufactured in different pharmaceutical plants in China are all based on the original formula as recorded in *Qing Dynasty Imperial Pharmacopeia of Patent Medicines* (*Qing Gong Nei Ting Fa Zhi Wan San Gao Dan Ge Yao Pei Ben*) with the possible omission of Ful Ursi or other ingredients. But Panacea Lozenges produced by manufacturers in Chengde and Wuhan are closest in composition to that used in the Qing imperial palace. This was largely because imperial remedies were kept secret. Panacea Lozenge has the action of clearing fire and relieving toxicity. It was applicable to dizziness due to sunstroke, sore throat, and nondescript boils or masses. It has been highly recommended by TCM practitioners and widely used in China.

## XXX.26. PASTE FOR ACTIVATING BLOOD AND CLEARING WIND

An imperial edict was presented to Longevity Pharmacy for one dose of Paste for Activating Blood and Clearing Wind (Huo Xue Qu Feng Gao) for Empress Dowager Cixi. The prescription was formulated by the imperial physicians Li Jun and Zhang Zhongyuan on the 26th day of the seventh month of the lunar calendar, with no information given as to the year.

*Ingredients*

| | |
|---|---|
| Radix Dedebouriellae  (Fang Feng) | 60 g |
| Fructus Viticis  (Man Jing Zi) | 30 g |
| Radix Angelicae Sinensis  (Dang Gui) | 90 g |
| Radix Astragali seu Hedysari  (Huang Qi) | 60 g |
| Ramulus Cinnamomi  (Gui Zhi) | 90 g |
| Rhizoma Ligustici Chuanxiong  (Chuan Xiong) | 60 g |
| Herba Menthae  (Bo He) | 30 g |
| Pericarpium Citri Reticulatae  (Chen Pi) | 30 g |
| Rhizoma Typhonii Gigantei  (Bai Fu Zi) | 15 g |
| Camphora  (Zhang Nao) | 15 g |
| Cortex Moudan Radicis  (Mu Dan Pi) | 30 g |
| Radix Paeoniae Lactiflorae  (Bai Shao) | 30 g |
| Caulis Spatholobi  (Ji Xue Teng) | 15 g |

The original records direct that the Rhizoma Thyphonii Gigantei and Camphora should be first ground into powder before mixing with the other ingredients. All were fried in two kilograms of sesame oil. After separating out the herbal residue, the remaining oily substance was further concentrated until its liquid fell like water drops in freezing weather. One kilogram of red lead and the powder from Rhizoma Typhonii Gigantei and Camphora were then added to make a paste suitable for external application.

*Comments*

Paste for Activating Blood and Clearing Wind was modified on the basis of combining Minor Decoction for Extending Life Expectancy (Xiao Xu Ming Fang) from the book entitled *Prescriptions Worth a Thousand Gold* (*Qian Jin Yao Fang*), and Angelicae Sinensis Decoction for Replenishing Blood (Dang Gui Bu Xue Gao) introduced by Li Dongyuan. The former was originally a prescription intended to be a comprehensive remedy for dealing with wind conditions, and most remedies for wind conditions were developed from this so-called Minor Decoction for Extending Life Expectancy from ancient times. Although Empress Dowager Cixi had chronic facial spasm, Radix Ephedrae and Semen Armenicacae were omitted since she had no exterior cold symptoms or signs. It was assumed that her chronic facial spasm resulted from invasion of exogenous pathogenic wind and was also related to her constitutional deficiency of nutrient blood. The therapeutic mechanism was based on the doctrine that "the treatment of chronic wind condition should be started by enriching blood, since normal circulation of blood would lead to spontaneous stopping of internal wind." Therefore, Radix Astragali seu Hedysari, Radix Angelicae Sinensis and Caulis Spatholobi were added to help form and nourish blood. Herba Menthae and Pericarpium Citri Reticulatae, ingredients of mild eliminating action, were applied to clear wind and dampness. The above two groups of modified ingredients enhanced the effect of activating blood and eliminating wind. Camphora, pungent and fragrant and wandering, was applied to clear unhygienic pathogenic factors. According to modern pharmaceutical studies, Camphora can mildly stimulate the local mucocutaneous membrane and thus promote local blood circulation. It was probably used here in consideration of her chronic facial spasm. The imperial physicians often had to work very hard to formulate an effective prescription.

## XXX.27. PASTE FOR CLEARING WIND-DAMP AND RESOLVING BLOOD STASIS

Paste for Clearing Wind-Damp and Resolving Blood Stasis (Qu Feng He Mai Tiao Qi Li Shi Hua Tan Gao) for Empress Dowager Cixi was carefully prepared by the imperial physicians Li Dechang, Quan Shun, Zhang Zhongyuan, Ye Cigao and a fifth whose name is not mentioned in the original records. It was prepared on the 19th day of the second month of the lunar calendar, with no information given as to the year.

*Ingredients*

| | |
|---|---|
| Rhizoma seu Radix Notopertygii  (Qiang Huo) | 60 g |
| Radix Angelicae Pubscentis  (Du Huo) | 60 g |
| Bombyx Batryticatus  (Jiang Can) | 90 g |
| Radix Clematis  (Wei Ling Xian) | 45 g |
| Radix Aconiti  (Chuan Wu) | 45 g |
| Rhizoma Curcumae Longae  (Jiang Huang) | 45 g |
| Retinervous Citri Fructus  (Ju Luo) | 60 g |
| Caulis Spatholobi  (Ji Xue Teng) | 90 g |
| Radix Gentianae Macrocephalae  (Qin Jiao) | 45 g |
| Ramulus Loranthi  (Sang Ji Sheng) | 60 g |
| Radix Angelicae Sinensis  (Dang Gui) | 60 g |
| Squama Manitis  (Chuan Shan Jia) | 60 g |
| Flos Carthami  (Hong Hua) | 60 g |
| Radix Dipsaci  (Xu Duan) | 60 g |
| Rhizoma Cyperi  (Xiang Fu) | 90 g |

| | |
|---|---|
| Resina Murrhae  (Mo Yao) | 45 g |
| Resina Olibani  (Ru Xiang) | 45 g |
| Zaocys  (Wu Shao She) | 45 g |
| Radix Ledebouriellae  (Fang Feng) | 60 g |
| Rhizoma Atractylodis  (Cang Zhu) | 60 g |
| Radix Paeoniae Rubra  (Chi Shao) | 60 g |
| Radix Linderae  (Tai Wu) | 60 g |
| Pericarpium Citri Reticulatae Viride  (Qing Pi) | 60 g |
| Rhizoma Pinelliae  (Ban Xia) | 60 g |
| Moschus  (She Xiang) | 15 g |

The original records state that the Rhizoma Curcumae Longae should be sliced before use. The Caulis Spatholobi, Resina Murrhae and Resina Olibani should be added in later for a shorter period of decocting. Raw Rhizoma Cyperi should be used. The Rhizoma Pinelliae should be prepared. The Moschus should be mixed in last. The above ingredients were well fried in five kilograms of sesame oil. After removing the herbal residue, the remaining oily substance was mixed with red lead to make the proper paste.

### Comments

The prescription was mainly composed of ingredients for eliminating wind and dampness, activating blood circulation and removing blood stasis, similar to those in Major Collateral Invigorating Pill (Da Huo Luo Dan). It was applied in conditions caused by stubborn phlegm and severe pathogenic wind attacking the channels and collaterals. Its application was to clear phlegm and disperse wind in treating Empress Dowager Cixi's chronic facial spasm.

## XXX.28. SYRUP FOR CLEARING DAMP-HEAT FROM MIDDLE JIAO

Syrup for Clearing Damp-Heat from Middle Jiao (Tiao Zhong Qing Re Hua Shi Gao) was prepared for Empress Dowager Cixi by the imperial physician Yao Baosheng on the 26th day of the fourth month of the lunar calendar, with no information given as to the year.

### Ingredients

| | |
|---|---|
| Poria  (Fu Ling) | 18 g |
| Cortex Moudan Radicis  (Mu Dan Pi) | 9 g |
| Rhizoma Atractylodis  (Cang Zhu) | 9 g |
| Herba Agastachis  (Huo Xiang) | 9 g |
| Cortex Magnoliae Officinalis  (Hou Po) | 6 g |
| Pericarpium Arecae  (Da Fu Pi) | 9 g |
| Rhizoma Coptidis  (Huang Lian) | 6 g |
| Radix Scutellariae  (Huang Qin) | 9 g |
| Fructus Amomi Kravahn  (Bai Kou Ren) | 9 g |
| Rhizoma Cyperi  (Xiang Fu) | 12 g |
| Radix Paeoniae Lactiflorae  (Bai Shao) | 18 g |
| Rhizoma Alismatis  (Ze Xie) | 12 g |

The original records state that the Poria and Fructus Amomi Kravahn should be ground into powder before use. The Rhizoma Atractylodis should be roasted until yellow. The Cortex Magnoliae Officinalis and Rhizoma Cyperi should be prepared. The Rhizoma Coptidis prepared in millet wine should be roasted until yellow and ground into powder and the Radix Scutellaraie roasted with millet wine. Raw Radix Paeoniae Lactiflorae should be used. The above ingredients were well decocted in water. After separating out the herbal residue, the remaining decoction was further concentrated and mixed with refined honey to make a syrup. Four spoonfuls of the syrup was taken each time with boiled water.

### Comments

Syrup for Clearing Damp-Heat from Middle Jiao as used in the Qing Dynasty imperial palace was essentially formed on the basis of Agastachis Powder for Rectifying *Qi* (Huo Xiang Zheng Qi San) by removing ingredients for relieving exterior symptoms and signs and increasing ingredients for clearing severe internal heat. It was applied to treat retention of dampness in the spleen and stomach accompanied by internal heat. Records concerning Empress Dowager Cixi's lifestyle say that she preferred sweet and rich food, which led to a gradual accumulation of internal dampness and heat. This caused poor function of the spleen in transforming and transporting, resulting in fluid retention in the body. Patent formulae in the form of syrup or paste were therefore often prepared for her.

## XXX.29. PRESCRIPTION FOR PACIFYING THE STOMACH AND RESOLVING PHLEGM-HEAT

Prescription for Pacifying the Stomach and Resolving Phlegm-Heat (He Zhong Hua Yin Re Fang) was carefully worked out by the imperial physicians Zhang Zhongyuan and Yao Baosheng for Empress Dowager Cixi on the seventh day of the fourth month of the lunar calendar. No information was given as to the year.

### Ingredients

| | |
|---|---|
| Poria  (Fu Ling) | 12 g |
| Rhizoma Atractylodis Macrocephalae  (Bai Zhu) | 6 g |
| Cortex Moudan Radicis  (Mu Dan Pi) | 4.5 g |
| Fructus Oryzae Germinature  (Gu Ya) | 9 g |
| Radix Coptidis  (Huang Lian) | 2.4 g |
| Rhizoma Cyperi  (Xiang Fu) | 6 g |
| Fructus Amomi  (Sha Ren) | 2.4 g |
| Massa Fermentata Medicinalis  (Shen Qu) | 6 g |
| Radix Codonopsis Pilosulae  (Dang Shen) | 6 g |
| Radix Glycyrrhizae  (Gan Cao) | 2.4 g |

The original records say that the Rhizoma Atractylodis Macrocephalae should be roasted until yellow, while the Fructus Oryzae Germinature and Massa Fermentata Medicinalis should be plain roasted. The Radix Coptidis prepared with ginger and the Fructus Amomi should be ground into powder. The Rhizoma Cyperi should be prepared before use. Seven pieces of Fructus Canarit ground in thin pieces and 1.2 grams of herbal Agastachis were taken as the main drugs.

*Comments*

Prescription for Pacifying the Stomach and Resolving Phlegm-Heat was modified on the basis of Extraordinary Merit Powder (Yi Gong San) and Six Gentlemen Decoction with Auchlandiae and Amomum (Xiang Sha Liu Jun Zi Tang). It was prescribed for such symptoms as poor appetite, fullness in the chest with profuse sputum, sour regurgitation and deficient type of gastric pain due to internal cold. The formula was mainly composed of aromatic drugs for resolving dampness, and bitter-tasting ingredients of warming property for drying the dampness. By adding in Radix Coptidis, Fructus Canarit and ingredients for increasing the appetite, additional therapeutic effects for clearing heat were obtained apart from that in promoting the spleen in drying dampness, activating *qi* and pacifying the stomach. It can also be recommended for swelling and pain in the throat due to heat retention in the stomach and lung.

## XXX.30. DECOCTION FOR REGULATING THE STOMACH AND CLEARING HEAT

Decoction for Regulating the Stomach and Clearing Heat (Qing Re Tiao Zhong Yin) was carefully prepared for Empress Dowager Cixi by the imperial physicians Zhang Zhongyuan and Yao Baosheng on the 25th day of the fifth month of the lunar calendar. No information was given as to the year.

*Ingredients*

| | |
|---|---|
| Folium Mori  (Sang Ye) | 9 g |
| Flos Chrysanthemi  (Ju Hua) | 9 g |
| Radix Scutellariae  (Huang Qin) | 6 g |
| Pericarpium Citri Reticulatae Rubra  (Ju Hong) | 3 g |
| Fructus Aurantii  (Zhi Ke) | 4.5 g |
| Massa Fermentata Medicinalis  (Shen Qu) | 9 g |
| Rhizoma Cyperi  (Xiang Fu) | 4.5 g |
| Radix Glycyrrhizae  (Gan Cao) | 3 g |

According to the original records, the Radix Scutellariae should be prepared with millet wine, the Fructus Aurantii roasted, and the Rhizoma Cyperi prepared. The above ingredients were decocted and the decoction taken while still warm. The next day the same formula but with three grams of Three Elixirs added and Massa Fermentata Medicinalis omitted was prescribed again.

*Comments*

Compared with Decoction for Clearing Heat and Resolving Dampness (Qing Re Hua Shi Yin), this prescription contained the same ingredients for clearing heat. However, ingredients for resolving dampness were replaced by those for promoting stomach function and relieving food retention. Thus the name Decoction for Regulating the Stomach and Clearing Heat. By referring to the prescription restructured by the imperial physicians Zhang Zhongyuan and Yao Baosheng on the 26th day of the fifth month of the lunar calendar in the same year, it was wiser to demonstrate actions by adding Three Elixirs and omitting Massa Fermentata Medicinalis.

## XXX.31. DECOCTION FOR CLEARING HEAT AND RESOLVING DAMPNESS

Decoction for Clearing Heat and Resolving Dampness (Qing Re Hua Shi Yin) was carefully formulated by the imperial physician Yao Baosheng around 5:00 - 7:00 p.m. on the 13th day of the 12th month of the lunar calendar, with no information given as to the year.

### Ingredients

| | |
|---|---|
| Flos Chrysanthemi  (Ju Hua) | 4.5 g |
| Folium Mori  (Sang Ye) | 9 g |
| Cortex Moudan Radicis  (Mu Dan Pi) | 4.5 g |
| Poria  (Fu Ling) | 12 g |
| Rhizoma Alismatis  (Ze Xie) | 4.5 g |
| Rhizoma Coptidis  (Huang Lian) | 2.4 g |
| Radix Glycyrrhizae  (Gan Cao) | 3 g |
| Fructus Aurantii  (Zhi Ke) | 4.5 g |

According to the original records, the Rhizoma Coptidis prepared with millet wine should be roasted until yellow and then ground into powder. The Fructus Aurantii should also be roasted until yellow before use. One piece of Medulla Junci Effusi was taken as the main drug.

### Comments

This prescription mainly consisted of ingredients of sweet flavour and cold property with the action of clearing dampness from the urinary tract. It apparently acted to clear heat and dampness without side-effects of drying the body fluid or over-consuming Yin. It was applicable to Yin deficiency syndrome with dampness. The Flos Chrysanthemi and Folium Mori were applied as the main ingredients. The Radix Coptidis was roasted with millet wine to maintain its medicinal property without retaining much bitter flavour. The prescription was thus formulated for clearing dampness and heat in the Upper Jiao. Most of the ingredients were of light quality, facilitating its purpose.

## XXX.32. YIN-NOURISHING SYRUP TO REGULATE MIDDLE JIAO AND RESOLVE EDEMA

Yin-Nourishing Syrup to Regulate Middle Jiao and Resolve Edema (Yang Yin Tiao Zhong Hua Yin Gao) was carefully worked out for Empress Dowager Cixi by the imperial physicians Zhang Zhongyuan and Yao Baosheng on the 20th day of the 11th month of the lunar calendar. No year was given.

### Ingredients

| | |
|---|---|
| Radix Panacis Quiquefloii  (Xi Yang Shen) | 9 g |
| Cinnabari-coated Poria  (Zhu Fu Ling) | 18 g |
| Semen Biotae  (Bai Zi Ren) | 12 g |
| Bulbus Fritillariae Cirrhosae  (Chuan Bei) | 9 g |
| Radix Angelicae Sinensis  (Dang Gui) | 12 g |
| Pericarpium Citri Reticulatae  (Chen Pi) | 9 g |
| Rhizoma Cyperi  (Xiang Fu) | 9 g |

| | |
|---|---|
| Massa Fermentata Medicinalis  (Shen Qu) | 12 g |
| Fructus Aurantii  (Zhi Ke) | 6 g |
| Fructus Crataegi  (Shan Zha) | 12 g |
| Radix Coptidis prepared with ginger  (Jiang Lian) | 4.5 g |

According to the original records the Radix Panacis Quiquefloii, Bulbus Fritillariae Cirrhosae and Radix Coptidis prepared with ginger should be ground, and the Rhizoma Cyperi should be prepared. The Massa Fermentata Medicinalis and Fructus Aurantii should be roasted and the Fructus Crataegi be roasted until yellow. The above ingredients were well decocted in water. After separating out the herbal residue, the remaining decoction was further concentrated and made in the form of syrup with refined honey.

### Comments

This prescription has the action of nourishing Yin, strengthening the spleen and clearing phlegm. Therapeutically, it bore the combined features of the Jade Syrup (Qiong Yu Gao) and Pill for Strengthening the Spleen (Jian Pi Wan) first recorded in *Standards for Syndrome Differentiation and Treatment* (*Zheng Zhi Zhun Shen*). It was indicated in conditions caused by poor functions of the spleen in transforming and transporting and heat retention in the lung and stomach. The clinical manifestations include excessive fire and lack of body fluid, dry cough, food retention, anorexia, and thirst. The normal condition of the spleen would ensure its regular transforming and transporting so that phlegm could not be formed. And thirst with desire for drinking could be relieved. This prescription was more appropriate for Yin deficiency accompanied by retention of phlegmatic fluid in the aged patients.

## XXX.33. PRESCRIPTION FOR TREATING WIND-COLD TYPE NUMBNESS

Prescription for Treating Wind-Cold Type Numbness (Zhi Feng Han Ma Mu Fang) was worked out by certain imperial physicians, with no information given as to the specific time.

### Ingredients

| | |
|---|---|
| Radix Aconiti  (Chuan Wu) | 18 g |
| Radix Aconiti Kusnezoffii  (Cao Wu) | 18 g |
| Radix et Rhizoma Rhei  (Da Huang) | 18 g |
| Radix Angelicae Sinensis  (Dang Gui) | 24 g |
| Radix Paeoniae Rubra  (Chi Shao) | 24 g |
| Radix Angelicae Dahuricae  (Bai Zhi) | 24 g |
| Fructus Forsythiae  (Lian Qiao) | 24 g |
| Radix Ampelopsis  (Bai Jian) | 24 g |
| Radix Linderae  (Wu Yao) | 24 g |
| Cortex Cinnamomi  (Rou Gui) | 24 g |
| Semen Momordica Cochinchinensis  (Mu Bie Zi) | 24 g |
| Ramulus Prunus Persica  (Tao Tiao) | 12 g |
| Ramulus Salix Babylonica  (Liu Tiao) | 12 g |
| Ramulus Sophorae  (Huai Tiao) | 12 g |

| Ramulus Mori  (Sang Tiao) | 12 g |
| Ramulus Ziziphi Jujuba  (Zao Tiao) | 12 g |

The above ingredients were soaked in one kilogram of sesame oil overnight and fried the following day until the herbal residue became yellow. After separating out the residue by using rice paper, 360 grams of red lead were added. The mixture was further processed until its drops fell like water drops in freezing weather. Then, 12 grams each of Resina Olibani and Resina Murrhae were added. After it was well mixed together, 3 grams of Resina Liguidambar Orientalis were finally added in.

### Comments

Most of the ancient prescriptions proposed for treating numbness due to wind-cold were composed of ingredients of warming property and dispersing actions, and largely based on the therapeutic principle of "using heat-property ingredients in treating cold-natured physical conditions" from *Yellow Emperor's Internal Medicine* (*Huang Di Nei Jing*). The underlying therapeutic priniciple was to stop pain by means of eliminating cold, and relieve numbness by activating the collaterals. What was unique concerning this prescription was the use of ingredients of cold property and bitter flavour, i.e. Radix et Rhizoma Rhei and Radix Ampelopsis for clearing heat. The paradox was that the ingredients for clearing damp-heat here also possessed action of promoting blood circulation and relieving blood stasis. Moreover, the adding of small amounts of cold-property ingredients for counterbalancing in fact enhanced the effect of warming the channels and eliminating cold. All the seemingly contradictory planning of ingredients was actually determined by the dominant syndrome. Also, Radix Angelicae Dahuricae, pungent, warming and drying, was used here to eliminate wind and dampness. Traditionally, it was generally applied in the treatment of headache. It also exhibited good therapeutic effect in the treatment of painful conditions due to invasion of wind-dampness. Such prescriptions demonstrate the rich experience of the imperial physicians.

## XXX.34. PASTE FOR CLEARING WIND AND ACTIVATING COLLATERALS

Paste for Clearing Wind and Activating Collaterals (Qu Feng Huo Luo Gao) was carefully worked out by the imperial physicians Zhuang Shouhe and Yao Baosheng on the 10th day of the seventh month of the lunar calendar, with no information given as to the year.

### Ingredients

| Agkistrodon Acutus  (Bai Hua She) | 1 |
| Scorpio  (Quan Xue) | 15 g |
| Bombyx Batryticatus  (Jiang Can) | 15 g |
| Rhizoma Typhonii Gigantei  (Bai Fu Zi) | 24 g |
| Radix Aconiti  (Chuan Wu) | 15 g |
| Herba Asari  (Xi Xin) | 15 g |
| Rhizoma seu Radix Notopterygii  (Qiang Huo) | 15 g |

| | |
|---|---|
| Herba Siegesbeckiae  (Xi Qian Cao) | 30 g |
| Arisaema cum Bile  (Dan Nan Xing) | 15 g |

The above ingredients were well fried in 750 grams of sesame oil. After separating out the herbal residue, the remaining oil was mixed with an adhesive to make the proper paste. Six grams of powdery Moschus were added when the paste was completely cool.

### Comments

Different from the previous Paste for Activating Blood and Clearing Wind (Huo Xue Qu Feng Gao, XXX. 26), this was mainly formulated for clearing pathogenic wind. Animal or insect ingredients were therefore used as the main ingredients to work deep into the channels and collaterals in search of pathogenic wind. Agkistrodon Acutus, due to its medicinal effect characterized by moving *qi* in channels, was applied for the various types of wind conditions. It was also used as a guiding drug to lead the herbal effect to the affected areas of the skin in order to treat wind conditions. As snakes like to eat photinia and live in underground holes with dirt and dampness, they possess poisonous and unhealthy properties that later become good for healing purposes. Being used as the prinicipal ingredient, it was believed to have the effect of searching wind from bones and tranquilizing patients from fright. Rhizoma Typhonii Gigantei and Radix Aconiti were used for clearing wind-cold and stopping pain. All other ingredients had the effect of clearing or subduing wind. TCM classics say that wind is characterized by constant moving and changes, and wind factor communicates with the liver. Most ingredients for clearing wind activate collaterals and promote blood circulation. It would be a misnomer for the remedy to be called Paste for Clearing Wind and Activating Collaterals. According to Qing Dynasty medical archives, Empress Dowager Cixi often received external application of the paste.

## XXX.35.  PASTE FOR SOOTHING TENDONS AND ACTIVATING COLLATERALS

Paste for Soothing Tendons and Activating Collaterals (Shu Jin Huo Luo Gao) was carefully prepared for Empress Dowager Cixi by the imperial physician Zhang Zhongyuan on the 24th day of the second month of the lunar calendar, with no information given as to the year.

### Ingredients

| | |
|---|---|
| Spica Prunellae  (Xia Ku Cao) | 9 g |
| Caulis Spatholobi  (Ji Xue Teng) | 15 g |
| Radix Tinosporae  (Jin Guo Lan) | 9 g |
| Cordyceps  (Dong Cong Xia Cao) | 12 g |
| Flos Lonicerae  (Jin Yin Hua) | 18 g |
| Fructus Forsythiae  (Lian Qiao) | 15 g |
| Ramulus Loranthi  (Sang Ji Sheng) | 18 g |
| Herba Erodii seu Geranii  (Lao Guan Cao) | 15 g |
| Resina Murrhae  (Mo Yao) | 9 g |
| Caulis Piperis Futokadurae  (Hai Feng Teng) | 9 g |

| | |
|---|---|
| Radix Angelicae Sinensis  (Dang Gui) | 12 g |
| Radix Paeoniae Lactiflorae  (Bai Shao) | 9 g |
| Rhizoma Ligustici Chuanxiong  (Chuan Xiong) | 6 g |
| Radix Rehmanniae  (Sheng Di Huang) | 9 g |
| Rhizoma seu Radix Notopterygii  (Qiang Huo) | 9 g |
| Radix Clematis  (Wei Ling Xian) | 9 g |
| Radix Angelicae Pubescentis  (Du Huo) | 9 g |
| Fructus Chaenomelis  (Mu Gua) | 9 g |
| Pericarpium Citri Reticulatae Rubra  (Ju Hong) | 9 g |
| Radix Curcumae  (Yu Jin) | 9 g |
| Rhizoma Pinelliae  (Ban Xia) | 9 g |
| Radix Glycyrrhizae  (Gan Cao) | 6 g |
| Moschus  (She Xiang) | 3 g |

The original directions require the Radix Curcumae to be ground before use. Powdery Moschus should be added later during processing. All the above ingredients were well fried in 1.5 kilograms of sesame oil. After separating out the herbal residue, the remaining oil was mixed with one kilogram of red lead to make the proper paste.

### Comments

This is a comprehensive prescription. Ingredients forming the Four Substances Decoction (Si Wu Tang) were used for nourishing blood. Ingredients for clearing wind were applied here for the purpose of soothing the liver. Those normally for nourishing Yin were used here for nourishing the liver. Ramulus ingredients were used for activating collaterals. Moschus, pungent and wondering, was applied for searching wind. The combined use of all these ingredients could heal the syndrome characterized by obstruction in the channels and collaterals. According to the health record of Empress Dowager Cixi, she often received the external application of the paste for her chronic facial spasm, which use was not contraindicated in chronic facial spasm.

## XXX.36.  PASTE FOR SOOTHING TENDONS AND ACTIVATING COLLATERALS PLUS

An imperial edict was delivered to Longevity Pharmacy to prepare one dose of Paste for Soothing Tendons and Activating Collaterals (Shu Jin Huo Luo Gao) on the 22nd day of the eighth month of the lunar calendar, with no information given as to the year.

### Ingredients

| | |
|---|---|
| Radix Angelicae Sinensis  (Dang Gui) | 15 g |
| Radix Paeoniae Rubra  (Chi Shao) | 12 g |
| Fructus Chaenomelis  (Mu Gua) | 18 g |
| Spica Prunellae  (Xia Ku Cao) | 18 g |
| Radix Bistortae  (Cao He Che) | 15 g |
| Resina Olibani  (Ru Xiang) | 12 g |
| Radix Tinosporae  (Jin Guo Lan) | 15 g |
| Arisaema cum Bile  (Dan Nan Xing) | 12 g |

| | |
|---|---|
| Radix Achyranthis Bidentatae  (Niu Xi) | 18 g |
| Flos Carthami  (Hong Hua) | 12 g |
| Bombyx Batryticatus  (Jiang Can) | 12 g |
| Rhizoma seu Radix Notopterygii  (Qiang Huo) | 15 g |
| Rhizoma Curcumae Longae  (Jiang Huang) | 12 g |
| Ramulus Cinnamomi  (Gui Zhi) | 18 g |
| Squama Manitis  (Chuan Shan Jia) | 12 g |
| Moschus  (She Xiang) | 3 g |

The original records say the Rhizoma Curcumae Longae should be sliced before use. Moschus was used only with special permission and was added last. The above ingredients were well fried in two kilograms of sesame oil. After separating out the herbal residue, the remaining oil was further concentrated until its drops fell like water drops in freezing weather. It was then mixed with 600 grams of red lead to make the proper paste. Moschus was added when the paste became completely cold. The ready paste was applied externally to the affected areas of the body.

### Comments

This prescription differed from the previous one in that Ramulus ingredients and those for nourishing blood and Yin were omitted and replaced by Flos Carthami, Radix Achyranthis Bidentatae, Bombyx Batryticatus, sliced Rhizoma Curcumae Longae, Ramulus Cinnamomi and Squama Manitis for activating blood, quelling wind and regulating channels and collaterals. Those with the strongest effect in quelling wind were Squama Manitis and Bombyx Batryticatus. It was again clear that the prescription was prepared in view of the chronic facial spasm of Empress Dowager Cixi.

## XXX.37.  FORMULA FOR TIGER BONE AND BEAR OIL PASTE

Formula for Tiger Bone and Bear Oil Paste (Xiong You Hu Gu Gao Pei Fang) was formulated with no record of the date.

### Ingredients

| | |
|---|---|
| Radix Polugomi Multifori  (He Shou Wu) | 15 g |
| Radix Aconiti Kusneziffii  (Cao Wu) | 15 g |
| Meretrix  (Wen Ge) | 15 g |
| Radix Dipsaci  (Xu Duan) | 15 g |
| Radix et Rhizoma Rhei  (Da Huang) | 15 g |
| Fructus Aurantii  (Zhi Ke) | 15 g |
| Fructus Gardeniae  (Zhi Zi) | 15 g |
| Radix Aconiti  (Chuan Wu) | 15 g |
| Rhizoma seu Radix Notopterygii  (Qiang Huo) | 15 g |
| Semen Persicae  (Tao Ren) | 15 g |
| Radix Sophorae Flavescentis  (Ku Shen) | 15 g |
| Radix Scutellariae  (Huang Qin) | 15 g |
| Herba Leonuri  (Yi Mu Cao) | 15 g |
| Caulis Piperis Futokadurae  (Hai Feng Teng) | 15 g |
| Cortex Dictamni Dasycarpi Radicis  (Bai Xian Pi) | 15 g |

Radix Clematis  (Wei Ling Xian)                                    15 g
Radix Scrophulariae  (Xuan Shen)                                   15 g
Radix Angelicae Dahuricae  (Bai Zhi)                               15 g
Herba Schizonepetae  (Jing Jie)                                    15 g
Pericarpium Citri Reticulatae Viride  (Qing Pi)                    15 g
Radix Rehmanniae  (Sheng Di Huang)                                 15 g
Rhizoma Ligustici  (Hao Ben)                                       15 g
Rhizoma Atractylodis  (Cang Zhu)                                   15 g
Flos Genkwa  (Yuan Hua)                                            15 g
Flos Lonicerae  (Jin Yin Hua)                                      15 g
Rhizoma Alpiniae Officinalis  (Gao Liang Jiang)                    15 g
Herba Artemisiae Capillaris  (Yin Chen)                            15 g
Herba Ephedrae  (Ma Huang)                                         15 g
Cortex Fraxini  (Qin Pi)                                           15 g
Radix Peucedani  (Qian Hu)                                         15 g
Radix Glycyrrhizae  (Gan Cao)                                      15 g
Cortex Phellodendri  (Huang Bai)                                   15 g
Rhizoma Anemarrhenae  (Zhi Mu)                                     15 g
Radix Linderae  (Wu Yao)                                           15 g
Squama Manitis  (Chuan Shan Jia)                                   15 g
Radix Achyranthis Bidentatae  (Niu Xi)                             15 g
Fructus Tribuli  (Ji Li)                                           15 g
Cortex Eucommiae  (Du Zhong)                                       15 g
Radix Polygale  (Yuan Zhi)                                         15 g
Herba Menthae  (Bo He)                                             15 g
Rhizoma Cimicifugae  (Sheng Ma)                                    15 g
Radix Ledebouriellae  (Fang Feng)                                  15 g
Semen Armenicacae  (Xin Ren)                                       15 g
Rhizoma Dio  (Shen Yao)                                            15 g
Rhizoma Alismatis  (Ze Xie)                                        15 g
Radix Angelicae Sinensis  (Dang Gui)                               15 g
Bulbus Fritillariae Cirhosae  (Bei Mu)                             15 g
Fructus Xanthii  (Cang Er Zi)                                      15 g
Rhizoma Cyperi  (Xiang Fu)                                         15 g
Radix Sanguisorbsae  (Di Yu)                                       15 g
Pericarpium Citri Reticulatae  (Chen Pi)                           15 g
Rhizoma Atractylodis Macrocephalae  (Bai Zhu)                      15 g
Arisaema cum Bile  (Dan Nan Xing)                                  15 g
Fructus Forsythiae  (Lian Qiao)                                    15 g
Rhizoma Coptidis  (Huang Lian)                                     15 g
Rhizoma Bletillae Striatae  (Bai Ji)                               15 g
Radix Angelicae Pubscentis  (Du Huo)                               15 g
Radix Paeoniae Lactiflorae  (Bai Shao)                             15 g
Semen Hydnocarpi  (Da feng Zi)                                     15 g
Radix Bupleuri  (Chai Hu)                                          15 g
Radix Platycodi  (Jie Geng)                                        15 g
Os Ursi  (Xiong Gu)                                               240 g
Os Tigris  (Hu Gu)                                                500 g
Ramulus Lorathi  (Shang Ji Sheng)                                   6 g

| | |
|---|---|
| Rhizoma Gastrodiae  (Tian Ma) | 30 g |
| Flos Carthami  (Hong Hua) | 30 g |
| Ramulus Prunus Persica  (Tao Tiao) | 5 |
| Ramulus Salix Babylonica  (Liu Tiao) | 5 |
| Ramulus Ulmus Pumila  (Yu Tiao) | 5 |
| Ramulus Sophorae  (Huai Tiao) | 5 |

The above ingredients were well fried in five kilograms of sesame oil. After separating out the herbal residue, the remaining oil was mixed with 2.5 kilograms of red lead to make the paste, to which were added 7.5 grams of Moschus, 7.5 grams of Borneoleum Syntheticum, 30 grams of Cortex Cinnamomi, 30 grams of Flos Caryophylli, 3 grams of melted Resina Draconis, 3 grams of Resina Olibani and 3 grams of Resina Murrhae.

### Comments

This prescription consists of a much greater number of ingredients in a wider range of categories than the last two. However, the main actions of the prescriptions are reinforcing the kidney, strengthening tendons and bones, activating blood circulation, resolving dampness and eliminating wind. It was believed the imperial formula for Tiger Bone and Bear Oil Paste (Hu Gu Xiong You Gao) was based on this one. The utensil for processing the Tiger Bone and Bear Oil Paste (Xiong You Hu Gu Gao) for Empress Dowager Cixi remains preserved by the Administrative Office for Unearthed Objects for exhibition at the Eastern Tombs where Empress Dowager Cixi was buried.

## XXX.38. FORMULA FOR TIGER BONE AND BEAR OIL PASTE PLUS

Formula for Tiger Bone and Bear Oil Paste Plus (Xiong You Hu Gu Gao You Fang) was carefully worked out by the imperial physicians Zhuang Shouhe and Li Dechang on the 22nd day of the 11th month of the lunar calendar in 1881.

### Ingredients

| | |
|---|---|
| Os Tigris  (Hu Gu) | 1 set |
| Cortex Cinnamomi  (Rou Gui) | 90 g |
| Resina Murrhae  (Mo Yao) | 150 g |
| Resina Olibani  (Ru Xiang) | 180 g |
| Radix Angelicae Sinensis  (Dang Gui) | 240 g |
| Crinis Carbonisatus  (Xue Yu) | 120 g |
| Oleum Ursi  (Xiong You) | 150 g |
| Sesame oil  (Xiang You) | 7.5 kg |
| Red lead  (Zhang Dan) | 3.75 kg |

According to the original records the Os Tigris should be soaked in water for seven days after which one day was spent cleaning the remaining meat on the bones. The bones were then dried in the sun for another day. This was followed by roasting the bones for two days. When they became crisp, the Radix Angelicae Sinensis and Crinis Carbonisatus were added to be roasted together with the tiger bones. After separating out the mixed residue, the remaining oily substance was mixed with Oleum Ursi for further concentration. When it was ready, the red lead was added to make the proper paste. The last procedure was to mix powdered Cortex Cinnamomi, Resina Olibani and Resina Murrhae into the paste.

### Comments

The prescription has the action of dispelling wind, consolidating the exterior of the body, activating blood and relieving pain. It was applied in Bi or Wei syndrome related to pathogenic wind-cold.

## XXX.39. MODIFIED FORMULA FOR TIGER BONE AND BEAR OIL PASTE

Modified Formula for Tiger Bone and Bear Oil Paste (Xiong You Hu Gu Gao Jia Jian Fang) was carefully prepared by the imperial physicians Zhuang Shouhe, Li Dechang and Dong Wenbin on the 11th day of the second month of the lunar calendar in 1883.

### Ingredients

| | |
|---|---|
| Os Tigris  (Hu Gu) | 1 set |
| Cortex Cinnamomi  (Rou Gui) | 90 g |
| Resina Olibani  (Ru Xiang) | 180 g |
| Resina Murrhae  (Mo Yao) | 150 g |
| Radix Angelicae Sinensis  (Dang Gui) | 240 g |
| Crinis Carbonisatus  (Xue Yu) | 120 g |
| Oleum Ursi  (Xiong You) | 150 g |
| Sesame oil  (Xiang You) | 7.5 kg |
| Red lead  (Zhang Dan) | 3.75 kg |
| Cortex Eucommiae  (Du Zhong) | 120 g |
| Rhizoma Cibotii  (Jin Mao Gou) | 120 g |
| Radix Morindae Officinalis  (Bai Ji Tian) | 90 g |
| Radix Dipsaci  (Xu Duan) | 120 g |
| Radix Angelicae Pubscentis  (Du Huo) | 90 g |

The preparation method was the same as above.

### Comments

This prescription was formed on the basis of Tiger Bone and Bear Oil Paste (Xiong You Hu Gu Gao) by adding Cortex Eucommiae, Rhizoma Cibotii, Radix Morindae Officinalis, Radix Dipsaci and Radix Angelicae Pubscentis for reinforcing the kidney. It showed remarkable effects in Wei syndrome of the bones and wind Bi syndrome due to kidney deficiency.

## XXX.40. NINE-*QI*-CAUSED PAIN RELIEVING PILL

Nine-*qi*-caused Pain Relieving Pill (Jiu Qi Nian Tong Fang) was formulated without information concerning the time.

### Ingredients

| | |
|---|---|
| Radix Angelicae Sinensis  (Dang Gui) | 120 g |
| Rhizoma Alpiniae Officinalis  (Gao Liang Jiang) | 120 g |
| Faeces Trogopterorum  (Wu Ling Zhi) | 120 g |

| | |
|---|---|
| Rhizoma Zedoariae  (E Zhu) | 120 g |
| Semen Arecae  (Bing Lang) | 120 g |
| Pericarpium Citri Reticulatae Viride  (Qing Pi) | 120 g |
| Rhizoma Corydalis  (Yuan Hu Suo) | 60 g |
| Radix Curcumae  (Yu Jin) | 60 g |
| Radix Auchlandiae  (Mu Xiang) | 60 g |
| Pericarpium Citri Reticulatae  (Chen Pi) | 60 g |
| Rhizoma Curcumae Longae  (Jiang Huang) | 60 g |
| Rhizoma Cyperi  (Xiang Fu) | 150 g |
| Radix Glycyrrhizae  (Gan Cao) | 45 g |

The above ingredients were processed into fine powder and mixed with vinegar to make the pills.

### Comments

Statements related to diseases or disorders caused by the nine types of *qi* date back to the chapter on pain in *Plain Questions* (*Su Wen*·"Ju Tong Lun"). This prescription was based on that recorded in *A Collection of Secret Prescriptions of Lu's Mansion* (*Lu Shi Jin Fang*) with modifications. It acts to regulate *qi* and stop pain, applicable to the various kinds of pain in the heart and epigastric region due to poor mechanism of *qi*. TCM holds that stagnation of *qi* gives rise to stasis of blood. It was for this reason that Radix Angelicae Sinensis, Faeces Trogopterorum and Rhizoma Corydalis were applied to assist the principal ingredients, i.e. those for regulating *qi*. According to Qing Dynasty imperial medical archives Nine-*qi*-caused Pain Relieving Pill was widely used, hinting at its proved therapeutic effects.

## XXX.41. PRESCRIPTION FOR UNIVERSAL BENEFIT PILL FOR DETOXIFICATION

Prescription for Universal Benefit Pill for Detoxification (Pu Ji Jie Wen Wan Fang) was formulated by the imperial physicians, with no information given concerning the specific date.

### Ingredients

| | |
|---|---|
| Herba Schizonepetae  (Jing Jie) | 120 g |
| Radix Scrophulariae  (Xuan Shen) | 240 g |
| Folium Isatidis  (Da Qing Ye) | 120 g |
| Fructus Arctii  (Niu Bang Zi) | 120 g |
| Radix Platycodi  (Jie Geng) | 120 g |
| Bombyx Batryticatus  (Jiang Can) | 120 g |
| Fructus Forsythiae  (Lian Qiao) | 150 g |
| Herba Menthae  (Bo He) | 90 g |
| Lasiophaera seu Calvatia  (Ma Bo) | 120 g |
| Flos Lonicerae  (Jin Yin Hua) | 150 g |
| Radix Sophorae Subprostratae  (Shan Dou Gen) | 120 g |
| Radix Glycyrrhizae  (Gan Cao) | 60 g |
| Radix Rehmanniae  (Sheng Di Huang) | 240 g |
| Radix Scutellariae  (Huang Qin) | 150 g |

Cortex Moudan Radicis  (Mu Dan Pi)                                    120 g

The original records say that the Bombyx Batryticatus should be roasted and the Cortex Moudan Radicis should be used without cores. The above ingredients were processed into fine powder and made into honey pills weighing nine grams each.

### Comments

This prescription was modified on the basis of the Universal Benefit Decoction for Detoxification (Pu Ji Xiao Du Yin) initiated by Li Dongyuan. Compared with another Universal Benefit Decoction for Detoxification (Pu Ji Xiao Du Yin) recorded in *Treatise on Differentiation and Treatments of Epidemic Febrile Diseases* (*Wen Bing Tiao Bian Lun*) with omission of Radix Bupleuri and Rhizoma Cimicifugae for sore throat caused by virulent pathogenic factors, this prescription offers stronger effect in clearing epidemic toxins. The therapeutic effect of nourishing Yin was also maintained in the process of clearing the toxins. Therapeutic results could be expected if it was applied in treating sore throat, retroauricular and preauricular pain, and swollen cheeks and infection with swelling in the head.

# XXX.42.  BOIL-INCLUSIVE EXTERNAL LOZENGE

Boil-inclusive External Lozenge (Qing Yu Ding) from *A Collection of Recommended Prescriptions* (*Liang Fang Ji Cheng*) was recorded in the imperial medical archives without any specific date.

### Ingredients

| | |
|---|---|
| Radix Cynanchi Atrati  (Bai Wei) | 30 g |
| Arisaema cum Bile  (Dan Nan Xing) | 30 g |
| Rhizoma Belancandae  (She Gan) | 30 g |
| Herba Asari  (Xi Xin) | 30 g |
| Radix Ledebouriellae  (Fang Feng) | 30 g |
| Rhizoma Alismatis  (Ze Xie) | 30 g |
| Rhizoma Coptidis  (Huang Lian) | 30 g |
| Radix Angelicae Dahuricae  (Bai Zhi) | 60 g |
| Scorpio  (Quan Xie) | 60 g |
| Venenum Bufonis  (Chan Su) | 60 g |
| Resina Draconis  (Xue Jie) | 60 g |
| Radix et Rhizoma Rhei  (Da Huang) | 60 g |
| Flos Lonicerae  (Jin Yin Hua) | 60 g |
| Caulis Akebiae  (Mu Tong) | 60 g |
| Fructus Gardeniae  (Zhi Zi) | 60 g |
| Spina Gleditsiae  (Ya Zao) | 60 g |
| Realgar  (Xiong Huang) | 120 g |
| Squama Manitis  (Chuan Shan Jia) | 75 g |
| Borneolum Syntheticum  (Bing Pian) | 1.5 g |
| Moschus  (She Xiang) | 0.9 g |
| Glycyrrhizae Uralensis Fish  (Gan Cao Shao) | 15 g |
| Flos Mume Albus  (Bai Mei Hua) | 90 g |
| Semen Oryzae Glutinosae  (Jiang Mi) | 120 g |

According to the original records, the Squama Manitis should be prepared before use. The Semen Oryzae Glutinosae should be used separately to make rice paste. The above ingredients were processed into fine powder together with Fructus Chaenomelis that was prepared with millet wine and made in the form of external lozenge of three grams each.

### Comments

The prescription was mainly made up of ingredients for clearing toxic heat. They were further assisted by the use of other ingredients for eliminating wind and dampness, activating blood, removing obstruction from channels and collaterals, cooling blood and stopping bleeding. It is applicable to the various sorts of boils, carbuncles and furuncles, insect bites as well as hemorrhoids. Referring to the case history of Empress Dowager Cixi, it should have been formulated for the treatment of her hemorrhoids and bloody stools. The nomenclature of the prescription means literally a lozenge for clearing fish mouth, or rather for clearing superficial ulcer shaped like fish mouth. According to old traditional Chinese medical jargon, so-called fish mouth referred to oozing ulcer in the inguinal groove. The ulcer would close when the body flexed and open when the body extended, thus acquiring the name fish-mouth ulcer. The truth is that it was most likely applied here for her diabrotic hemorrhoids. Imperial physicians made the lozenge for external application for that purpose. It not only cleared toxic heat, but it also cooled the blood and stopped bleeding. It is a pity that there was no written record about its actual use, as it would be difficult to predict now whether it was effective or not.

## XXX.43. TOXIN-ERADICATING EXTERNAL LOZENGE

The prescription for Toxin-eradicating External Lozenge (Ba Du Ding) from *A Collection of Recommended Prescriptions* (*Liang Fang Ji Cheng*) was presented without any specific date.

### Ingredients

| | |
|---|---|
| Rhizoma Bletillae Striatae (Bai Ji) | 30 g |
| Radix Ampelopsis (Bai Lian) | 30 g |
| Arisaema cum Bile (Dan Nan Xing) | 60 g |
| Spina Gleditsiae (Ya Zao) | 45 g |
| Radix Trichosanthis (Tian Hua Fen) | 45 g |
| Rhizoma Belamcadae (She Gan) | 45 g |
| Radix Angelicae Dahuricae (Bai Zhi) | 60 g |
| Scorpio (Quan Xue) | 90 g |
| Realgar (Xiong Huang) | 15 g |
| Squama Manitis (Chuan Shan Jia) | 75 g |
| Venenum Bufonis (Chan Su) | 30 g |
| Resina Draconis (Xue Jie) | 60 g |
| Borneolum Syntheticum (Bing Pian) | 1.5 g |
| Moschus (She Xiang) | 0.9 g |
| Herba Asari (Xi Xin) | 30 g |
| Radix et Rhizoma Rhei (Da Huang) | 60 g |
| Caulis Akebiae (Mu Tong) | 30 g |

| | |
|---|---|
| Rhizoma Coptidis  (Huang Lian) | 60 g |
| Fructus Gardeniae  (Zhi Zi) | 60 g |
| Flos Lonicerae  (E Bao Hua) | 60 g |
| Radix Ledebouriellae  (Fang Feng) | 30 g |
| Rhizoma Alismatis  (Ze Xie) | 30 g |
| Glycyrrhiza Uralensis Fish  (Gan Cao Shao) | 1.5 g |
| Flos Mume Albus  (Bai Mei Hua) | 90 g |
| Resina Olibani  (Ru Xiang) | 60 g |
| Resina Murrhae  (Mo Yao) | 60 g |
| Semen Oryzae Glutinosae  (Jiang Mi) | 120 g |

The original records require that the Squama Manitis should be prepared before use. The Fructus Gardeniae should be roasted and the Semen Oryzae Glutinosae ground into fine powder and made separately into rice paste. The above ingredients were processed into fine powder and made in the form of lozenge weighing three grams each, together with Fructus Chaenomelis prepared with millet wine.

*Comments*

Toxin-eradicating External Lozenge, a highly recommended remedy for detoxifying, clearing purulence and stopping pain, is applicable in all kinds of boils, carbuncles and furuncles. A large number of ingredients in the prescription have the action of clearing toxic heat and purulence and promoting the growth of muscle. It is generally suitable for boils due to excessive toxic fire. Caution must be taken should patients with skin boils already have deficiency of antipathogenic *qi*.

## XXX.44. WATER PALACE EXTERNAL LOZENGE

The prescription for Water Palace External Lozenge (Kan Gong Ding) from *A Collection of Recommended Prescriptions* (*Liang Fang Ji Cheng*) was presented with no information concerning the specific time.

*Ingredients*

| | |
|---|---|
| Old ink  (Gu Mo) | 30 g |
| Rhizoma Picrorhizae  (Hu Huang Lian) | 6 g |
| Fel Ursi  (Xiong Dan) | 9 g |
| Moschus  (She Xiang) | 1.5 g |
| Acacia Catechu  (Er Cha) | 6 g |
| Borneolum Syntheticum  (Bing Pian) | 2.1 g |
| Calculus Bovis  (Niu Huang) | 0.9 g |

The above ingredients were ground into powder and mixed with mainly pig bile and a small amount of ginger juice, rhubarb infusion and concentrated vinegar to make 1.5-gram lozenges. The lozenge was ground in water and applied externally with a brush to the local lesions.

*Comments*

Water Palace External Lozenge, a very effective external application, was applied for various boils in their early stage as manifested by local erythema, swelling and pain, for erysipelas due to severe damp-heat, and for nameless, inflammatory swellings. Its external application is also suitable for hemorrhoids, for instance, for a patient complaining of severe pain due to hemorrhoids, three to five external applications in the local area being capable of completely relieving the pain. It was very appropriate for Empress Dowager Cixi because she often suffered from fistulae and hemafecia due to hemorrhoids.

The external lozenge was originally named after one of the branches of the Chinese Eight Trigrams. Water corresponds to the branch of the Eight Trigrams, known as Kan in Chinese pronunciation. Located in the north, it dominates water and corresponds to the kidney. *Plain Questions* (*Su Wen*) says, "The kidney is in charge of defecation and urination." It should therefore be effective for use in treating fistulae. By analyzing the herbal properties of the ingredients, cold property ingredients were used to clear heat, namely using water to subdue fire. This is one of the therapeutic principles often applied in traditional Chinese medicine. Its nomenclature implies that the application of the remedy would help its actions in alleviating heat, cooling blood, resolving purulent masses and relieving swelling.

## XXX.45.  FIRE PALACE EXTERNAL LOZENGE

The prescription for Fire Palace External Lozenge (Li Gong Ding) from *A Collection of Recommended Prescriptions* (*Liang Fang Ji Cheng*) was presented without any information concerning the specific time.

*Ingredients*

| | |
|---|---|
| Resina Draconis  (Xue Jie) | 9 g |
| Cinnabari  (Zhu Sha) | 6 g |
| Chalcanthitum  (Dan Fan) | 9 g |
| Old ink  (Gu Mo) | 30 g |
| Venenum Bufonis  (Chan Su) | 9 g |
| Moschus  (She Xiang) | 4.5 g |

The above ingredients were ground into powder and made into the form of water-bound lozenge of 1.5 grams each, coated with Cinnabari for external application.

*Comments*

Fire Palace External Lozenge was applied in the treatment of a very severe type of boils in the initial stage marked by erythema and swelling without apparent abscess. Some might be taken as malignant growth nowadays. It was also applied for furuncles, scabies, acute pyogenic infections of the perineum and carbuncles resulting from toxic heat invasion. It was also indicated in insect or animal bites. Regarding the Eight Trigrams in association with the nomenclature of the remedy as Fire Palace External Lozenge (Li Gong Ding), fire corresponds to Li in the Eight Trigrams. Li is located in the south. Fire corresponds to the heart. *Plain Questions* says, "The onset of possible boils or carbuncles is related to fire in the heart channel." This external lozenge can thus be applied to various types of boils or ulcer due to pathogenic heat or fire.

## XXX.46.  INSTANT MEASLES PRESCRIPTION

An imperial edict was passed to Longevity Pharmacy to prepare six doses of Instant Measles Prescription (Ling Ying Sha Yao Fang) on the 14th day of the fifth month of the lunar calendar, with no information given as to the year.

### Ingredients

| | |
|---|---:|
| Rhizoma Atractylodis  (Cang Zhu) | 1.12 kg |
| Radix et Rhizoma Rhei  (Da Huang) | 3 kg |
| Flos Caryophylli  (Ding Xiang) | 216 g |
| Rhizoma Gastrodiae  (Tian Ma) | 576 g |
| Herba Ephedrae  (Ma Huang) | 1.2 kg |
| Cinnabari  (Zhu Sha) | 3 kg |
| Venenum Bufonis  (Chan Su) | 162 g |
| Moschus  (She Xiang) | 180 g |
| Radix Glycyrrhizae  (Gan Cao) | 884 g |

The original records state that special permission was required for using Moschus. The above ingredients were processed in fine powder to be made as Cinnabari-coated pills.

### Comments

Instant Measles Prescription was formed on the basis of Enriching Pill for Emergencies (Bei Ji Wan) from *Empirical Prescriptions of Huizhi Mansion* (*Hui Zhi Tang Jing Yan Fang*). It is indicated in sunstroke manifested by coma, vomiting, diarrhea, colicky abdominal pain and acute measles. Because of its wide range of indications, it was used as patent medicine for emergency cases in the imperial palace. Empress Dowager Cixi often took it in summer. The administration of the pill in the imperial palace varied according to different conditions. For sunstroke with manifestations of dizziness and vertigo, colicky abdominal pain, coma and measles, two pills were first ground into the powder and blown into nose. Then, six pills were taken with mixed well and river water, or just cold water. For sudden onset of abdominal pain, muscular spasm due to direct attack of pathogenic cold, or cholera with cold hands and feet, unproductive vomiting and diarrhea due to dry cholera, the above-mentioned administration of the pills was simply repeated. For elimination of filthy pathogenic factors, three pills were chewed in the mouth so that pathogenic heat could not invade the body. For the treatment of various boils or insect bites, the pills were processed into powder and mixed with top-quality alcohol for local rubbing. For infantile undeveloped smallpox manifested by fullness and suffocating appearance, and windstroke in aged patients due to wind-phlegm, the pills were taken orally together with Medulla Junci Effuci soup or cold water. For acute infantile convulsion with locked jaws, four to five pills were ground into powder for blowing into the nose. In the meantime, soup prepared with the pills was taken orally in order to resuscitate the patient. For sudden loss of consciousness, powder ground from the pill was blown into the nose or taken orally and would hopefully resuscitate the patient. Although it was a remedy largely proposed for the treatment of measles, it did cover a wide range of indications and could therefore be justifiably called Instant Resuscitating Pill.

## XXX.47.  THREE-YELLOW WAX-COATED PILL

One dose of Three-yellow Wax-coated Pill (San Huang Bao La Wan) was prescribed with no information given as to the time.

### Ingredients

| | |
|---|---|
| Resina Garciniae  (Teng Huang) | 60 g |
| Concretio Silicea Bambusae  (Tian Zhu Huang) | 60 g |
| Radix Euphorbiae Pekinensis  (Da Ji) | 30 g |
| Radix Angelicae Sinensis  (Dang Gui) | 30 g |
| Calculus Bovis  (Nie Huang) | 30 g |
| Herba Artemisia Anomala  (Liu Ji Lu) | 30 g |
| Moschus  (She Xiang) | 30 g |
| Succinum  (Hu Po) | 30 g |
| Realgar  (Xiong Huang) | 15 g |
| Resina Draconis  (Xue Jie) | 15 g |
| Acacia Catechu  (Er Cha) | 15 g |
| Resina Olibani  (Ru Xiang) | 15 g |
| Borneolum Syntheticum  (Bing Pian) | 15 g |
| Hydragyrum  (Shui Yin) | 15 g |

The above ingredients were processed into fine powder and mixed with 360 grams of yellow bees wax to make pills of three grams each.

### Comments

The prescription for Three-yellow Wax-coated Pill originated from *Golden Mirror of Medical Tradition* (*Yi Zong Jin Jian*). Its nomenclature was associated with Resina Garciniae, Concretio Silicea Bambusae and Realgar, because each of these ingredients bears the pronunciation of yellow in Chinese. Due to its actions in eliminating stasis, generating new muscle, stopping pain, resolving phlegm and clearing boils, it has always been regarded as an important patent medicine in TCM surgery. The pill can be prescribed for both oral administration and external application. Externally, it could be mixed with sesame oil and applied in various types of boils by spreading the mixture with a feather. The medicine should be kept away from fire. Internally, it was applied for clearing stubborn sputum, reserving vital energy, dissolving toxins, activating channels and collaterals, restoring bones and tendons and removing blood stasis. It is also indicated in traumatic injuries, lumbar sprain, over-strain or tetanus, or amenorrhea, retention of placenta, hemiplegia or even malignant boils. However, in the initial course of the treatment, intake of cold or raw food, fruits, strong alcoholic drinks or any food that might induce attacks of old diseases should be avoided. This prescription was formed out of profound technical considerations and was highly valued in the imperial palace. Empress Dowager Cixi sometimes granted permission to use the medicine for imperial ministers besides using it herself.

# XXX.48.  MIGHTY PILL

An imperial edict was passed to Longevity Pharmacy to prepare one dose of Mighty Pill (Wu Wei Wan), also known as Glowworm Pill (Ying Huo Wan) on the sixth day of the seventh month of the lunar calendar, with no information given as to the year.

### Ingredients

| | |
|---|---|
| Luciola Vitticollis  (Ying Huo Chong) | 30 g |
| Herba Huchnera Cruciata  (Gui Jian Yu) | 30 g |
| Fructus Tribuli  (Ci Ji Li) | 30 g |
| Realgar  (Xiong Huang) | 60 g |
| Auripigmentum  (Ci Huang) | 60 g |
| Cornu Antelopis  (Ling Yang Jiao) | 45 g |
| Chlorite  (Meng Shi) | 60 g |
| Iron Hammer Handle  (Tie Chui Bing) | 45 g |

According to the original records, the Cornu Antelopis and Chlorite should be calcined. The part of the iron hammer handle wrapped by iron should be burnt. The above ingredients were ground into fine powder and mixed with a proper amount of red lead, eggs and a piece of cockscomb. They were mashed and ground into fine particles and made into pills the size of almonds. Five pills were placed in a red triangular silk bag to be worn on the right arm to guard against evil factors. For those who served in the army, the small bag should be worn in the lumbar region. For those living at home, the bag could be hung at the top of the door. Miraculous effects were believed to result.

### Comments

There is a legend about Mighty Pill that in the Han Dynasty (206 BC-AD 220) there was a very famous army commander whose name was Liu Zinan, leading a large number of troops fighting against Mongols on the frontier. During one of the battles in the 12th year of the Ever Peace Era, he was wearing a Mighty Pill bag on the battlefield when enemy arrows were flying at him like heavy rain. Instead of knocking him down, the arrows all dropped to the ground in front of his horse. The Mongols found it magic. Later on, when Liu's followers were also wearing this kind of bag to fight against enemy troops, nobody was ever injured. The medicine was believed to have the effect of avoiding tragedy. As to the actions of the ingredients included in the bag, it was found that Herba Huchnera Cruciata, Realgar, Auripigmentum and Iron Hammer Handle all had the effect of clearing toxic heat, refreshing the mind and bringing resuscitation. According to *Comprehensive Discussion on Febrile Disease* (*Shang Han Zong Bing Lun*) by Pang Anshi, Mighty Pill was applied for wiping out epidemic diseases and preventing their spreading. Apparently, the effect of the medicine in turning down shooting arrows was a fairy tale by Commander Liu Zinan's admirers. Empress Dowager Cixi used it in the seventh month of the lunar calendar in 1895 for the purpose of clearing summer heat.

## XXX.49. BLETILLAE STRIATAE EXTERNAL LOZENGE

The prescription for Bletillae Striatae External Lozenge (Bai Ding Zi) from *A Collection of Recommended Prescriptions* (*Liang Fang Ji Cheng*) was presented for Empress Dowager Cixi with no information as to the time.

### Ingredients

| | |
|---|---|
| Bai Jiang Dan (patent powder) 12 g | |
| Silver powder (Yin You) | 6 g |
| Calcitum (Han Shui Shi) | 6 g |
| Human urine sendiment (Ren Zhong Bai) | 6 g |

The above ingredients were prepared in fine powder and mixed with Bletillae Striatae paste to make external lozenges of the usual size. It is not for oral administration. The lozenge was normally mixed with old vinegar and spread on the affected parts of the body with a feather brush. Further spreading of the medicine would not be done until the applied areas became dry. It was believed to have the effect of resolving toxins.

### Comments

All four ingredients were white in colour. They were made in the form of lozenges with Bletillae Striatae. Thus, in Chinese, it was called the white lozenge. Bai Jiang Dan is a patent powder meant for external application in TCM. It consists of Cinnabari, Realgar, Hydrargyrum, Borax, Niter, Sodium Chloride and Alumen. Bletillae Striatae External Lozenge (Bai Ding Zi) is indicated in boils, multiple abscess, subcutaneous nodules, malignant carbuncles in the initial stage, ear polyps and nodules of the external auditory meatus.

## XXX.50. VENENUM BOFONIS EXTERNAL LOZENGE

The prescription for Venenum Bufonis External Lozenge (Chan Su Ding) from *A Collection of Recommended Prescriptions* (*Liang Fang Ji Cheng*) was presented with no information concerning the time.

### Ingredients

| | |
|---|---|
| Realgar (Xiong Huang) | 240 g |
| Cinnabari (Zhu Sha) | 30 g |
| Snail (Wo Niu) | 60 g |
| Borneolum Syntheticum (Bing Pian | 3 g |
| Venenum Bufonis (Chan Su) | 1.5 g |

The above ingredients were ground into fine powder and made into Cinnabari-coated lozenges.

### Comments

Venenum Bufonis External Lozenge was applied for lumbodorsal cellulitis, furuncles, carbuncles in the nape, breast abscess, nameless inflammatory swellings, malignant carbuncles and various kinds of insect bites. In the philosophy of TCM, the onset of boils, carbuncles or furuncles is related to stagnant *qi* and blood and derangement between the nutrient and defensive systems. Here, the lozenge was also mixed with old vinegar for local application. Venenum

Bufonis, poisonous, has the action of relieving toxicity and swelling. According to modern pharmacological studies, it can promote cardiac function and release parahormones, clear toxicity and promote blood circulation. It has therefore been recommended as a high-quality drug in general surgery. Furthermore, this Venenum Bufonis Lozenge is different from either Venenum Bufonis Pill (Chan Su Wan) as recorded in *Standards for Syndrome Differentiation and Treatments* (*Zheng Zhi Zhun Shen*) or Venenum Bufonis Cake (Chan Su Bing) as recorded in *Complete Works on External Therapies* (*Yang Yi Da Quan*). Caution should be taken in using any of these drugs.

## XXX.51. MIRACULOUS COLLATERAL-ACTIVATING PILL

An order was sent from Longevity Pharmacy to prepare one dose of Miraculous Collateral-activating Pill (Shen Xiao Huo Luo Dan) for Empress Dowager Cixi on the fifth day of the fourth month of the lunar calendar, with no information given as to the year.

*Ingredients*

| | |
|---|---|
| Os Tigris  (Hu Gu) | 15 g |
| Arisaema cum Bile  (Dan Nan Xing) | 24 g |
| Radix Ledebouriellae  (Fang Feng) | 18 g |
| Rhizoma Pinelliae  (Ban Xia) | 18 g |
| Rhizoma seu Radix Notopterygii  (Qiang Huo) | 18 g |
| Rhizoma Ligustici Chuanxiong  (Chuan Xiong) | 18 g |
| Scoprio  (Quan Xue) | 18 g |
| Exocarpium Citri Grandis  (Guang Hong) | 18 g |
| Rhizoma Atractylodis  (Cang Zhu) | 18 g |
| Bulbus Fritellariae Cirhosae  (Chuan Bei) | 18 g |
| Rhizoma Typhonii Gigantei  (Bai Fu Zi) | 18 g |
| Radix Angelicae Pubescentis  (Du Huo) | 18 g |
| Ramulus Cinnamomi  (Gui Zhi) | 18 g |
| Radix Angelicae sinensis  (Dang Gui) | 18 g |
| Radix Linderae  (Wu Yao) | 18 g |
| Rhizoma Acori Graminei  (Shi Chang Pu) | 18 g |
| Herba Ephedrae  (Ma Huang) | 18 g |
| Calculus Bovis  (Niu Huang) | 5 g |
| Lignum Aquilariae Resinatum  (Cheng Xiang) | 14 g |
| Radix Aconiti Praeparatae  (Fu Zi) | 9.5 g |
| Ramulus Uncariae cum Uncis  (Gou Teng) | 30 g |
| Radix Angelicae Dahuricae  (Bai Zhi) | 30 g |
| Radix Achyranthis Bidentatae  (Niu Xi) | 30 g |
| Rhizoma Gastrodiae  (Tian Ma) | 5 g |
| Moschus  (She Xiang) | 3 g |
| Borneolum Syntheticum  (Bing Pian) | 4.6 g |
| Resina Liquidambar Orientalis  (Su He You) | 30 g |
| Bombyx Batryticatus  (Jiang Can) | 30 g |

The above ingredients were ground into powder and mixed with honey to make wax-coated pills of six grams each.

*Comments*

Miraculous Collateral-activating Pill was composed of 30 ingredients. It was formed on the basis of Collateral-activating Pill (Huo Luo Dan) from *Complete Records of Holy Benevolence* (*Shen Ji Zong Lu*), and had the action of soothing the liver, activating blood, eliminating dampness and resolving phlegm. It was indicated in all kinds of wind conditions and wind Bi syndromes manifested by painful joints involving the shoulders, lumbar region and knees, deviation of the mouth and eyes, paralysis of the body, and muscular spasm.

The main action of the prescription was to activate the channels and collaterals. Smooth channels and collaterals will ensure the normal circulation of both *qi* and blood so that Bi syndrome caused by the invasion of wind, cold and dampness can be removed. Activating collaterals virtually means activating the circulation of blood. Normal circulation of blood will lead to the spontaneous calming of internal wind. This prescription was therefore applied in the treatment of numbness of the limbs, muscular spasm, and painful joints. Based on this prescription, imperial physicians often made more modified prescriptions in an attempt to treat Empress Dowager Cixi's facial spasm. For example, according to the health records of Empress Dowager Cixi on the 18th day of the fifth month of the lunar calendar in 1901, the imperial physicians Quan Shun and Zhang Zhongyuan took her pulse and found that the Empress had "a wiry and slightly rapid pulse in the liver area, but a deep and slippery one in the lung and spleen areas," "tired eyes and occasional twitching eyelids." They believed it "to be caused by stagnation of liver *qi* and phlegm-damp." Here the prescription was also based on Collateral-activating Pill. Pills prepared according to this prescription can be given regularly to patients over 40 years of age even though they were healthy. One pill was taken each time with millet wine, boiled water or tea. Because of its actions in activating blood and removing obstructions from channels and collaterals, anyone who takes it regularly is believed to be free from wind diseases for life.

## XXX.52. MODIFIED MIRACULOUS COLLATERAL-ACTIVATING PILL

One dose of Modified Miraculous Collateral-activating Pill (Jia Jian Shen Xiao Huo Luo Dan) was prescribed for Empress Dowager Cixi by the imperial physicians Quan Shun and Zhang Zhongyuan on the 10th day of the fourth month of the lunar calendar in 1902.

*Ingredients*

| | |
|---|---|
| Arisaema cum Bile  (Dan Nan Xing) | 6 g |
| Radix Ledebouriellae  (Fang Feng) | 4.5 g |
| Radix Peucedani  (Qian Hu) | 4.5 g |
| Rhizoma et Radix Notopterygii  (Qiang Huo) | 4.5 g |
| Scorpio  (Quan Xie) | 4.5 g |
| Pericarpium Citri Reticulatae Rubra  (Ju Hong) | 6 g |
| Rhizoma Atractylodis  (Cang Zhu) | 4.5 g |
| Radix Curcumae  (Yu Jin) | 4.5 g |
| Rhizoma Typhonii Gigantei  (Bai Fu Zi) | 4.5 g |

| | |
|---|---|
| Radix Angelicae Sinensis  (Dang Gui) | 4.5 g |
| Radix Linderae  (Wu Yao) | 4.5 g |
| Rhizoma Cyperi  (Xiang Fu) | 4.5 g |
| Radix Poria  (Fu Ling) | 6 g |
| Rhizoma Acori Graminei  (Shi Chang Pu) | 4.5 g |
| Herba Ephedrae  (Ma Huang) | 6 g |
| Calculus Bovis  (Niu Huang) | 2.4 g |
| Radix Aconiti Praeparatae  (Fu Zi) | 2.4 g |
| Ramulus Uncariae cum Uncis  (Gou Teng) | 9 g |
| Resina Liquidambar Orientalis  (Su He You) | 3 g |
| Rhizoma Gastrodiae  (Tian Ma) | 3 g |
| Moschus  (She Xiang) | 1.2 g |
| Borneolum Syntheticum  (Bing Pian) | 1.2 g |
| Radix Angelicae Dahuricae  (Bai Zhi) | 4.5 g |
| Bombyx Batryticatus  (Jiang Can) | 9 g |
| Radix Rehmanniae  (Sheng Di Huang) | 9 g |
| Radix Paeoniae Lactiflorae  (Bai Shao) | 9 g |
| Cornu Antelopis  (Ling Yang Jiao) | 6 g |

The original records state that the Rhizoma Atractylodis, Bombyx Batryticatus and Radix Paeoniae Lactiflorae should be roasted and the Rhizoma Cyperi prepared. The above ingredients were ground into fine powder and mixed with refined honey to make wax-coated pills of three grams each.

### Comments

Modified Miraculous Collateral-activating Pill (Jia Jian Shen Xiao Huo Luo Dan) was formulated on the basis of Miraculous Collateral-activating Pill (Shen Xiao Huo Luo Dan) minus Os Tigris, Bulbus Fritillariae Cirhosae, Radix Angelicae Pubescentis, Ramulus Cinnamomi, Rhizoma Pinelliae and Lignum Aquilariae Resinatum, but plus Radix Rehmanniae Praeparatae, Radix Paeoniae Lactiflorae, Radix Curcumae and Cornu Antelopis. It was also proposed to treat Empress Dowager Cixi for her facial spasm. In the prescription, ingredients from Four Substances Decoction (Si Wu Tang) were applied to nourish blood. Those consisting of Two Cures Decoction (Er Chen Tang) were used for resolving phlegm, and Bombyx Batryticatus and Scorpio for subduing wind. Other ingredients were added for eliminating wind and dampness, soothing liver wind, nourishing the liver, relaxing tendons and activating collaterals. It was therefore a proper remedy for Empress Dowager Cixi in the treatment of her chronic facial spasm and twitching of eyelids.

## XXX.53. PRESCRIPTION FOR PREVENTING EPIDEMICS

Two doses of Prescription for Preventing Epidemics (Bi Wen Fang) were ordered for preparation on the 24th day of the first month of the lunar calendar, with no information given as to the year.

### Ingredients

| | |
|---|---|
| Realgar  (Xiong Huang) | 240 g |
| Herba Huchnera Cruciata  (Gui Jian Yu) | 500 g |

| Radix Codopsis Pilosulae  (Dan Shen) | 500 g |
| Semen Phaseoli  (Chi Xiao Dou) | 500 g |

The above ingredients were made into pills the size of Chinese parasol tree seeds.

### Comments

Prescription for Preventing Epidemics, consisting of four ingredients, was based on the Pill for Preventing Epidemics (Bi Wen Dan) from the book *Bao's New Compilation of Proved Recipies* (*Bao Xiang'ao Yan Fang Xin Bian*). The original formula contained many ingredients, but the one applied in the imperial palace had only four, which was of great pharmaceutical significance. Specifically, Realgar resolves toxins, kills parasites and clears foul pathogenic factors. Herba Huchnera Cruciata, whose wood bears another name in Chinese that is phonetically pronounced as Gou Gu, has the effect of treating severe pain resulting from a heart condition, according to the book *Cui's Empirical Formulas* (*Cui Shi Fang*). It can also remove blood stasis and regulate channels and collaterals. And there have been reports in recent years of using it in treating cancer patients. Radix Codopsis Pilosulae activates blood, and Semen Phaseoli eliminates toxins and dampness. The combined use of the four ingredients offers a stronger therapeutic effect in eradicating various sorts of toxins. It was therefore used for preventing epidemics. Small in the number of ingredients, the prescription had very concentrated actions. Its clinical value should not be ignored.

## XXX.54.  PILL FOR PREVENTING EPIDEMICS PLUS

Pill for Preventing Epidemics Plus (Bi Wen Dan You Fang) was prepared for imperial use, with no information given as to the time.

There was a sudden and rapid occurrence of severe epidemics in the spring that year which worsened in the lunar fourth and fifth months. An untimely change of weather with rising temperature led to epidemics from the south spreading north. It was so severe that there were no surviving sick. It was very fortunate that we had access to information about Pill for Preventing Epidemics (Bi Wen Dan). The pill was remarkably effective despite its ordinary and simple ingredients. It therefore should be recommended for emergency use in epidemics.

### Ingredients

| Radix Glycyrrhizae  (Gan Cao) | 30 g |
| Rhizoma Atractylodis  (Cang Zhu) | 30 g |
| Herba Asari  (Xi Xin) | 30 g |
| Resina Olibani  (Ru Xiang) | 30 g |

The above ingredients were ground into fine powder and mixed with 250 grams of dried date pulp to make small cakes the size of Arillus Longan. They were then smoked over burning charcoal before use to ensure that no disaster would occur for three days in a whole family. For the preparation of the cakes in different seasons, 30 grams of Gypsum Fibrosum were added in the summer and 1.5 grams of Cinnabari added in winter. No modification of the prescription was required in spring or autumn. All good-hearted people should help advocate the use of the herbal cake for the well-being and health of all and for unforgettable praiseworthy conduct.

## Comments

The prescription is made up of common ingredients. Its outstanding therapeutic effect was probably associated with the way the cakes were prepared by smoking. Both Herba Asari and Resina Olibani, rich in volatile oil, help resolve epidemic toxins, eliminate swelling and tranquilize patients. The smoked herbal cake with Radix Glycyrrhizae for relieving toxins, and the Rhizoma Atractylodis for eliminating dampness can stop the spread of epidemics. Prescribing the Pill for Preventing Epidemics Plus (Bi Wen Dan You Fang) gave clear evidence that official postive measures were taken by the government for the prevention of infectious epidemic diseases in the Qing Dynasty.

# XXX.55. FIRST ELIXIR POWDER FOR RESUSCITATION

Five doses of First Elixir Powder for Resuscitation (Hui Sheng Di Yi Xian Dan) were prepared for Empress Dowager Cixi on the seventh day of the fourth month of the lunar calendar, with no information given as to the year.

## Ingredients

| | |
|---|---|
| Eupolyphaga seu Steleopnaga (Tu Bie Chong) | 15 g |
| Pyritum (Zi Ran Tong) | 9 g |
| Resina Olibani (Ru Xiang) | 6 g |
| Resina Draconis (Xue Jie) | 6 g |
| Cinnabari (Zhu Sha) | 6 g |
| Moschus (She Xiang) | 3 g |
| Radix Angelicae Sinensis (Dang Gui) | 30 g |

The original records direct that the Pyritum should be prepared with vinegar, while the Resina Draconis and Cinnabari should be ground in water. Moschus should be used only with special permission. The Radix Angelicae Sinensis should be roasted with millet wine.

## Comments

There are altogether seven ingredients in this prescription. All are drastic ingredients for removing stagnation. Conventionally only prescriptions of mild actions could be recommended for the imperial use. In fact, imperial physicians sometimes formed prescriptions in line with symptoms and signs of a given disease or a syndrome, not just in consideration of whether the proposed remedies would be of mild actions or not. Even an imperial figure like Empress Dowager Cixi would have to take prescriptions that were thought to be "as fearful as tigers and wolves" if she contracted a critical disease. The old name for this prescription was Imperial First Elixir Powder for Resuscitation from Trauma (Nei Fu Die Da Hui Sheng Di Yi Dan). It acts to heal bone fractures, activate blood and relieve pain. It was indicated in various kinds of traumatic injuries and wounds from knives and spears, from falling and stumbling, contusion, and stabbing, abrasion and sports injuries accompanied by severe pain. Today, the patent medicine Powder for Traumatic Injuries (Di Da Dan) made in Tianjin is based on this prescription. It was recommended to Empress Dowager Cixi because medicines for activating blood and resolving blood stasis applied in traumatic injuries were also effective in treating certain gynecological conditions. She had menstrual complaints in her youth. In her later years she suffered from diabetes, plus a frequent rash of skin conditions. Although ingredients in this prescription had drastic effect in removing stagnation, the primary consideration was how to treat her physical illness, not only to conform to conventional belief.

## Part Two
# MEDICAL PRESCRIPTIONS WRITTEN FOR EMPEROR GUANGXU WITH COMMENTARY

## I. REGENERATION PRESCRIPTIONS

### I.1. ANCIENT PRESCRIPTION FOR LONGEVITY AND REPRODUCTION

Ancient Prescription for Longevity and Reproduction (Gu Fang Chang Chun Yi Shou Guang Si Fang) was carefully prepared for Emperor Guangxu by the imperial physicians Zhuang Shouhe and Li Dechang on the 29th of the eighth month of the lunar calendar, with no information given as to the year.

*Ingredients*

| | |
|---|---|
| Radix Asparagi  (Tian Men Dong) | 15 g |
| Radix Ophiopogonis  (Mai Men Dong) | 15 g |
| Radix Rehmanniae Praeparatae  (Shu Di Huang) | 15 g |
| Rhizoma Dio  (Shan Yao) | 15 g |
| Radix Achyranthis Bidentatae  (Niu Xi) | 15 g |
| Radix Rehmanniae  (Sheng Di Huang) | 15 g |
| Cortex Eucommiae  (Du Zhong) | 15 g |
| Fructus Corni  (Shan Zhu Yu) | 15 g |
| Poria  (Fu Ling) | 15 g |
| Semen Biotae  (Bai Zi Ren) | 15 g |
| Radix Morindae Officinalis  (Ba Ji Tian) | 15 g |
| Radix Auchlandiae  (Mu Xiang) | 15 g |
| Pericarpium Zanthoxyli  (Chuan Jiao) | 7.5 g |
| Rhizoma Alismatis  (Ze Xie) | 7.5 g |
| Rhizoma Acori Graminei  (Shi Chang Pu) | 7.5 g |
| Radix Polygonati  (Yuan Zhi) | 7.5 g |
| Semen Cuscutae  (Tu Si Zi) | 30 g |
| Herba Cistanchis  (Rou Cong Rong) | 30 g |
| Fructus Lycii  (Gou Qi Zi) | 12 g |
| Fructus Rubi  (Fu Pen Zi) | 12 g |
| Cortex Lycii Radicis  (Di Gu Pi) | 12 g |

According to the original records, the kernel in both the Radix Asparagi and Radix Ophiopogonis should be discarded. Neither the Radix Rehmanniae nor the Radix Rehmanniae Praeparatae should be prepared in iron utensils. The Pericarpium Zanthoxyli should be roasted before use. The Cortex Eucommiae should be roasted in salty water and the oily substance in the Semen Biotae should be extracted before use. The above ingredients were processed into powder and made into pills together with refined honey. Twelve grams of the pills were taken each time with slightly salty water.

### Comments

This prescription has the action of nourishing the kidney, reinforcing the spleen, nourishing the heart and moistening the lung. It was modified on the basis of Incompatible Dioscoreae Pill (Wu Bi Shan Yao Wan) from *Imperial Grace Formulary of the Tai Ping Era (Tai Ping Hui Min He Ju Ji Fang)*, and Five Seeds Pill for Promoting Reproduction (Wu Zi Yan Zong Wan) from *Standards for Syndrome Differentiation and Treatment (Zheng Zhi Zhun Sheng)*. The Semen Biotae and Radix Polygonati were added for calming the heart and mind, the Rhizoma Acori Graminei for nourishing the heart, the Radix Auchlandiae and Pericarpium Zanthoxyli for regulating the *qi* mechanism, and the Cortex Lycii Radicis for clearing the heat of deficiency.

In his early youth, Emperor Guangxu suffered from a number of illnesses. Lingering and complicated diseases made his body constitution poor. According to his own complaints, he had "tinnitus, seminal emission in dreams, flare-up of deficient fire, and cold sensation in the lower limbs," "chronic cough, difficulty in swallowing food after taking a few mouthfuls, and fullness in the chest and diaphragm." Referring to his health records in the first month of the lunar calendar in 1899, he often complained of "sore throat." Based on the above analysis, it is clear that the imperial physicians Zhuang Shouhe and Li Dechang made the prescription specially for coping with Emperor Guangxu's deficiency of the heart and kidney. Since he had premature ejaculation, the Semen Plantaginis from the original Five Seeds Pill for Promoting Reproduction was omitted. In consideration of the fact that Fructus Schisandrae and Halloysitum Rubrum are of strong astringent flavour and constraining property, they were omitted in the prescription modification. This prescription is virtually a tonifying remedy despite the fact that part of its nomenclature, phonetically pronounced "guang si," means to produce many offspring.

## I.2. EUGENIC KIDNEY-REINFORCING PLASTER

The specific lunar time concerning the preparation of Eugenic Kidney-reinforcing Plaster (Yu Lin Gu Ben Gao) remains unknown.

### Ingredients

| | |
|---|---:|
| Cortex Eucommiae  (Du zhong) | 120 g |
| Radix Rehmanniae Praeparatae  (Shu Di Huang) | 120 g |
| Radix Aconiti Praeparatae  (Fu Zi) | 120 g |
| Herba Cistanchis  (Rou Cong Rong) | 120 g |
| Radix Achyranthis Bidentatae  (Niu Xi) | 120 g |
| Fructus Psoraleae  (Bu Gu Zhi) | 120 g |
| Radix Scrophulariae  (Xu Duan) | 120 g |
| Cortex Cinnamomi  (Rou Gui) | 120 g |
| Radix Glycyrrhizae  (Gan Cao) | 120 g |
| Radix Rehmanniae  (Sheng Di Huang) | 45 g |
| Fructus Illicii Veri  (Da Hui Xiang) | 45 g |

| | |
|---|---|
| Fructus Foenuculi  (Xiao Hui Xiang) | 45 g |
| Semen Cuscutae  (Tu Si Zi) | 45 g |
| Fructus Litseae Cubebae  (She Chuang Zi) | 45 g |
| Semen Gastrodiae  (Tian Ma) | 45 g |
| Lignum Cercis Chinensis  (Zi Shao Hua) | 45 g |
| Cornu Cervi  (Lu Jiao) | 45 g |
| Sheep kidney  (Yang Yao) | 1 pair |
| Halloysitum Rubrum  (Chi Shi Zhi) | 30 g |
| Os Draconis  (Long Gu) | 30 g |

These ingredients were well fried in four kilograms of sesame oil. After separating out the herbal residue, 1.44 kilograms of red lead were added, followed by adding respectively 30 grams of Realgar, Flos Caryophylli, Resina Olibani, Lignum Aquilariae Resinatum and Resina Murrhae, plus one gram of Moschus and 1.5 grams of Actilolitum.

### Comments

According to *Documents of Imperial Prescriptions from the First History Archives of China*, "Eugenic Kidney-reinforcing Plaster is believed to be an empirical prescription," though it is more convincing to believe that it was formed by a Qing Dynasty imperial physician. Although Eugenic Kidney-reinforcing Plasters from different sources of TCM all carry a footnote saying that it was originally from the collections of the imperial prescriptions of the Qing Dynasty, the actual ingredients vary. The formula introduced here according to the imperial records of medicine was believed "to have unquestionable effect in strengthening reproductive function." Also, "sustained use of the plaster by either men or women will help produce sufficient *qi* and blood, lustrous complexion and black lustrous hair. Users will have strong body constitution, especially strong kidney essence for reproduction."

The actual instructions for application are as follows: A woman should have it applied on the umbilicus, while a man should have it on bilateral Shenshu (UB 23) and Dantian, an area near Qihai (CV 6). The plasters are fixed by a bandage of terry cloth so that they will not move. The plasters were changed every half a month. Imperial medical records also say, "Anybody who is patient enough to use it lifelong will always have an agile physical body and still look quite young despite advanced age." It is obvious that the above is an over-statement; however, analysis of the ingredients shows that the formula does have the action of reinforcing the kidney, consolidating kidney essence, warming channels and collaterals and eliminating cold. Generally speaking, male infertility can be caused by any such factors as no production of sperm, impotence, premature ejaculation, an insufficient number of active sperms, or sperm growth retardation. According to the medical records of 1907, "Emperor Guangxu had a serious problem of seminal emission for some 20 years, amounting to more than 10 times monthly." "He even had seminal emission without dreams, nor was his penis erect. The semen was dilute in quality. And there had been chronic deficient cold in his lower abdomen." It is assumed that the effect in strengthening reproduction mainly lies in the action of warming the kidney and consolidating kidney essence. Only when impotence is cured can the kidney essence be replenished and the aim of achieving reproduction be reached. In the late Qing Dynasty when the imperial regime was declining, the imperial family was in decline as well. Many records are found concerning the use of the plaster by Emperor Guangxu, showing his desire for offspring to carry on the dynasty.

# II.  LONGEVITY PRESCRIPTION

## II.1.  HEART-NOURISHING AND LONGEVITY PILL

The lunar time concerning the preparation of Heart-nourishing and Longevity Pill (Yang Xin Yan Ling Yi Shou Dan) was not available in the original records.

### Ingredients

| | |
|---|---|
| Radix Poria  (Fu Shen) | 15 g |
| Semen Codopsis Pilosulae  (Dan Shen) | 12 g |
| Radix Paeoniae Lactiflorae  (Bai Shao) | 12 g |
| Cortex Moudan Radicis  (Dan Pi) | 9 g |
| Radix Angelicae Sinensis  (Dang Gui) | 15 g |
| Rhizoma Ligustici Chuanxiong  (Chuan Xiong) | 6 g |
| Radix Rehmanniae  (Sheng Di Huang) | 12 g |
| Radix Bupleuri  (Chai Hu) | 9 g |
| Rhizoma Cyperi  (Xiang Fu) | 12 g |
| Fructus Gardeniae  (Shan Zhi Zi) | 9 g |
| Radix Scutellariae  (Huang Qin) | 9 g |
| Pericarpium Citri Reticulatae  (Chen Pi) | 9 g |
| Rhizoma Atractylodis Macrocephalae  (Bai Zhu) | 6 g |
| Fructus Aurantii  (Zhi Ke) | 12 g |
| Semen Ziziphi Spinosae  (Suan Zao Ren) | 12 g |
| Semen Biotae  (Bai Zi Ren) | 12 g |

The original records state that the Semen Biotae, Fructus Gardeniae, Rhizoma Atractylodis Macrocephalae, Fructus Aurantii and Semen Ziziphi Spinosae should be roasted before use, while the Radix Rehmanniae should be roasted with millet wine. The above ingredients were processed into fine powder and made into pills with refined honey the size of mung beans. Nine grams of the pills were taken with boiled water each time.

### Comments

This prescription has the action of nourishing the heart, calming the mind, reinforcing kidney Yin and regulating the liver and spleen. It was mainly suggested for nourishing the heart and calming the mind though it was also claimed to have the effect of extending life expectancy. Emperor Guangxu was crowned when he was still a child, with Empress Dowager Cixi attending to state affairs from behind a curtain. He suffered from a number of illnesses when he was very young. During the Reform Movement of 1898 he was imprisoned by Empress Dowager Cixi for opposing her in the movement. Being greatly concerned whether he would live or die in prison, he started to have deficiency of both the heart and kidney as well as disharmony between spleen and liver. His health records carry the following, "Restlessness with easy sweating, poor sleep at night, tinnitus, nightmares which often woke him up," and "dreaming of fighting, occasional premature ejaculation, soreness in the lumbar region and knees especially when he sat for long periods, mental vagueness with disturbed mind on hard work, spontaneous laughing without apparent reasons, occasional murmuring to himself, and poor appetite." As days went by, the above symptoms and signs became worse. Although this prescription was suggested for both Empress Dowager Cixi and Emperor Guangxu, it was meant to help her extend life expectancy, while for him it was to dispel chronic illnesses that caused him to suffer for so many years of his life.

# III. TONICS

## III.1. REINFORCED LOQUAT SYRUP

This prescription for Reinforced Loquat Syrup (Jia Wei Pi Pa Gao) was presented for the imperial use on the 17th day of the third month of the lunar calendar, with no information given as to the year.

*Ingredients*

| | |
|---|---|
| Folium Eriobotryae (Pi Pa Ye) | 60 leaves |
| Honey (Feng Mi) | 1/2 cup |
| Semen Nelumbinis (Lian Zi) | 120 g |
| Pear (Li) | 2 |
| Fructus Jujubae (Da Zao) | 240 g |

According to the original records, either dry or fresh loquat leaves were suitable. However, they could be omitted if cough was not a complaint. Large pears with deep navel depressions were peeled and chopped before use. Honey should be well boiled, or omitted if stools were loose.

Loquat leaves were first well boiled with river water in an iron utensil, followed by filtering the fluid through a piece of fine silk. Loquat leaf residue was discarded. Small pear pieces, dates and lotus seeds were then put into the decocting utensil. Loquat liquid was poured into the utensil to cover the ingredients well. The mixture was decocted for five minutes and then stirred again before it was further decocted for another five minutes. The syrup was preserved in porcelain for oral administration at leisure, but warmed for use. Among all the ingredients, only the dates were peeled while they were still quite warm.

This remedy was recommended for treating deficiency of *qi* and blood manifested by emaciation, weakness and soreness of the four limbs, general lassitude, soreness in the lumbar region and back, and poor appetite. It was also suggested for all types of deficiency conditions.

*Comments*

The ingredients introduced here are different from those of the loquat syrup available in the market. Loquat syrup manufactured in certain places in China, such as that made in Shenyang, has the same ingredients as that described above.

But the processing is much simpler than this imperial one. This is probably due to the fact that this prescription was specially prepared for Emperor Guangxu. When Emperor Guangxu was some 25 years old, he often felt general lassitude and soreness in the lumbar region and back when he sat for any length of time. He also suffered from "dry cough and sore throat."

Loquat syrup has the action of moistening the lung and strengthening the spleen. Its recommended use for Emperor Guangxu would mean that the syndrome agreed with the remedy. Sustained use of the syrup also helps one benefit from its tonifying effect.

## III.2.  KIDNEY-YIN REINFORCING PILL

The prescription for Kidney-Yin Reinforcing Pill (Yi Yin Gu Ben Wan) was prepared for Emperor Guangxu on the seventh day of the intercalary fourth month of the lunar calendar in 1906.

### Ingredients
| | |
|---|---|
| Radix Rehmanniae Praeparatae  (Shu Di Huang) | 24 g |
| Cortex Moudan Radicis  (Mu Dan Pi) | 9 g |
| Fructus Corni  (Shan Zhu Yu) | 12 g |
| Rhizoma Dio  (Shan Yao) | 12 g |
| Poria  (Fu Ling) | 15 g |
| Rhizoma Alismatis  (Ze Xie) | 9 g |
| Fructus Rosae Laevigata  (Jin Yin Zi) | 15 g |
| Semen Cuscutae  (Tu Si Zi) | 15 g |

The above ingredients were ground into fine powder and made into pills together with refined honey the size of mung beans. The pill was taken with rice congee.

### Comments

This prescription was formed on the basis of Bolus of Six Drugs Including Rehmanniae (Liu Wei Di Huang Wan) plus Fructus Rosae Laevigata and Semen Cusoutae. Bolus of Six Drugs Including Rehmanniae, a traditional remedy for moistening and reinforcing kidney Yin, is applied in the treatment of conditions due to kidney Yin deficiency and flare-up of the deficiency fire. It is actually the main prescription for "strengthening the lord of water, i.e. the kidney, so as to sedate deficiency fire due to kidney Yin deficiency," an idea advocated by the ancient physician Wang Taiyi. Semen Cuscutae, reinforcing both kidney and liver, has the effect of strengthening kidney Yang, especially for solving such problems as impotence, seminal emission, dizziness and vertigo. Fructus Rosae Laevigata, strong in astringent flavour, was used here for treating premature ejaculation due to kidney deficiency. It is fairly reasonable to assume that this prescription was especially for consolidating the Emperor's kidney essence.

## III.3.  KIDNEY-YIN REINFORCING PILL PLUS

The prescription for Kidney-Yin Reinforcing Pill Plus (Yi Yin Gu Ben Wan You Fang) was carefully prepared by the imperial physicians Quan Shun and

Zhong Xun on the 10th day of the 10th month of the lunar calendar, with no information given as to the year.

*Ingredients*

| | |
|---|---|
| Radix Rehmanniae Praeparatae  (Shu Di Huang) | 120 g |
| Fructus Corni  (Shan Zhu Yu) | 60 g |
| Cortex Moudan Radicis  (Dan Pi) | 60 g |
| Poria  (Fu Ling) | 120 g |
| Rhizoma Atractylodis Macrocephalae  (Bai Zhu) | 60 g |
| Semen Cuscutae  (Tu Si Zi) | 60 g |
| Rhizoma Coptidis  (Huang Lian) | 1.5 g |
| Cortex Cinnamomi  (Rou Gui) | 1 g |
| Semen Euryales  (Qian Shi) | 60 g |
| Herba Dendrobii  (Shi Hu) | 15 g |
| Concha Ostreae  (Mu Li) | 24 g |
| Radix Nelumbinis  (Lian Xu) | 60 g |
| Radix Paeoniae Lactiflorae  (Bai Shao) | 120 g |
| Rhizoma Dio  (Shan Yao) | 120 g |
| Radix Ophiopogonis  (Mai Men Dong) | 24 g |

The original records state that the Rhizoma Atractylodis Macrocephalae and Rhizoma Dio should be roasted before use. The former should be prepared with powdery earth for roasting. The Concha Ostreae should be burnt on a fire before use, while the kernel of the Radix Ophiopogonis should be discarded.

*Comments*

This prescription was also primarily based on Bolus of Six Drugs Including Rehmanniae (Liu Wei Di Huang Wan) by omitting Rhizoma Alismatis since it was normally used against constipation. The whole prescription focused on reinforcing kidney Yin. At the same time, it was modified according to actions and indications of Golden Lock Pill for Preserving Kidney Essence (Jin Suo Gu Jing Wan) in an attempt to consolidate kidney essence. Some of the ingredients were copied from Pill for Heart and Spleen Harmony (Jiao Tai Wan) for the purpose of regaining the harmony between heart and kidney and treating anxiety. The prescription also contains some ingredients for reinforcing the spleen in consideration of the function of the Middle Jiao. Around the year 1904, the health records for Emperor Guangxu included the following descriptions, "restlessness, irritability with sweating, easily disturbed sleep at night," "shortness of breath, reluctant speech, and poor appetite" in addition to "occasional premature ejaculation." The prescription jointly prepared by the imperial physicians Quan Shun and Zhong Xun was made precisely according to the actual condition of Emperor Guangxu, rather than what its nomenclature indicates in terms of reinforcing and consolidating kidney Yin.

## III.4. FORMULA FOR REINFORCING YIN AND TREATING CHRONIC DEFICIENCY

Formula for Reinforcing Yin and Treating Chronic Deficiency (Yi Yin Zhi Lao Fang) was recorded without indication of specific time.

### Ingredients

| | |
|---|---|
| Radix Panacis Quiquefloii (Xi Yang Shen) | 120 g |
| Semen Astragali Complanati (Tong Xi Li) | 120 g |
| Rhizoma Alismatis (Ze Xie) | 45 g |
| Radix Rehmanniae Praeparatae (Shu Di Huang) | 360 g |
| Rhizoma Dio (Shan Yao) | 180 g |
| Radix Ophiopogonis (Mai Men Dong) | 90 g |
| Radix Paeoniae Lactiflorae (Bai Shao) | 90 g |
| Os Draconis (Long Gu) | 60 g |
| Fructus Chaenomelis (Mu Gua) | 60 g |
| Radix Poria (Fu Shen) | 150 g |
| Concha Ostreae (Mu Li) | 60 g |
| Herba Lycopodii (Shen Jin Cao) | 45 g |
| Radix Polygalae (Yuan Zhi) | 2.4 g |
| Cortex Moudan Radicis (Mu Dan Pi) | 4.5 g |
| Radix Glycyrrhizae (Gan Cao) | 2.4 g |
| Radix Angelicae Sinensis (Dang Gui) | 9 g |
| Semen Cuscutae (Tu Si Zi) | 90 g |
| Radix Nelumbinis (Lian Xu) | 90 g |

According to the original records, the Radix Paeoniae Lactiflorae, Fructus Chaenomelis and Herba Lycopodii should be roasted with millet wine. The Semen Astragali Complanati and Radix Angelicae Sinensis should be washed in millet wine. Both Concha Ostreae and Os Draconis should be burnt on fire before use. The pulp in the centre of the Radix Poria was kept as part of the ingredient while the kernel in the Radix Polygalae was omitted. The Radix Glycyrrhizae should be processed before use. The above ingredients were ground into powder and mixed with refined honey and made into pills the size of Chinese parasol-tree seeds.

This prescription was prepared especially for chronic deficiency syndrome, disharmony between heart and kidney, and all types of Yin deficiency conditions. It had remarkable effects in nourishing Yin, relaxing tendons, and strengthening Yang. On the 12th day of the 12th month of the lunar calendar, the same prescription was modified by omitting Rhizoma Alismatis and Fructus Mume, but adding powdered Radix Puerariae, Fructus Gardeniae, Medulla Junci Effusi, Talcum and Cinnabari.

### Comments

This prescription, reinforcing both *qi* and Yin and bringing harmony between the heart and kidney, embodies the main actions of Pulse Activating Infusion (Sheng Mai Yin) and Bolus of Six Drugs Including Rehmanniae (Liu Wei Di Huang Wan). Emperor Guangxu suffered from a number of illnesses when he was young. Both his health records and his remains unearthed some years ago proved that he was quite thin. It is most credible that he had such diseases as pulmonary tuberculosis and tuberculosis of the lumbar region. Furthermore, he suffered from pain in the lumbar region and hips, plus the chronic problem of seminal emission. Therefore, his condition would be in the category of general chronic deficiency in terms of TCM. Referring to *Synopsis of Prescriptions of the Golden Chamber (Jin Gui Yao Lue)*, the priniciple of treatment appended to the general chronic deficiency syndrome, i.e. Lao syndrome in TCM, is to reinforce the spleen and kidney. Yet the prescription introduced here was suggested to work more in bringing the harmony between heart and kidney. It was of course determined according to the actual condition of Emperor Guangxu. The prescription can also serve as a reference for proposed treatment for general chronic deficiency syndrome.

# IV. PRESCRIPTIONS FOR PROMOTING HAIR GROWTH AND PREVENTING HAIR LOSS

## IV.1. HAIR GROWTH FORMULA

Hair Growth Formula (Ling Fa Yi Zhang Fang) was recorded without information concerning the specific time.

### Ingredient

Radix Ziziphus Jujubae  (Zao Shu Gen)                                1 metre

The original records state that the Radix Ziziphus Jujubae growing towards the east should be used. It was placed in a steamer and steamed until the liquid flowed out at both ends and collected. Rubbing this liquid on the hair promoted its growth.

### Comments

Empress Dowager Cixi often used it during her lifetime. In 1980, the tomb where Emperor Guangxu was buried was opened to the public, and viewers saw the hair of the late Emperor still long and black though he died many years before. He died in middle age, but his hair remained black despite his emaciated body that had been afflicted with many illnesses. It is not unreasonable to believe that his black hair was enriched by the use of the formula.

## IV.2. HAIR GROWTH FORMULA PLUS

Hair Growth Formula Plus (Ling Fa Yi Zhang Fang You) was recorded without information concerning the specific time.

### Ingredients

Folium Mori  (Sang Ye)
Folium Cannabis Sativa  (Ma Ye)

The above ingredients were decocted for shampoo. Washing the hair with the liquid seven times could make it grow a metre long.

### Comments

Empress Dowager Cixi often used this formula during her lifetime. Whether it could make the hair grow incredibly long or not still remains a riddle. It might have been somewhat effective since everyone in the imperial palace used it for promoting hair growth. The claim in the original text, "washing the hair with the liquid seven times could make the hair grow a metre long" was obviously poppycock.

## IV.3. HAIR LOSS PREVENTION FORMULA

Hair Loss Prevention Formula (Ling Fa Bu Luo Fang) was recorded without information concerning the specific time.

### Ingredients

| | |
|---|---|
| Semen Torreyae  (Fei Zi) | 3 |
| Juglandis  (He Tao) | 3 |
| Cacumen Biotae  (Ce Bai Ye) | 30 g |

The above ingredients were ground fine and soaked in snow water, the medicinal liquid being used for combing the hair.

### Comments

This is one of the formulas Empress Dowager Cixi preferred to use for her own hair. Hair in TCM, also known as part of blood, is the outward manifestation of the kidney. "On the Nature of Remote Antiquity" ("Shang Gu Tian Zhen Lun") in *Plain Questions* (*Su Wen*) says, "When kidney *qi* is rich and strong, hair can grow and teeth remain solid." Hair loss is mainly the consequence of deficiency of blood and kidney *qi*. The prescription introduced here has the action of cooling blood, nourishing the kidney and moistening dryness. The formula could be effective.

# V.  MEDICINAL SHAMPOOS

## V.1. MEDICINAL SHAMPOO I

The prescription for Medicinal Shampoo I (Xi Tou Fang Yi) was carefully prepared by the imperial physicians Fan Yimei and Tong Chenhai for Emperor Guangxu on the eighth day of the first month of the lunar calendar, with no information given as to the year.

### Ingredients

| | |
|---|---|
| Rhizoma Gastrodiae  (Tian Ma) | 4.5 g |
| Folium Mori  (Sang Ye) | 4.5 g |
| Herba Menthae  (Bo He) | 4.5 g |
| Radix Angelicae Dahuricae  (Bai Zhi) | 4.5 g |
| Radix Ledebouriellae  (Fang Feng) | 4.5 g |
| Rhizoma seu Radix Notopterygii  (Qiang Huo) | 3 g |
| Flos Lonicerae  (Jin Yin Hua) | 3 g |
| Pericarpium Zanthoxyli  (Chuan Jiao) | 1.8 g |

The above ingredients were mixed and decocted. The filtered liquid was used for shampoo.

### Comments

Emperor Guangxu very often chose to use these medicinal shampoos which are two prescriptions for external therapy. Since 1903, Emperor Guangxu often suffered from headache and dizziness. According to his own accounts, his headache was caused by neglecting to wear a cap in cold weather. He also said, "Wind-cold entered my head when it was freezing cold, leading to the onset of frequent headache." Based on the analysis of more than 10 shampoo remedies collected here, most of the ingredients were used for clearing the head, brightening the vision, and eliminating wind-cold. The ones that were commonly applied include Herba Menthae, Radix Gastrodiae, Radix Angelicae Dahuricae, Radix Ledebouriellae, Rhizoma seu Radix Notopterygii, Flos Lonicerae, Folium Mori and Pericarpium Zanthoxyli. Some of the ingredients were modified according to the changes of symptoms and signs. In extant records of Emperor Guangxu's daily life, medicated shampoos were occasionally recorded. They may have been effective in relieving the Emperor's headache and dizziness.

In the prescription, Radix Gastrodiae was used for dealing with headache and dizziness caused by liver Yin deficiency. Herba Menthae and Folium Mori were used for sedating liver fire, brightening the vision and eliminating wind. Flos Lonicerae was used for dispelling toxic heat and eliminating wind-heat. Radix Angelicae Dahuricae, Radix Ledebouriellae and Rhizoma seu Radix Notopterygii were applied for clearing wind-cold from the superficial portion of the body and stopping pain. Among all these ingredients, only Pericarpium Zanthoxyli, pungent and warm, was used for eliminating cold and dampness, warming the Middle Jiao and stopping pain. Its use was on the one hand to produce better action in pungent warming and on the other to help eliminate dampness and sedate pain in the four limbs. Subsequent prescriptions all originated from this one, with certain modifications of ingredients.

## V.2. Medicinal Shampoo II

The prescription for Medicinal Shampoo II (Xi Tou Fang Er) was carefully prepared by the imperial physician Tong Chenhai late in the evening on the 15th day of the first month of the lunar calendar, with no information given as to the year.

*Ingredients*

| | |
|---|---|
| Rhizoma seu Radix Notopterygii (Qiang Huo) | 3 g |
| Herba Menthae (Bo He) | 3 g |
| Rhizoma Ligustici (Hao Ben) | 4.5 g |
| Flos Chrysanthemi (Ju Hua) | 4.5 g |
| Flos Lonicerae (Jin Yin Hua) | 3 g |
| Radix Ledebouriellae (Fang Feng) | 4.5 g |
| Radix Gastrodiae (Tian Ma) | 3 g |
| Pericarpium Zanthoxyli (Chuan Jiao) | 1.8 g |

The above ingredients were first decocted, then filtered before the shampoo was ready for washing the head.

*Comments*

This prescription was modified on the basis of the previous one by omitting Folium Mori and Radix Angelicae Dahuricae, and adding Rhizoma Ligustici and Flos Chrysanthemi. Such a modification was aimed at strengthening its effect in clearing wind-heat from the head and eyes.

## V.3. MEDICINAL SHAMPOO III

The prescription for Medicinal Shampoo III (Xi Tou Fang San) was carefully prepared by the imperial physician Tong Chenhai on the 25th day of the second month of the lunar calendar. No information was given as to the year.

### Ingredients

| | |
|---|---|
| Herba Menthae  (Bo He) | 3 g |
| Flos Chrysanthemi  (Ju Hua) | 4.5 g |
| Radix Gastrodiae  (Tian Ma) | 4.5 g |
| Radix Ledebouriellae  (Fang Feng) | 6 g |
| Folium Mori  (Sang Ye) | 6 g |
| Gypsum Fibrosum  (Shi Gao) | 12 g |
| Pericarpium Zanthoxyli  (Chuan Jiao | 2.1 g |
| Flos Lonicerae  (Jin Yin Hua) | 6 g |

The original records stipulate that frosted Folium Mori and raw Gypsum Fibrosum should be used. The above ingredients were decocted and filtered and the shampoo was ready for washing the head.

### Comments

This prescription was formed on the basis of Medicinal Shampoo I (Xi Tou Fang Yi) by omitting Radix Angelicae Dahuricae and Rhizoma seu Radix Notopterygii, but adding Flos Chrysanthemi and Gypsum Fibrosum. Obviously, Tong Chenhai believed that the first medicinal shampoo was somewhat too strong, pungent, and hot. He intended here to use Flos Chrysanthemi, pungent and cool, for relieving superficial symptoms and signs, and Gypsum Fibrosum with its sweet flavour and cold property to relieve muscle pain. The above changes were made to prevent over-dispersing, which would not be appropriate for Emperor Guangxu's body, whose constitution was typically Yin-deficient.

## V.4. MEDICINAL SHAMPOO IV

The prescription for Medicinal Shampoo IV (Xi Tou Fang Si) was carefully prepared by the imperial physician Tong Chenhai for Emperor Guangxu on the 13th day of the third month of the lunar calendar, with no information given as to the year.

### Ingredients

| | |
|---|---|
| Folium Mori  (Sang Ye) | 4.5 g |
| Flos Chrysanthemi  (Ju Hua) | 4.5 g |
| Radix Angelicae Dahuricae  (Bai Zh | 6 g |
| Herba Menthae  (Bo He) | 4.5 g |
| Flos Lonicerae  (Jin Yin Hua) | 6 g |
| Rhizoma seu Radix Notopterygii  (Qiang Huo) | 3 g |
| Fructus Viticis  (Man Jing Zi) | 3 g |
| Fructus Forsythiae  (Lian Qiao) | 3 g |

The original recipe calls for frosted Folium Mori to be used. The Fructus Viticis should be ground into powder before use. The above ingredients were decocted and filtered, and the shampoo was ready for washing the head.

### Comments

This prescription was formed on the basis of Medicinal Shampoo I (Xi Tou

Fang Yi) by omitting Radix Gastrodiae, Radix Ledebouriellae and Pericarpium Zanthoxyli, while adding Flos Chrysanthemi, Fructus Viticis and Fructus Forsythiae. The main intention of the modification was still to prevent the over strong effect from pungent warming ingredients. Radix Gastrodiae is normally used to treat patients for dizziness due to Yin deficiency. According to the analysis of ingredients in this prescription, the use of Radix Gastrodiae was for dealing with headache and was thus also omitted.

## V.5. MEDICINAL SHAMPOO V

The prescription for Medicinal Shampoo V (Xi Tou Fang Wu) was carefully prepared for Emperor Guangxu by the imperial physician Tong Chenhai on the 13th day of the third month of the lunar calendar, with no information given as to the year.

*Ingredients*

| | |
|---|---|
| Flos Chrysanthemi (Ju Hua) | 4.5 g |
| Herba Menthae (Bo He) | 4.5 g |
| Radix Ledebouriellae (Fang Feng) | 6 g |
| Flos Lonicerae (Jin Yin Hua) | 6 g |
| Radix Angelicae Dahuricae (Bai Zhi) | 6 g |
| Pericarpium Zanthoxyli (Chuan Jiao | 2.1 g |
| Gypsum Fibrosum (Shi Gao) | 9 g |
| Rhizoma seu Radix Notopterygii (Qiang Huo) | 3 g |

The original records require that raw Gypsum Fibrosum be used. The above ingredients were decocted and filtered for making the medicinal shampoo.

*Comments*

This prescription was modified on the basis of Medicinal Shampoo I (Xi Tou Fang Yi) by omitting Radix Gastrodiae and Folium Mori, while adding Gypsum Fibrosum and Flos Chrysanthemi. It was thus formed in an attempt to relieve superficial symptoms and signs by using pungent cooling ingredients, stop general aching and eliminate pathogenic heat. Also, the date of this prescription was the same as that recorded in Medicinal Shampoo Four (Xi Tou Fang Si). The two were probably prepared in different years.

## V.6. MEDICINAL SHAMPOO VI

The prescription for Medicinal Shampoo VI (Xi Tou Fang Liu), functioning in clearing heat and wind, was prepared by the imperial physician Fan Yimei late in the evening on the third day of the fourth month of the lunar calendar, with no information given as to the year.

*Ingredients*

| | |
|---|---|
| Folium Mori (Sang Ye) | 12 g |
| Flos Chrysanthemi (Ju Hua) | 6 g |
| Radix Angelicae Dahuricae (Bai Zhi | 6 g |
| Radix Paeoniae Rubra (Chi Shao) | 6 g |
| Herba Menthae (Bo He) | 3 g |

| Radix Scutellariae  (Huang Qin) | 4.5 g |
| Folium Phyllostachyos  (Zhu Ye) | 3 g |
| Radix Gastrodiae  (Tian Ma) | 3 g |

The original recipe calls for frosted Folium Mori and roasted Radix Paeoniae Rubra. The Radix Scutellariae should be prepared with millet wine. The above ingredients were decocted and filtered, and the shampoo was ready for washing the head.

### Comments

This prescription was formed on the basis of Medicinal Shampoo I (Xi Tou Fang Yi) by omitting Radix Ledebouriellae, Rhizoma seu Radix Notopterygii, Flos Lonicerae and Pericarpium Zanthoxyli, while adding Flos Chrysanthemi, Radix Paeoniae Rubra, Radix Scutellariae and Folium Phyllotachyos. The name of the prescription in the original script was Medicinal Shampoo for Eliminating Wind-Heat (Hua Feng Qing Re Xi Tou Fang). What deserves mentioning is the use of Folium Phyllostachyos in the prescription. It was probably for achieving better effect in clearing heat and calming restlessness. This prescription was prepared by the imperial physician Fan Yimei around midnight when the Emperor was most likely to have a severe attack of headache, dizziness and vertigo and the imperial physician would be summoned to make the prescription immediately. These medicinal shampoos were apparently effective.

## V.7. MEDICINAL SHAMPOO VII

The prescription for Medicinal Shampoo VII (Xi Tou Fang Qi) was carefully prepared by the imperial physician Tong Chenhai on the second day of the seventh month of the lunar calendar, with no information as to the year.

### Ingredients

| Rhizoma seu Radix Notopterygii  (Qiang Huo) | 3 g |
| Radix Ledebouriellae  (Fang Feng) | 3 g |
| Fructus Viticis  (Man Jing Zi) | 3 g |
| Radix Angelicae Dahuricae  (Bai Zhi) | 4.5 g |
| Flos Lonicerae  (Jin Yin Hua) | 4.5 g |
| Folium Mori  (Sang Ye) | 3 g |
| Gypsum Fibrosum  (Shi Gao) | 12 g |
| Cortex Moudan Radicis  (Dan Pi) | 6 g |

According to the original recipe the Gypsum Fibrosum should be used raw. The above ingredients were decocted and filtered for use in washing the head.

### Comments

This prescription was formed on the basis of Medicinal Shampoo I (Xi Tou Fang Yi) by omitting Radix Gastrodiae, Herba Menthae and Pericarpium Zanthoxyli, while adding Fructus Viticis, Gypsum Fibrosum and Cortex Moudan Radicis. Cortex Moudan Radicis was used here to reinforce the effect of the shampoo in activating blood circulation and cooling blood.

## V.8.  MEDICINAL SHAMPOO VIII

The prescription for Medicinal Shampoo VIII (Xi Tou Fang Ba) was carefully prepared by the imperial physician Tong Chenhai for Emperor Guangxu on the 17th day of the 11th month of the lunar calendar, with no information given as to the year.

*Ingredients*

| | |
|---|---|
| Radix Gastrodiae  (Tian Ma) | 6 g |
| Radix Ledebouriellae  (Fang Feng) | 6 g |
| Radix Angelicae Dahuricae  (Bai Zhi) | 6 g |
| Herba Menthae  (Bo He) | 4.5 g |
| Fructus Forsythiae  (Lian Qiao) | 6 g |
| Gypsum Fibrosum  (Shi Gao) | 12 g |
| Pericarpium Zanthoxyli  (Chuan Jiao) | 3 g |
| Radix Puerariae  (Ge Gen) | 6 g |

The original records say that green Fructus Forsythiae and raw Gypsum Fibrosum should be used. The above ingredients were decocted and filtered and the shampoo was then ready for use.

*Comments*

This prescription was formed on the basis of Medicinal Shampoo I (Xi Tou Fang Yi) by omitting Folium Mori, Rhizoma seu Radix Notopterygii and Flos Lonicerae, while adding Gypsum Fibrosum, Fructus Viticis and Radix Puerariae. The modification was apparently intended to strengthen the effect of clearing heat from the head and eyes.

## V.9.  MEDICINAL SHAMPOO IX

The prescription for Medicinal Shampoo IX (Xi Tou Fang Jiu), i. e. the prescription for eliminating wind and stopping headache, was carefully prepared by the imperial physician Fan Yimei for Emperor Guangxu on the 29th day of the 12th month of the lunar calendar, with no information given as to the year.

*Ingredients*

| | |
|---|---|
| Radix Notopterygii  (Qiang Huo) | 4.5 g |
| Rhizoma Ligustici Chuanxiong  (Chuan Xiong) | 6 g |
| Radix Angelicae Dahuricae  (Bai Zhi) | 6 g |
| Rhizoma Ligustici  (Hao Ben) | 6 g |
| Radix Gastrodiae  (Tian Ma) | 3 g |
| Folium Mori  (Sang Ye) | 4.5 g |
| Flos Chrysanthemi  (Ju Hua) | 3 g |
| Herba Menthae  (Bo He) | 3 g |

The above ingredients were decocted and filtered to prepare the remedy for washing the head.

*Comments*

This prescription was formed on the basis of Medicinal Shampoo I (Xi Tou Fang Yi) by omitting Radix Ledebouriellae, Flos Lonicerae and Pericarpium Zanthoxyli, while adding Rhizoma Ligustici, Flos Chrysanthemi and Rhizoma

Ligustici Chuanxiong. The prescription would thus have the effect of eliminating wind and stopping headache. Rhizoma Ligustici Chuanxiong, pungent and warming, was used for activating blood circulation and relieving *qi* stagnation. It is usually prescribed for relieving pain.

## V.10. MEDICINAL SHAMPOO X

The prescription for Medicinal Shampoo X (Xi Tou Fang Shi) was carefully prepared for Emperor Guangxu by the imperial physician Tong Chenhai around one o'clock in the morning on the 27th day of the ninth month of the lunar calendar, with no information given as to the year.

### Ingredients

| | |
|---|---|
| Rhizoma seu Radix Notopterygii  (Qiang Huo) | 6 g |
| Radix Ledebouriellae  (Fang Feng) | 6 g |
| Flos Chrysanthemi  (Ju Hua) | 6 g |
| Herba Schizonepetae  (Jing Jie Sui) | 6 g |
| Flos Lonicerae  (Jin Yin Hua) | 6 g |
| Pericarpium Zanthoxyli  (Chuan Jiao) | 2.4 g |
| Herba Menthae  (Bo He) | 4.5 g |
| Fructus Forsythiae  (Lian Qiao) | 6 g |
| Bombyx Batryticatus  (Jiang Can) | 3 g |
| Folium Perillae  (Zi Su Ye) | 3 g |

The above ingredients were decocted and filtered in preparing the remedy for washing the head.

### Comments

This prescription was also based on Medicinal Shampoo I (Xi Tou Fang Yi). Here, Radix Angelicae Dahuricae, Folium Mori and Radix Gastrodiae were omitted from the original formula, while Flos Chrysanthemi, Fructus Forsythiae, Herba Schizonepetae, Folium Perillae and Bombyx Batryticatus were added. The main purpose of the modification was to help eliminate wind, clear heat and stop pain.

## V.11. MEDICINAL SHAMPOO XI

The prescription for Medicinal Shampoo XI (Xi Tou Fang Shi Yi) was carefully prepared for Emperor Guangxu around one to three o'clock in the afternoon on the 12th day of the ninth month of the lunar calendar, with no information given as to the year.

### Ingredients

| | |
|---|---|
| Bombyx Batryticatus  (Jiang Can) | 12 g |
| Radix Ledebouriellae  (Fang Feng) | 30 g |
| Radix Angelicae Dahuricae  (Bai Zhi) | 24 g |
| Herba Menthae  (Bo He) | 21 g |
| Rhizoma seu Radix Notopterygii  (Qiang Huo) | 30 g |
| Rhizoma Ligustici Chuanxiong  (Chuan Xiong) | 30 g |
| Rhizoma Ligustici  (Hao Ben) | 30 g |
| Radix Paeoniae Rubra  (Chi Shao) | 30 g |

| | |
|---|---|
| Radix Stephaniae Tetrandrae  (Fang Ji) | 24 g |
| Periostracum Cicadae  (Chan Tui) | 24 g |
| Flos chrysanthemi  (Ju Hua) | 30 g |
| Herba Schizonepetae  (Jing Jie Sui) | 30 g |

### Comments

This prescription was formed on the basis of Medicinal Shampoo X (Xi Tou Fang Shi) by omitting Flos Lonicerae, Pericarpium Zanthoxyli, Folium Perillae and Fructus Forsythiae, while adding Rhizoma Ligustici, Radix Paeoniae Rubra, Rhizoma Ligustici Chuanxiong, Radix Stephaniae Tetrandrae, Periostracum Cicadae and Radix Angelicae Dahuricae. This modification was made to strengthen the effect of activating blood and dispersing wind.

# VI. PRESCRIPTIONS FOR HEADACHE

## VI.1. CHRYSANTHEMI AND LIGUSTICI CHUANXIONG TEA

Information concerning the specific time of preparing Chrysanthemi and Ligustici Chuanxiong Tea (Chuan Ju Cha Tiao San) is not given in the original document.

### Ingredients

| | |
|---|---|
| Herba Schizonepetae  (Jing Jie) | 6 g |
| Radix Ledebouriellae  (Fang Feng) | 6 g |
| Rhizoma Ligustici Chuanxiong  (Chuan Xiong) | 6 g |
| Flos Chrysanthemi  (Ju Hua) | 9 g |
| Herba Asari  (Xi Xin) | 1.5 g |
| Radix Angelicae Dahuricae  (Bai Zhi) | 6 g |
| Rhizoma Astractylodis Macrocephalae  (Bai Zhu) | 6 g |
| Herba Menthae  (Bo He) | 2.4 g |
| Radix Glycyrrhizae  (Gang Cao) | 2.4 g |

The original records state that the Rhizoma Atractylodis Macrocephalae should be roasted before use. The above ingredients were ground into fine powder and taken three to six grams each time with weak tea.

### Comments

This prescription, which originated from *Imperial Grace Formulary of the Tai Ping Era* (*Tai Ping Hui Min He Ju Ji Fang*), has the actions of eliminating pathogenic wind and stopping pain. It was applied in the treatment of nasal obstruction, headache and severe paroxysmal headache of lingering nature due to invasion of exogenous pathogenic wind-cold.

## VI.2. HEADACHE PLASTER

The prescription for Headache Plaster (Tie Tou Zhi Tong Fang) was prepared around three to five o'clock in the afternoon on the 24th day of the ninth month of the lunar calendar, with no information given concerning the year.

### Ingredients

| | |
|---|---|
| Herba Schizonepetae  (Jing Jie Sui) | 7.5 g |
| Squama Manitis  (Chuan Shan Jia) | 4.5 g |
| Radix Angelicae Dahuricae  (Bai Zhi) | 7.5 g |
| Os Draconis  (Long Gu) | 4.5 g |
| Scorpio  (Quan Xue) | 3 g |
| Eupolyphagaseu steleophaga  (Di Bie Chong) | 3 g |
| Spina Gleditsiae  (Ya Zao) | 4.5 g |
| Borneolum Syntheticum  (Bing Pian) | 0.9 g |
| Bombyx Batryticatus  (Jiang Can) | 3 g |
| Herba Menthae  (Bo He) | 1.5 g |

The original records call for the Squama Manitis to be roasted and the Scorpio detoxicated before use. The Borneolum Syntheticum was added later. The above ingredients were ground into fine powder and made into paste together with honey. The paste was evenly stirred before it was spread onto pieces of cloth to be plastered at the bilateral Taiyang extra acupuncture points.

### Comments

This prescription has the action of dispersing pathogenic wind, removing obstruction from channels and collaterals, activating blood circulation and stopping pain. According to official writings recording the daily life of Emperor Guangxu around 1904, his dizziness and headache were caused by his not wearing a small hat, indicating that his headache and dizziness probably resulted from invasion of wind-cold. The Emperor was given this external plaster in addition to oral administration of internal decoctions. It should be pointed out that the prescription contains a large proportion of sea shell or insect ingredients which could cause skin allergy and should therefore be provided with caution. As Emperor in the late Qing Dynasty, respected by the whole nation, that he should have to wear plasters on his temporal regions shows how strongly he wished to be rid of his lingering headache and dizziness. The plaster may have been effective in relieving his headache.

## VI.3. THE EMPEROR'S HERBAL BATH REMEDY I

The Emperor's Herbal Bath Remedy I (Huang Shang Xi Yao Fang Yi) was carefully prepared for Emperor Guangxu by the imperial physician Yang Shifen around five to seven o'clock in the afternoon of the fifth day of the seventh month of the lunar calendar, with no information given as to the year.

### Ingredients

| | |
|---|---|
| Radix Angelicae Dahuricae  (Bai Zhi) | 4.5 g |
| Periostracum Cicadae  (Chan Tui) | 3 g |
| Rhizoma Ligustici  (Hao Ben) | 4.5 g |
| Radix Platycodi  (Ku Gen) | 6 g |
| Herba Menthae  (Bo He) | 3 g |
| Pericarpium Citri Reticulatae Rubra (Ju Luo) | 3 g |

The above ingredients were boiled in a suitable amount of water for herbal steaming and bathing.

*Comments*

Characterized by an ascending and upward dispersing property, this prescription is good for eliminating wind-heat and stopping headache.

## VI.4.  THE EMPEROR'S HERBAL BATH REMEDY II

The Emperor's Herbal Bath Remedy II (Huang Shang Xi Yao Fang Er) was carefully prepared by the imperial physician Tong Chenhai aroung five to seven o'clock in the afternoon on the 29th day of the 11th month of the lunar calendar, with no information given as to the year.

*Ingredients*

| | |
|---|---:|
| Folium Mori  (Sang Ye) | 4.5 g |
| Ledebouriellae  (Fang Feng) | 4.5 g |
| Herba Menthae  (Bo He) | 3 g |
| Radix Gastrodiae  (Tian Ma) | 3 g |
| Fructus Forsythiae  (Lian Qiao) | 4.5 g |
| Flos Lonicerae  (Jin Yin Hua) | 3 g |
| Gypsum Fibrosum  (Shi Gao) | 9 g |
| Pericarpium Zanthoxyli  (Chuan Jiao) | 1.8 g |

The original records require that raw Gypsum Fibrosum and green Fructus Forsythiae should be used. All the ingredients were boiled in a suitable amount of water for herbal steaming and bathing.

*Comments*

This prescription follows the therapeutic principles for clearing heat and eliminating wind at the same time. The imperial physician Tong Chenhai made this prescription in an attempt to treat the Emperor for his headache due to wind-heat invasion. Pericarpium Zanthoxyli is effective also in dealing with itching due to eczema, in addition to its effect in stopping local pain.

## VI.5.  THE EMPEROR'S HERBAL BATH REMEDY III

The Emperor's Herbal Bath Remedy III (Huang Shang Xi Yao Fang San) was carefully prepared by the imperial physician Tong Chenhai around 11 o'clock in the morning to one o'clock in the afternoon on the second day of the 11th month of the lunar calendar, with no information given concerning the year.

*Ingredients*

| | |
|---|---:|
| Radix Angelicae Dahuricae  (Bai Zhi) | 6 g |
| Radix Ledebouriellae  (Fang Feng) | 4.5 g |
| Radix Puerariae  (Ge Gen) | 4.5 g |
| Radix Gastrodiae  (Tian Ma) | 3 g |
| Flos Lonicerae  (Jin Yin Hua) | 6 g |
| Gypsum Fibrosum  (Shi Gao) | 9 g |
| Pericarpium Zanthoxyli  (Chuan Jiao) | 3 g |
| Resina Olibani  (Ru Xiang) | 3 g |

The original recipe calls for raw Gypsum Fibrosum and powdered Resina Olibani to be used. The above ingredients were boiled in a suitable amount of water for herbal steaming and bathing.

### Comments

This prescription also has the action of eliminating wind and dampness, clearing heat and stopping pain. The combined use of Radix Angelicae Dahuricae and Radix Puerariae was to treat the Emperor for his frontal headache. What should be pointed out in particular is the selection of Flos Lonicerae and Gypsum Fibrosum as ingredients in winter without any warnings of contraindications. This shows that imperial physicians stuck to the principle of choosing ingredients according to clinical manifestations while trying to work out a prescription in the process of syndrome differentiation.

## VI.6. HERBAL BATH REMEDY FOR CLEARING WIND-HEAT

Herbal Bath Remedy for Clearing Wind-Heat (Qu Feng Qing Re Xi Yao Fang) was carefully worked out by the imperial physician Fan Yimei for Emperor Guangxu on the 19th day of the 11th month of the lunar calendar, with no information given concerning the year.

### Ingredients

| | |
|---|---|
| Radix Ledebouriellae (Fang Feng) | 9 g |
| Rhizoma Ligustici Chuanxiong (Chuan Xiong) | 6 g |
| Radix Angelicae Dahuricae (Bai Zhi) | 6 g |
| Herba Menthae (Bo He) | 3 g |
| Folium Mori (Sang Ye) | 6 g |
| Flos Chrysanthemi (Ju Hua) | 4.5 g |
| Radix Gastrodiae (Tian Ma) | 3 g |

The above ingredients were boiled in water for washing the head.

### Comments

This prescription is similar to both Ligustici Chuanxiong Headache Powder (Chuan Xiong Cha Tiao San) recorded in *Imperial Grace Formulary of the Tai Ping Era* (Tai Ping Hui Min He Ju Ji Fang) and Ligustici Chuanxiong Pill (Chuan Xiong Wan) recorded in *A Collection of Distinguished Prescriptions* (*Ben Shi Fang*). This external remedy was applied for severe headache, migraine, blurring of vision and dizziness. Rhizoma Ligustici Chuanxiong is "a *qi*-moving ingredient among those that normally activate blood." Its therapeutic effect "can rise to the head and descend to the sea of blood." It has the action of activating blood, resolving blood stasis, eliminating wind and stopping pain. Pharmaceutical studies prove that 10% Radix Ligustici Chuanxiong extract can help suppress brain activities and paralyze the central nervouse system. This also explains why it has tranquilizing, analgesic and anti-spasm effect. The ancient remedy Radix Ligustici Chuanxiong Powder, composed of Radix Ligustici Chuanxiong itself plus Radis Gastrodiae, can also be applied in the treatment of headache and dizziness due to upward disturbance of liver wind. Therefore, this prescription worked out by the imperial physician Fan Yimei was appropriate for Emperor Guangxu's condition.

## VI.7.  HERBAL BATH REMEDY FOR CLEARING WIND AND EASING NUMBNESS

Herbal Bath Remedy for Clearing Wind and Easing Numbness (Qu Feng Juan Ma Xi Yao Fang) was carefully worked out by the imperial physician Zhao Wenkui on the third day of the ninth month of the lunar calendar, with no information given as to the year.

*Ingredients*

| | |
|---|---|
| Radix Gastrodiae  (Tian Ma) | 6 g |
| Radix Ledebouriellae  (Fang Feng) | 6 g |
| Radix Angelicae Dahuricae  (Bai Zhi) | 6 g |
| Bombyx Batryticatus  (Jiang Can) | 6 g |
| Herba Menthae  (Bo He) | 4.5 g |
| Rhizoma Ligustici  (Hao Ben) | 6 g |
| Radix Angelicae Sinensis  (Dang Gui) | 9 g |

The original records direct that the Bombyx Batryticatus should be roasted before use. The above ingredients were boiled and filtered in preparing the remedy for external washing.

*Comments*

In the late years of his life, Emperor Guangxu often had dizziness, vertigo, headache and tinnitus. This prescription was formulated precisely for these symptoms. Radix Gastrodiae, the superb ingredient for quelling wind, is also called the wind-quelling plant. Pharmaceutical studies show that Radix Gastrodiae extract has noted effects in resisting metrazol paroxysmal convulsions, sedating pain, controlling epilepsy and promoting bile secretion. The use of Bombyx Batryticatus and Radix Angelicae Sinensis in the prescription was for the purpose of eliminating wind while activating blood. Radix Angelicae Dahuricae, Rhizoma Ligustici and Herba Menthae were added in order to deal with headache, dizziness and blurring of vision. It contains only seven ingredients, demonstrating how careful an imperial physician was in preparing a prescription for the Emperor.

# VII.  PRESCRIPTIONS FOR DIZZINESS AND VERTIGO

## VII.1.  PILL FOR RESOLVING PHLEGM AND CONTROLLING DIZZINESS

Pill for Resolving Phlegm and Controlling Dizziness (Hua Tan Qing Xuan Wan) was carefully prepared by the imperial physicians Zhang Zhongyuan, Quan Shun and Zhong Yuan on the 11th day of the ninth month of the lunar calendar, with no information given concerning the year.

*Ingredients*

| | |
|---|---|
| Rhizoma Pinelliae  (Ban Xia) | 60 g |
| Poria  (Fu Ling) | 30 g |
| Fructus Aurantii  (Zhi Ke) | 15 g |

| | |
|---|---|
| Natrii Sulfas Exsiccatus  (Xuan Min Fen) | 9 g |
| Arisaema cum Bile  (Dan Nan Xing) | 15 g |

The original records say that both the Rhizoma Pinelliae and Arisaema cum Bile should be processed, while the Fructus Aurantii should be roasted before use. All the ingredients were ground into fine powder and mixed with Massa Fermentata Medicinalis paste to make pills the size of mung beans. Six grams of the pills were taken in the morning and evening with rice congee.

*Comments*

In TCM, dizziness and vertigo are often mentioned together as "xuan" and "yun." The former refers to a dizzy sensation with blurring of vision while the latter refers to dizziness accompanied by a general revolving sensation. Factors accounting for the onset of dizziness and vertigo are of either an excessive or a deficient nature. The former is usually due to the deficiency of Yin and blood while the latter is due to phlegm or fire. Emperor Guangxu himself suffered from deficiency of the spleen and stomach as well as subsequent poor transformation and transportation. The accumulation of dampness thus caused phlegm to obstruct the Middle Jiao and poor mechanism of *qi* in ascending and descending, leading to dizziness and vertigo. Ancient practitioners of TCM often claimed that phlegm was in all cases responsible for dizziness and vertigo.

The prescription introduced here was modified on the basis of Phlegm-repelling Decoction (Dao Tan Tang). Natrii Sulfas Exsiccatus was added to increase the effect of clearing heat, eliminating pathogenic water, and resolving phlegm and dampness. Dizziness and vertigo would be cured when the *qi* mechanism of descending and ascending in the Middle Jiao returns to harmony.

## VII.2. PILL FOR PACIFYING MIDDLE JIAO AND EASING DIZZINESS

Pill for Pacifying Middle Jiao and Easing Dizziness (He Zhong Zhi Xuan Wan) was carefully prepared by the imperial physicians Zhuang Shouhe and Zhong Xun for Emperor Guangxu on the ninth day of the seventh month of the lunar calendar, with no information given as to the year.

*Ingredients*

| | |
|---|---|
| Flos Inullae  (Xuan Fu Hua) | 9 g |
| Radix Gastrodiae  (Tian Ma) | 4.5 g |
| Rhizoma Ligustici Chuanxiong  (Chuan Xiong) | 6 g |
| Flos Chrysanthemi  (Ju Hua) | 12 g |
| Radix Angelicae Sinensis  (Dang Gui) | 12 g |
| Radix Paeoniae Lactiflorae  (Bai Shao) | 9 g |
| Radix Rehmanniae  (Sheng Di Huang) | 12 g |
| Radix Panacis Quiquefloii  (Xi Yang Shen) | 12 g |
| Rhizoma Atractylodis Macrocephalae  (Bai Zhu) | 9 g |
| Poria  (Fu Ling) | 12 g |
| Pericarpium Citri Reticulatae  (Chen Pi) | 6 g |
| Radix Glycyrrhizae  (Gan Cao) | 3 g |

According to the original records the Rhizoma Atractylodis Macrocephalae should be roasted and the Radix Glycyrrhizae processed for use. The Radix Paeoniae Lactiflorae should be prepared with millet wine. All ingredients were ground into powder and made into honey pills the size of mung beans. Three grams of pills were taken each time with boiled water before sleep.

## Comments

This prescription was modified on the basis of Eight Treasures Decoction (Ba Zhen Tang). Its original ingredients were copied here to reinforce *qi* and blood, the root cause of the condition. The Pericarpium Citri Reticulatae and Flos Inullae were added to strengthen the spleen, resolve phlegm and rectify the reversed *qi*. The Flos Chrysanthemi and Radix Gastrodiae were used to soothe the liver and ease dizziness and vertigo. The combination of the Radix Gastrodiae and Rhizoma Ligustici Chuanxiong bears the therapeutic property of Radix Gastrodiae Pill (Tian Ma Wan) as recorded in *Prescriptions Helping the Ordinary* (*Pu Ji Fang*). The two can be applied to treat patients for headache, dizziness and vertigo due to phlegm-wind. The name of the pill is therefore appropriate.

## VII.3. PRESCRIPTION FOR LIVER *QI* STAGNATION DIZZINESS

Prescription for Liver *Qi* Stagnation Dizziness (Gan Jue Tou Yun Fang) was prepared for Emperor Guangxu on the 23rd day of the 11th month of the lunar calendar. No information was given as to the year or the imperial physician who prepared the prescription.

### Ingredients

| | |
|---|---|
| Ramulus Uncariae cum Uncis  (Gou Teng) | 3 g |
| Pericarpium Citri Reticulatae  (Chen Pi) | 3 g |
| Rhizoma Pinelliae  (Ban Xia) | 3 g |
| Radix Ophiopogonis  (Mai Men Dong) | 4.5 g |
| Poria  (Fu Ling) | 4.5 g |
| Gypsum Fibrosum  (Shi Gao) | 4.5 g |
| Radix Angelicae Sinensis  (Dang Shen) | 4.5 g |
| Flos Chrysanthemi  (Ju Hua) | 4.5 g |
| Radix Ledebouriellae  (Fang Feng) | 4.5 g |
| Radix Glycyrrhizae  (Gan Cao) | 2.4 g |
| Rhizoma Zingiberis Recens  (Sheng Jiang) | 7 slices |

The above ingredients were prepared as decoction for oral administration.

## Comments

The dizziness quoted here refers to that caused by failure of the liver in maintaining free flow of *qi*. According to the analysis of the ingredients, it should be a prescription for dealing with dizziness and vertigo due to derangement of *qi* between the liver and stomach as well as the subsequent upward disturbance of liver *qi* by phlegm. Specifically, Rhizoma Pinelliae and Pericarpium Citri Reticulatae were used to wipe out the dampness, resolve phlegm, regulate *qi* and pacify the stomach. The Gypsum Fibrosum and Radix Ophiopogonis were applied to nourish Yin and sedate fire. The Ramulus Uncariae cum Uncis and Radix

Glycyrrhizae were used to soothe the liver and quell wind. The Radix Ledebour-iellae was applied to enhance the effect of the decoction in eliminating wind and dampness. In fact, the ingredients in this prescription are intended to cope with conditions of both the liver and stomach. As for Emperor Guangxu's condition, this prescription was appropriate. His deficient Middle Jiao, however, should limit the use of Gypsum Fibrosum of a cooling property.

# VIII. PRESCRIPTION FOR FACIAL EDEMA

## VIII.1. FACIAL EDEMA PRESCRIPTION

The original records provide no name of the imperial physician who formu-lated the prescription, nor the specific lunar time.

*Ingredients*

| | |
|---|---|
| Radix Angelicae Sinensis  (Dang Gui) | 3 g |
| Herba Schizonepetae  (Jing Jie) | 15 g |
| Radix Ledebouriellae  (Fang Feng) | 15 g |
| Radix Gentianae Macrophyllae  (Qin Jiao) | 9 g |
| Fructus Forsythiae  (Lian Qiao) | 15 g |
| Flos Lonicerae  (Jin Yin Hua) | 15 g |
| Radix Coptidis  (Huang Lian) | 9 g |
| Radix Glycyrrhizae  (Gan Cao) | 30 g |

The above ingredients were soaked in five to six bowls of water to be decocted until two to three bowls of concentrated decoction remained. This was used to compress and wash the face.

*Comments*

This prescription has the action of eliminating wind and dampness and clearing pathogenic heat. The remedy was prepared for facial edema due to invasion of dampness and wind into the facial region. It remains to be seen whether it is effective.

# IX. OPHTHALMOLOGICAL PRESCRIPTIONS

## IX.1. HEAD-CLEARING AND EYE COMPRESS REMEDY

Head-clearing and Eye Compress Remedy (Qing Shang Zhi Tong Xun Mu Fang) was carefully prepared by the imperial physician Zhao Wenkui for Emperor Guangxu, on the 29th day of the first month of the lunar calendar, with no information given as to the year.

*Ingredients*

| | |
|---|---|
| Flos Chrysanthemi  (Ju Hua) | 6 g |
| Folium Mori  (Sang Ye) | 6 g |
| Herba Menthae  (Bo He) | 3 g |
| Radix Paeoniae Rubra  (Chi Shao Yao) | 9 g |

| Fructus Leonuri  (Chong Wei Zi) | 6 g |
| Bombyx Batryticatus  (Jiang Can ) | 6 g |

The original recipe says the Bombyx Batryticatus should be roasted before use. The above ingredients were boiled in water for compressing the eyes.

### Comments

Eye problems bothered Emperor Guangxu for many years. Around 1899 to 1904, references to his eye condition were seen here and there in his health records. In the second month of the lunar calendar of 1899, his health records stated "There was still congestion in the eyes, blurring of vision, especially in the left eye, and occasional swelling in the eyelids." As late as 1904, similar words were found in his health records. Judging from the symptoms and signs recorded in the Emperor's medical records, he might have suffered from a type of chronic conjunctivitis. Several prescriptions for external washing were prepared in an attempt to treat this chronic eye condition. As many as 15 such prescriptions were selected in this book. Basically, they can be divided into four categories, i. e. prescriptions for eliminating wind and heat, for sedating liver fire, activating blood and clearing heat, for soothing the liver, regulating *qi* and sedating fire, and for reinforcing Yin, sedating Yang, eliminating wind, and clearing heat and compressing the eyes.

Although this prescription is entitled Head-clearing and Eye Compress Remedy, it was actually aimed at eliminating wind, clearing heat, nourishing the liver and brightening the vision. The Bombyx Batryticatus was used for eliminating wind and relieving eye congestion. The Fructus Leonuri, functioning in cooling the liver and brightening the vision, was used here for eye conditions due to blood stasis. Radix Paeoniae Rubra, entering into the liver channel, is particularly good at sedating liver fire and treating eye conditions. The above ingredients are characterized by fragrance and ascending properties, and were thus used for hot-compressing the eyes in Emperor Guangxu's case.

## IX.2. EYEWASH REMEDY FOR CLEARING LIVER FIRE AND RELIEVING PAIN

Eyewash Remedy for Clearing Liver Fire and Relieving Pain (Qing Gan Ding Tong Xi Mu Fang) was carefully prepared by the imperial physician Zhao Wenkui for Emperor Guangxu on the 25th day of the ninth month of the lunar calendar, with no information given as to the year.

### Ingredients

| Bombyx Batryticatus  (Jiang Can) | 6 g |
| Herba Menthae  (Bo He) | 1.8 g |
| Radix Paeoniae Rubra  (Chi Shao) | 6 g |
| Flos Carthami  (Hong Hua) | 3 g |
| Herba Equiseti Hiemalis  (Mu Zei Cao) | 3 g |
| Nux Prinsepiae  (Rui Ren) | 4.5 g |
| Cortex Fraxini  (Qin Pi) | 6 g |

The original recipe calls for the Bombyx Batryticatus to be roasted before use. The above ingredients were boiled in water for local eyewashing.

*Comments*

The remedy nomenclature actually implies its therapeutic properties. Bombyx Batryticatus eliminates wind and disperses mass. Radix Paeoniae Rubra clears heat and activates blood circulation. Herba Menthae clears wind-heat. Herba Equiseti Hiemalis eliminates heat, subdues fire and brightens the vision. Cortex Fraxini clears heat from the liver and also brightens the vision. The combination of these ingredients tends to clear heat, subdue fire, cool blood and relieve toxic heat.

## IX.3.  EYEWASH REMEDY FOR CLEARING HEAT AND BRIGHTENING VISION

Eyewash Remedy for Clearing Heat and Brightening Vision (Qing Re Ming Mu Xi Yao Fang) was carefully worked out by the imperial physician Tong Chenhai for Emperor Guangxu around seven to nine o'clock in the evening on the 27th day of the fifth month of the lunar calendar, with no information given as to the year.

*Ingredients*

| | |
|---|---:|
| Flos Chrysanthemi  (Ju Hua) | 4.5 g |
| Herba Menthae  (Bo He) | 2.4 g |
| Radix Paeoniae Rubra  (Chi Shao) | 6 g |
| Radix Gentianae  (Long Dan Cao) | 4.5 g |
| Fructus Tribuli Terrestris  (Bai Ji Li) | 6 g |
| Bombyx Batryticatus  (Jiang Can) | 4.5 g |

The above ingredients were boiled in water for local steaming and washing p.r.n.

*Comments*

This prescription was formed on the basis of Head-clearing and Eye-compress Remedy (Qing Shang Zhi Tong Xun Mu Fang) by omitting Folium Mori and Fructus Leonuri, while adding Radix Gentianae and Fructus Tribuli Terrestris. Fructus Tribuli Terrestris entering into the liver channel brightens the vision and eliminates wind. This is also a modified prescription according to the first one in this chapter.

## IX.4.  EYEWASH REMEDY FOR REMOVING STASIS AND BRIGHTENING VISION

Eyewash Remedy for Removing Stasis and Brightening Vision (Xiao Yu Ming Mu Xi Yao Fang) was carefully prepared by the imperial physician Zhao Wenkui for Emperor Guangxu on the third day of the ninth month of the lunar calendar without any information as to the year.

*Ingredients*

| | |
|---|---:|
| Herba Equiseti Hiemalis  (Mu Zei Cao) | 3 g |
| Radix Paeoniae Rubra  (Chi Shao) | 6 g |
| Flos Carthami  (Hong Hua) | 3 g |
| Nux Prinsepiae  (Rui Ren) | 6 g |
| Flos Eriocauli  (Gu Jing Cao) | 3 g |

Natrii Sulfas Exsiccatus  (Xuan Ming Fen)                            4.5 g

The original records require the Nux Prinsepiae to be ground into powder, then all the above ingredients were boiled for local compress and washing.

### Comments

The explanation of the prescription is similar to the previous one. The only difference is in the use of Natrii Sulfas Exsiccatus. In this prescription, it was applied externally to the local area. Because of its pungent salty aroma, it has the action of clearing heat and subduing fire. According to the record in *Folk Remedies* (Jian Bian Fang), compressing it on a piece of beancurd and extracting the liquid for use as eye drops can treat patients for congestion in the eye. Modern studies prove that the fluid from its main element $Na_2SO_4$ produces good anti-swelling and pain-relieving effects, especially that of promoting lymph formation in case of infectious trauma.

## IX.5.  PRESCRIPTION FOR SUBDUING LIVER FIRE AND BRIGHTENING VISION

Prescription for Subduing Liver Fire and Brightening Vision (Qing Gan Yi Huo Ming Mu Fang) was carefully prepared by the imperial physician Zhao Wenkui for Emperor Guangxu on the seventh day of the 12th month of the lunar calendar, with no information given as to the year.

### Ingredients

| | |
|---|---|
| Fructus Leonuri  (Chong Wei Zi) | 6 g |
| Cortex Fraxini  (Qin Pi) | 6 g |
| Radix Paeoniae Rubra  (Chi Shao) | 4.5 g |
| Pericarpium Citri Reticulatae Viride (Qing Pi) | 6 g |
| Natrii Sulfas Exsiccatus  (Xuan Ming Fen) | 3 g |
| Herba Equiseti Hiemalis  (Mu Zei Cao) | 3 g |
| Nux Prinsepiae  (Rui Ren) | 6 g |

The above ingredients were boiled in water for external washing and hot compress.

### Comments

This prescription has the action of clearing toxic heat, eliminating wind and brightening the vision. Cortex Fraxini, bitter and pungent, was used to soothe the liver and disperse stagnant *qi*, preventing stagnant liver *qi* from turning into heat. The therapeutic principle adopted here is one for dealing with the root cause of the condition.

## IX.6.  EYE-COMPRESS REMEDY FOR CLEARING LIVER FIRE AND BRIGHTENING VISION

Eye-compress Remedy for Clearing Liver Fire and Brightening Vision (Qing Gan Ming Mu Xun Xi Fang) was carefully prepared by the imperial physician Zhao Wenkui for Emperor Guangxu on the first day of the fifth month of the lunar calendar in 1903.

*Ingredients*

| | |
|---|---|
| Herba Equiseti Hiemalis  (Mu Zei Cao) | 6 g |
| Radix Paeoniae Rubra  (Chi Shao) | 6 g |
| Flos Carthami  (Hong Hua) | 3 g |
| Folium Mori  (Sang Ye) | 3 g |
| Bombyx Batryticatus  (Jiang Can) | 6 g |
| Herba Chloranthus Spicatus  (Zhu Lan Cha) | 3 g |

The original records state that frosted Folium Mori and roasted Bombyx Batryticatus should be used. The above ingredients should be boiled for external hot compress and washing.

*Comments*

The characteristics of this prescription is that ingredients for promoting blood circulation were added to those for eliminating wind, clearing heat and brightening the vision. According to studies carried out in different areas of China, the therapeutic principle known as activating blood and resolving blood stasis has an anti-inflammatory effect in the treatment of various types of inflammation. This therapeutic principle has also been reported in the treatment of conjunctivitis. It is therefore apparent that combining ingredients for activating blood and resolving blood stasis is a superior way of forming prescriptions which distinguished the imperial physicians from other current practitioners of TCM.

## IX.7. HERBAL WASH FOR ELIMINATING HEAT AND BRIGHTENING VISION

Herbal Wash For Eliminating Heat and Brightening Vision (Qing Jie Ming Mu Xi Yao Fang) was carefully prepared by the imperial physician Yang Jihe on the 10th day of the fifth month of the lunar calendar, with no information given as to the year.

*Ingredients*

| | |
|---|---|
| Herba Menthae  (Bo He) | 4.5 g |
| Fructus Viticis  (Man Jing Zi) | 6 g |
| Radix Ledebouriellae  (Fang Feng) | 6 g |
| Radix Coptidis  (Huang Lian) | 6 g |
| Radix Gentianae  (Long Dan Cao) | 6 g |
| Pericarpium Citri Reticulatae Viride  (Qing Pi) | 9 g |
| Rhizoma Ligustici Chuanxiong  (Chuanxiong) | 9 g |
| Folium Mori  (Sang Ye) | 12 g |

The original recipe calls for the Pericarpium Citri Reticulatae Viride to be roasted. The Radix Coptidis and Radix Gentianae should be prepared with millet wine and the Fructus Viticis and Radix Coptidis made into powder. The above ingredients were well boiled in water for local compress and washing.

*Comments*

In this prescription, the Herba Menthae and Folium Mori were used for clearing heat and eliminating wind. The Fructus Viticis and Radix Ledebouriellae were used for their pungent, warming properties in promoting the dispersal of pathogenic factors. The Rhizoma Ligustici Chuanxiong was used for regulating the function of the liver and promoting blood circulation. The Pericarpium Citri Reticulatae Viride was used for strengthening the spleen and regulating *qi*. The Radix Gentianae was used for clearing damp-heat from the liver and gallbladder. The Radix Coptidis, bitter and cold, was used for purging toxic heat, eliminating dryness and heat. The main element of Radix Coptidis is berberine with its strong effect in resisting and killing bacteria. According to reports, lower concentrations of coptisine may resist cocci, bacilli and protozoa while high concentrations are effective in killing bacteria. Clinically, Radix Coptidis decoction has been reported to have good effects in the treatment of purulent infections. The Radix Coptidis should be roasted with millet wine to help achieve better ascending effects. *Entrance to Medicine* (*Yi Xue Ru Men*) says, "Radix Coptidis roasted with millet wine helps its medicinal effect to rise to the head, eyes and tongue." The combination of Radix Coptidis with other ingredients in the prescription strengthens the therapeutic effect in clearing heat from the upper part of the body and brightening the vision. According to *Orthodox Explanation to Materia Medica* (*Ben Cao Zheng Yi*), Radix Coptidis in the treatment of "eye conditions must be combined with ingredients that have the effect of eliminating wind and subduing fire," but this may only be a claim based on personal experience.

## IX.8. EYEWASH REMEDY I

Eyewash Remedy I (Xi Mu Fang Yi) was recorded without indicating the time or the name of the imperial physician who formulated it.

*Ingredients*

| | |
|---|---|
| Radix Ledebouriellae  (Fang Feng) | 4.5 g |
| Herba Menthae  (Bo He) | 2.4 g |
| Flos Chrysanthemi  (Ju Hua) | 6 g |
| Folium Mori  (Sang Ye) | 3 g |
| Radix Paeoniae Rubra  (Chi Shao) | 6 g |

The above ingredients were well boiled in water for local washing.

*Comments*

This prescription was modified on the basis of Head-clearing and Eye-compress Remedy (Qing Shang Zhi Tong Xun Mu Fang) by omitting Fructus Leonuri and adding Radix Ledebouriellae that has the action of eliminating wind and dampness, and clearing wind from the facial area. *The Pearl Pocket* (*Zhen Zhu Nang*) says, "Radix Ledebouriellae has the effect of dispersing stagnant *qi* in the facial region and eyes, and dispelling remaining stagnant *qi* in the channels and collaterals." The reason for using Radix Ledebouriellae was therefore to reinforce the effect of the prescription in dispelling dampness.

## IX.9. EYEWASH REMEDY II

Eyewash Remedy II (Xi Mu Fang Er) was carefully prepared for Emperor Guangxu by the imperial physician Yang Shifen on the third day of the intercalary third month of the lunar calendar in 1903.

*Ingredients*

| | |
|---|---:|
| Folium Mori  (Sang Ye) | 3 g |
| Rhizoma Cyperi  (Xia Ku Cao) | 3 g |
| Periostracum Cicadae  (Chan Tui) | 3 g |
| Folium Menthae  (Bo He Ye) | 1.5 g |
| Herba Equiseti Hiemalis  (Mu Zei Cao) | 3 g |
| Flos Chrysanthemi  (Ju Hua) | 3 g |
| Radix Angelicae Dahuricae  (Bai Zhi) | 3 g |
| Radix Angelicae Sinensis  (Dang Gui) | 4.5 g |

The original records say that frosted Folium Mori, and Radix Angelicae Sinensis processed with millet wine should be used. The above ingredients were well boiled in water for local washing and compress.

*Comments*

This prescription was also modified according to the principle of clearing wind-heat and dampness. Rhizoma Cyperi, bitter and pungent in flavour but cold in property, helps to clear heat and relieve congestion of the eye, purge fire from the liver channel and promote vision. It was used for treating painful eyes due to liver fire. Radix Angelicae Dahuricae, pungent and warm, disperses wind-cold from the superficial portion of the body, clears nasal obstruction and stops pain. Periostracum Cicadae clears nephelium and brightens the vision. Radix Angelicae Sinensis, commonly believed to be an ingredient for nourishing blood and promoting its circulation, was used here for reinforcing blood and removing obstruction from the channels and collaterals. All of the ingredients, plus Folium Mori, Flos Chrysanthemi and Herba Menthae together achieve the aim of clearing wind-heat, removing nephelium and promoting vision.

## IX.10. EYEWASH REMEDY III

Eyewash Remedy III (Xi Mu Fang San) was carefully prepared by the imperial physician Tong Chenhai around nine to 11 o'clock on the eighth day of the fifth month of the lunar calendar in 1903.

*Ingredients*

| | |
|---|---:|
| Folium Mori  (Sang Ye) | 2.4 g |
| Herba Menthae  (Bo He) | 2.4 g |
| Bombyx Batryticatus  (Jiang Can) | 3 g |
| Nux Prinsepiae  (Rui Ren) | 3 g |
| Radix Paeoniae Rubra  (Chi Shao) | 4.5 g |
| Semen Celosiae  (Qing Xiang Zi) | 2.4 g |

The original records say that the Nux Prinsepiae should be made into powder before use. Folium Mori should be frosted. The above ingredients were well boiled in water for local compress and washing.

*Comments*

This prescription was formed on the basis of modifying ingredients from Head-clearing and Eye-compress Remedy (Qing Shang Zhi Tong Xun Mu Fang) by omitting Fructus Leonuri and Flos Chrysanthemi while adding Semen Celosiae and Nux Prinsepiae. Semen Celosiae, a main ingredient for treating eye conditions, has the effect of promoting eyesight and clearing nephelium. Nux Prinsepiae, sweet and cold, has the effect of eliminating wind, dispersing heat, nourishing the liver and brightening the vision. *The Original Classics* (*Ben Jing*) says, "Nux Prinsepiae, brightening the vision, is indicated in eye congestion, painful eyes and lacrimation." *Elementary Comments on Materia Medica* (*Ben Cao Meng Quan*) claims Nux Prinsepiae "is applied only in treating various eye conditions." Being effective in the treatment of congestion of eyes, eye swelling, nephelium covering the pupil, and blurring of vision.

## IX.11. EYEWASH REMEDY IV

Eyewash Remedy IV (Xi Mu Fang Si) was carefully prepared by the imperial physician Yang Shifen around seven to nine o'clock on the second day of the ninth month of the lunar calendar in 1903.

*Ingredients*

| | |
|---|---|
| Folium Mori  (Sang Ye) | 6 g |
| Flos Chrysanthemi  (Ju Hua) | 3 g |
| Bombyx Batryticatus  (Jiang Can) | 6 g |
| Herba Menthae  (Bo He) | 2.4 g |
| Semen Cassiae  (Cao Jue Ming) | 3 g |
| Radix Paeoniae Lactiflorae  (Bai Shao) | 6 g |
| Pericarpium Citri Reticulatae Rubra  (Ju Luo) | 3 g |
| Radix Angelicae Sinensis  (Dang Gui) | 6 g |

According to the original records, the Folium Mori should be used frosted. The above ingredients were boiled for local compress and washing.

### Comments

This prescription was formed by using mainly pungent dispersing ingredients that have the effect of eliminating pathogenic wind, plus ingredients for soothing the liver, reinforcing Yin, promoting blood circulation and removing obstruction. It was also modified on the basis of Head-clearing and Eye-compress Remedy (Qing Shang Zhi Tong Xun Mu Fang).

## IX.12. EYEWASH REMEDY V

Eyewash Remedy V (Xi Mu Fang Wu) was carefully prepared by the imperial physician Tong Chenhai on the 22nd day of the 11th month of the lunar calendar, with no information given as to the year.

*Ingredients*

| | |
|---|---|
| Flos Chrysanthemi  (Ju Hua) | 3 g |
| Herba Menthae  (Bo He) | 2.1 g |
| Radix Paeoniae Rubra  (Chi Shao) | 3 g |
| Bombyx Batryticatus  (Jiang Can) | 3 g |
| Flos Eriocauli  (Gu Jing Cao) | 3 g |
| Flos Lonicerae  (Jin Yin Hua) | 3 g |
| Nux Prinsepiae  (Rui Ren) | 4.5 g |

Gypsum Fibrosum  (Shi Gao)                                    6 g

The original recipe calls for raw Gypsum Fibrosum to be used. The above ingredients were well boiled in water for local compress and washing.

### Comments

This prescription was formed on the basis of Head-clearing and Eye-compress Remedy (Qing Shang Zhi Tong Xun Mu Fang) by omitting Fructus Leonuri and Folium Mori while adding Flos Eriocauli for clearing wind-heat. Gypsum Fibrosum was used here to eliminate heat, while Nux Prinsepiae was to clear dampness from the urinary tract. The combination of the two should also help to clear pathogenic heat.

## IX.13. EYEWASH REMEDY VI

Eyewash Remedy VI (Xi Mu Fang Liu) was carefully prepared by the imperial physician Tong Chenhai around seven to nine o'clock on the sixth day of the 12th month of the lunar calendar, with no information given concerning the year.

### Ingredients
Folium Mori  (Sang Ye)                                        3 g
Flos Chrysanthemi  (Ju Hua)                                 4.5 g
Radix Paeoniae Rubra  (Chi Shao)                             6 g
Nux Prinsepiae  (Rui Ren)                                   4.5 g

According to the original records, the Folium Mori should be used frosted. The above ingredients were well boiled in water for local compress and washing.

### Comments

Although the number of ingredients in this prescription is quite small, the selection is quite reasonable as the ingredients have the effect of eliminating wind-heat and nourishing the liver. A prescription for eye washing and compress does not necessarily need to include many ingredients.

## IX.14. EYEWASH REMEDY VII

Eyewash Remedy VII (Xi Mu Fang Qi) was carefully prepared by the imperial physician Ren Xigen for Emperor Guangxu around seven to nine o'clock on the 25th day of the first month of the lunar calendar, with no information given as to the year.

### Ingredients
Pericarpium Citri Reticulatae Viride  (Qing Pi)             3 g
Natrii Sulfas Exsiccatus  (Xuan Ming Fen)                   3 g
Cortex Phellodendri  (Huang Bai)                             6 g
Radix Ledebouriellae  (Fang Feng)                           3 g
Flos Chrysanthemi  (Ju Hua)                                 3 g
Rhizoma Picrorhizae  (Hu Huang Lian)                       2.4 g

The above ingredients were well boiled for local washing and compress.

### Comments

This prescription has the action of clearing heat, eliminating wind, soothing the liver, promoting bile excretion, nourishing kidney Yin and brightening the vision. Rhizoma Picrorhizae was used for clearing heat. According to *Newly Revised Canon of Materia Medica* (*Xin Xiu Ben Cao*), Rhizoma Picrorhizae has the effect of "reinforcing the liver and gallbladder, and brightening the vision." Cortex Phellodendri nourishes Yin and subdues fire. The combination of Rhizoma Picrorhizae and Cortex Phellodendri helps to clear the internal heat due to Yin deficiency.

## IX.15.  EYEWASH REMEDY VIII

Eyewash Remedy VIII (Xi Mu Fang Ba) was carefully prepared by the imperial physician Ren Xigen for Emperor Guangxu, with no information given concerning the time.

*Ingredients*

| | |
|---|---|
| Bombyx Batryticatus  (Jiang Can) | 6 g |
| Flos Chrysanthemi  (Ju Hua) | 3 g |
| Pericarpium Citri Reticulatae Viride  (Qing Pi) | 4.5 g |
| Natrii Sulfas Exsiccatus  (Xuan Ming Fen) | 3 g |

The above ingredients were well boiled in water for local compress and washing.

*Comments*

The Bombyx Batryticatus in this prescription clears wind-heat, while the Flos Chrysanthemi nourishes the liver and brightens vision. Natrii Sulfas Exsiccatus clears heat and subdues fire. Pericarpium Citri Reticulatae Viride soothes the liver and relieves *qi* stagnation. The grouping of ingredients here is very appropriate and significant.

## IX.16.  EYE COMPRESS REMEDY

Eye Compress Remedy (Xun Mu Fang) was prepared carefully by the imperial physician Zhao Wenkui for Emperor Guangxu on the 24th day of the 11th month of the lunar calendar, with no information given concerning the time.

*Ingredients*

| | |
|---|---|
| Concha Margaritifere Usta  (Zhen Zhu Mu) | 18 g |
| Fructus Schisandrae  (Wu Wei Zi) | 6 g |
| Magnetitum  (Ci Shi) | 18 g |
| Flos Chrysanthemi  (Ju Hua) | 18 g |
| Folium Mori  (Sang Ye) | 6 g |
| Haematitum  (Dai Zhe Shi) | 9 g |

The original writings require that the Concha Margaritifera Usta should be raw, the Folium Mori frosted and the Magnetitum and Haematitum fried. The above ingredients were roasted with vinegar for eye compress whenever necessary.

*Comments*

The combination of ingredients in this prescription is very considered and appropriate. Folium Mori and Flos Chrysanthemi eliminate wind and clear heat from the Upper Jiao. According to *Great Ming Dynasty Materia Medica* (*Ri Hua Zi Ben Cao*), Fructus Schisandrae promotes eyesight. Modern pharmaceutical studies prove that it does actually promote eyesight for those with or without eye disease; it also improves vision. The main chemical element in Haematitum is $Fe_2O_3$, which soothes the liver and sedates the abnormal rising of *qi*. According to the record from *Ren Zhai Zhi Internal Medicine Formula* (*Ren Zhai Zhi Zhi Fang*), two portions of Haematitum and one portion of Gypsum Fibrosum, turned into powder and finally made into soft paste to be spread respectively at the inner and outer canthuses as well as at the temporal regions, can help patients with congestion of the eye and clouded pupil due to nephelium. The combination of Concha Margaritiferae Usta, Magnetitum and Massa Fermentata Medicinalis, processed in pill form and known as Magnetitum and Concha Margaritiferae Usta Pill (Ci Zhu Wan) according to *Prescriptions Worth a Thousand Gold* (*Qian Jin Yao Fang*), is indicated in blurring of vision and dizzy sensation. The chemical element of Magnetitum is $Fe_3O_4$. Again, according to *The Great Ming Dynasty Materia Medica* (*Ri Hua Zi Ben Cao*), Magnetitum was used for treating poor vision. According to the book *Amplification on Materia Medica* (*Ben Cao Yan Yi*), Magnetitum was applied for deafness, kidney deficiency and blurring of vision. Concha Margaritiferae Usta, mainly consisting of $Na_2CO_3$, has the action of soothing the liver and sedating hyperactivity of liver Yang. According to the records in *New Reference for Diet Therapy* (*Yin Fa Xin Can*), Magnetitum has the effect of dealing with accumulation of pathogenic heat and eye conditions. According to recent reports, some professionals applied Concha Margaritiferae Usta as the chief ingredient plus Rhizoma Atractylodis and Radix Ginseng prepared in decoction form for the treatment of some eye conditions such as lenticular opacity and optic nerve atrophy. This prescription is on the whole typical of minerals, shells and plant ingredients in combination.

## IX.17.  EYE COMPRESS REMEDY I

Eye Compress Remedy I (Xun Xi Fang Yi) was carefully prepared for Emperor Guangxu by the imperial physician Zhao Wenkui on the 23rd day of the 11th month of the lunar calendar, with no information given as to the year.

### Ingredients

| | |
|---|---|
| Flos Chrysanthemi  (Ju Hua) | 6 g |
| Folium Mori  (Sang Ye) | 6 g |
| Nux Prinsepiae  (Rui Ren) | 6 g |
| Radix Paeoniae Rubra  (Chi Shao) | 6 g |
| Flos Eriocauli  (Gu Jing Cao) | 6 g |

The above ingredients were boiled in water for local compress and washing.

### Comments

This prescription is a modification of the previous one, with a still smaller number of ingredients. As Zhao Wenkui served as an imperial physician in the late

Qing Dynasty, it may be assumed that this prescription was prepared for Emperor Guangxu around 1904.

## IX.18.  EYE COMPRESS REMEDY II

Eye Compress Remedy II (Xun Xi Fang Er) was prepared for Emperor Guangxu, with no information given as to the time.

*Ingredients*

| | |
|---|---|
| Flos Chrysanthemi  (Ju Hua) | 9 g |
| Folium Mori  (Sang Ye) | 9 g |
| Radix Ledebouriellae  (Fang Feng) | 9 g |
| Flos Eriocauli  (Gu Jing Cao) | 9 g |
| Concha Haliotidis  (Shi Jue Ming) | 9 g |
| Radix Paeoniae Rubra  (Chi Shao) | 9 g |
| Herba Menthae  (Bo He) | 3 g |
| Nux Prinsepiae  (Rui Ren) | 9 g |
| Bombyx Batryticatus  (Jiang Can) | 6 g |
| Folium Calmelliae Sinensis  (Cha Ye) | 9 g |
| Radix Scutellariae  (Huang Qin) | 9 g |

According to the original records, the Folium Mori should be frosted and the Bombyx Batryticatus roasted. The above ingredients were boiled for local compress and washing.

*Comments*

Careful reading of the prescription reveals that most of the ingredients are those normally applied for eye disorders. Folium Mori clears heat from the liver channel and brightens the vision. According to ancient TCM literature such remedies as Folium Mori and Radix Ephedrae Pill (Sang Ma Wan) and Rehmanniae Pill with Fructus Lyoli and Flos Chrysanthemi (Ji Ju Di Huang Wan) existed. Flos Eriocauli and Radix Ledebouriellae processed into fine powder are effective in treating nephelium. Nux Prinsepiae nourishes the liver and brightens the vision. It was used in combination with Folium Mori and Flos Chrysanthemi in the treatment of congestion and swelling of the eye. The imperial physicians' prescriptions clearly indicate that Emperor Guangxu had suffered from eye conditions due to wind-heat invasion.

# X.  PRESCRIPTIONS FOR NASAL CONDITIONS

## X.1.  BLUE CLOUD POWDER

Blue Cloud Powder (Bi Yun San) was carefully prepared by the imperial physicians Fan Shaoxiang and Xiao Tingjian for Emperor Guangxu on the 27th day of the 10th month of the lunar calendar, with no information given as to the year.

*Ingredients*

| | |
|---|---|
| Herba Menthae  (Bo He) | 3 g |

| | |
|---|---|
| Flos Chrysanthemi (Ju Hua) | 3 g |
| Rhizoma Ligustici Chuanxiong (Chuan Xiong) | 3 g |
| Radix Angelicae Dahuricae (Bai Zhi) | 3 g |
| Herba Centipedae (E Er Bu Shi Cao) | 0.9 g |
| Indigo Naturalis (Qing Dai) | 0.9 g |
| Borneolum Syntheticum (Bing Pian) | 0.6 g |

The original records require that the Herba Menthae should be grown in the south. The above ingredients were processed into fine powder and filtered for very gentle nasal inhalation.

*Comments*

This prescription was also presented for treating Empress Dowager Cixi's recurrent nasal condition. The only difference is that it did not include Herba Asari and Scorpio, but did include Borneolum Syntheticum and Flos Chrysanthemi. According to the health records of Empress Dowager Cixi she suffered from facial spasm. In her prescription, therefore, Scorpio was used for stopping wind and releasing spasm, while Herba Asari was for eliminating wind-cold and stopping pain.

Emperor Guangxu's situation was different. He had constitutional Yin deficiency. His health records state, "Occasional dryness and pain in the left nasal cavity, unpleasant nasal smell or occasional black thread-like substance in the nasal discharge." The above record shows that he had chronic retention of damp-heat in the Upper Jiao. This was why fragrant Borneolum Syntheticum was used for clearing heat and stopping pain. Flos Chrysanthemi clears wind-heat, nourishes the liver and brightens the vision. This prescription also serves as an example of forming a prescription on the basis of syndrome differentiation in accordance with symptoms and signs.

## X.2. RED JADE OINTMENT

Red Jade Ointment (Hong Yu Gao) was carefully prepared by the imperial physicians Zhu Kun, Men Dingao, Yang Jihe and Zhong Xun on the 25th day of the 11th month of the lunar calendar in 1899.

*Ingredient*

| | |
|---|---|
| Red Jade Oinment (Hong Yu Gao) | 3 g |

*Comments*

With a jade toothpick spread a tittle of the ointment inside the nasal cavity.

*Comments*

Red Jade Ointment, an ointment for external application, can be found in the records of the imperial hospital prescriptions. It consisted of Radix Angelicae Sinensis (30 g), Flos Carthami (9 g), Radix Paeoniae Rubra (9 g), Rhizoma Bletillae Striatae (9 g) and Radix Ledebouriellae (9 g). The above ingredients were fried in 500 grams of sesame oil until they became burnt yellow. The residue was separated out. This was followed by adding 60 grams of yellow wax, 30 grams of mixture from Cinnabari and Hydrargyrum, and 15 grams of Resina Olibani. The paste was used for treating syphilis and furuncles of all sizes. Ingredients in this prescription promote muscle growth in the affected areas, relieve pain and inflammation, stop itching, relieve swelling, and clear toxic boils.

According to health records of Emperor Guangxu on the 25th day of the 11th month of the lunar calendar in 1899, the imperial physicians Zhu Kun, Men Dingao, Yang Jihe and Zhong Xun were allowed to diagnose the Emperor's condition. The prescription formed by the physicians was similar to that introduced here. Nevertheless, the case history of Emperor Guangxu also contained "dryness and pain in the nose with occasional black thread-like substance in the nasal discharge." The indications of this prescription also cover these symptoms and signs. It is therefore assumed that the two prescriptions were actually made on the same day.

## X.3.  NASAL DISCHARGE CLEARING REMEDY

Nasal Dischareg Clearing Remedy (Tou Nao Wen Yao Fang) was prepared by the imperial physician Zhang Zhongyuan for Emperor Guangxu on the sixth day of the sixth month of the lunar calendar.

### Ingredients
| | |
|---|---|
| Usonae  (Song Luo Cha) | 6 g |
| Pedicellus Melo  (Gua Di) | 3 g |
| Borneolum Syntheticum  (Bing Pian) | 0.8 g |

The above ingredients were processed into fine powder for nasal inhalation in order to clear the nasal cavity.

### Comments
Usonae used in the prescription is also known as Nuluo. *The Book of Songs* (*Shi Jing*) says, "Usonae is a parasitic plant known as Nuluo or Niao that grows on pine trees." *The Lament* (*Li Sao*) also records a plant that grows side by side with another called Pili in Chinese language. Usonae, bitter and sweet, can subdue liver fire, disperse wind and relieve toxicity. Pedicellus Melo, bitter and cold, has the effect of resolving nasal polyp according to writings in *Additional Records* (*Bie Lu*). *The Great Ming Dynasty Materia Medica* (*Ri Hua Zi Ben Cao*) also mentions its application in treating nasal obstruction due to exogenous invasion of cold or heat. Borneolum Syntheticum, cool and bitter, removes obstruction from nasal cavity and brightens vision. It is often used in the treatment of nasal polyp. All three have the effect of removing obstruction from the nasal cavity and must have been effective.

# XI.  MOUTHWASH REMEDIES

## XI.1.  MOUTHWASH REMEDY I FOR CLEARING GASTRIC HEAT

Mouthwash Remedy for Clearing Gastric Heat I (Qing Wei Shu Kou Fang Yi) was prepared on the 13th day of the fifth month of the lunar calendar, with no information given concerning the year.

### Ingredients

| | |
|---|---|
| Radix Rehmanniae  (Sheng Di Huang) | 18 g |
| Radix Paeoniae Rubra  (Chi Shao) | 6 g |
| Herba Menthae  (Bo He) | 3 g |
| Natrii Sulfas Exsiccatus  (Xuan Ming Fen) | 3 g |
| Pollen Typhae  (Pu Huang) | 3 g |
| Flos Carthami  (Hong Hua) | 3 g |
| Resina Olibani  (Ru Xiang) | 3 g |
| Herba Violae  (Zi Hua Di Ding) | 3 g |
| Radix Angelicae Dahuricae  (Bai Zhi) | 3 g |

The original recipe calls for raw Pollen Typhae to be used. The above ingredients were boiled in water for rinsing the mouth.

### Comments

Mouth rinsing plays an important role in maintaining oral hygiene. *The Book of Rites* (*Li Ji*) says, "Rinse the mouth with salty water when roosters crow early in the morning." People in ancient times understood well the significance of good oral hygiene in preventing oral diseases. Almost all mouthwash remedies contained medicinal ingredients. In addition to maintaining oral cleanliness, these remedies at the same time and more importantly had therapeutic effects. In TCM theory the mouth maintains a close relationship with the internal Zang-Fu organs. For instance, teeth are related to the kidney while gums are related to the stomach and large intestine. The spleen opens into the mouth while the heart opens into the tongue. According to the health records of Emperor Guangxu, there may have occurred "broken blisters on the left palate, occasional visible specks of blood during oral rinsing, a foreign-body sensation in the throat, forming of blisters on the left side of the throat, slight soreness on that side, and some difficulty in chewing and swallowing food," and "toothache on the left side." The above description indicates that Emperor Guangxu suffered from such conditions as oral ulcer, periodontitis and chronic pharygitis. Most of his mouthwash remedies therefore had the action of clearing gastric heat.

In this prescription, Gypsum Fibrosum was used as the main ingredient to clear stomach fire. Natrii Sulfas Exsiccatus was added to strengthen that effect. Herba Menthae, with pungent flavour and cooling property, according to *Concise Materia Medica for Emergencies* (*Ben Cao Bei Yao*), is useful in treating disorders of the mouth, eye, ear and throat. Flos Carthami, Radix Paeoniae Rubra and Pollen Typhae can all activate blood and promote menstruation. At the same time, they have the effect of clearing toxic heat. According to contemporary pharmaceutical studies, most blood-activating ingredients have anti-inflammatory effects. It is true that this prescription is effective in clearing fire from the gastrointestinal system, relieving toxic heat and activating blood. It should be mentioned that mouthwash remedies are applied only for mouthwashing. Analysis should be made by combining the local and general conditions in order to understand the principles involved.

Three ingredients, namely Resina Olibani, Herba Violae and Radix Angelicae Dahuricae in the prescription were added by Emperor Guangxu himself as the characters with a Chinese brush-pen in the original bore much resemblance. Emperor Guangxu suffered from many ailments which helped him understand certain TCM principles. He had the habit of correcting the prescriptions presented by imperial physicians, and his health records show a number of changes in prescriptions or ingredients. In this prescription these four ingredients were added in light of symptoms and signs, for Resina Olibani and Herba Violae are far from pleasant, and some were not sure whether he would like them or not. Perhaps, after long illness, he used these ingredients in hatred of his illnesses.

## XI.2. MOUTHWASH REMEDY II FOR CLEARING GASTRIC HEAT

Mouthwash Remedy II for Clearing Gastric Heat (Qing Wei Shu Kou Fang Er) was carefully prepared by the imperial physician Zhao Wenkui for Emperor Guangxu on the eighth day of the ninth month of the lunar calendar, with no information given as to the year.

*Ingredients*

| | |
|---|---|
| Gypsum Fibrosum  (Shi Gao) | 9 g |
| Radix Paeoniae Rubra  (Chi Shao) | 6 g |
| Flos Carthami  (Hong Hua) | 3 g |
| Table salt  (Shi Yan) | 6 g |
| Pollen Typhae  (Pu Huang) | 0.9 g |
| Plumula Nelumbinis  (Lian Xin) | 3 g |

The original recipe calls for raw Gypsum Fibrosum and Pollen Typhae to be used. The Pollen Typhae should be packed for preparation. The above ingredients were boiled for mouthwash.

*Comments*

This prescription has the effect of clearing stomach fire, activating blood and promoting menstruation. Table salt relieves toxic heat. It also enters into the kidney channel and is good for teeth. According to *Treatise on Differentiation and Treatment of Epidemic Febrile Diseases* (*Wen Bin Tiao Bian Lun*), "Plumula Nelumbinis, sweet, salty and bitter, may work into the heart through the kidney and bring heart fire down to the kidney though it enters the kidney channel only. In return, Plumula Nelumbinis can also help take kidney water up to purge heart fire." Plumula Nelumbinis thus harmonizes the heart and kidney. Analysis of the prescription reveals that attention was paid to the relationship between the mouth and stomach, as well as the heart and kidney. This comprehensive approach is beneficial in treatment.

## XI.3. MOUTHWASH REMEDY FOR RELIEVING GUM SWELLING

Mouthwash Remedy for Relieving Gum Swelling (Xiao Zhong Shu Kou Fang) was carefully prepared by the imperial physician Zhao Wenkui, with no information given as to the specific time.

*Ingredients*

| Pollen Typhae  (Pu Huang) | 6 g |
| Flos Carthami  (Hong Hua) | 4.5 g |
| Radix Angelicae Sinensis  (Dang Gui) | 4.5 g |
| Resina Murrhae  (Mo Yao) | 6 g |
| Table salt  (Shi Yan) | 12 g |

The original records say that raw Pollen Typhae and fine roots of Angelicae Sinensis should be used. The above ingredients were boiled for rinsing the mouth.

### Comments

Gum swelling is usually caused by toxic heat and stasis. This prescription was intended basically to relieve swelling by means of removing heat and stasis, focusing on activating blood and removing obstruction from channels and collaterals. The underlying principle was that blood stasis would be removed when blood circulation was activated to normal so that swelling disappeared. Also, table salt, having the effect of relieving heat and fortifying teeth, can help relieve swelling and stop pain.

## XI.4. MOUTHWASH REMEDY FOR CLEARING GASTRIC HEAT AND RELIEVING GUM SWELLING

Mouthwash Remedy for Clearing Gastric Heat and Relieving Gum Swelling (Qing Wei Xiao Zhong Shu Kou Fang) was carefully prepared by the imperial physician Zhao Wenkui on the seventh day of the eighth month of the lunar calendar, with no information given as to the year.

### Ingredients

| Pollen Typhae  (Pu Huang) | 3 g |
| Radix Paeoniae Rubra  (Chi Shao) | 6 g |
| Flos Carthami  (Hong Hua) | 3 g |
| Fructus Forsythiae  (Lian Qiao) | 6 g |
| Gypsum Fibrosum  (Shi Gao) | 12 g |
| Table salt  (Shi Yan) | 6 g |

According to the original records, raw Pollen Typhae and Gypsum Fibrosum should be used. The Pollen Typhae should be packed for preparation. The above ingredients were boiled for rinsing the mouth.

### Comments

The main action of this prescription lies in activating blood and clearing toxic heat.

## XI.5. MOUTHWASH REMEDY I

Mouthwash Remedy I (Shu Kou Fang Yi) was carefully prepared by the imperial physician Zhao Wenkui on the fourth day of the ninth month of the lunar calendar, with no information given as to the year.

### Ingredients

| Gypsum Fibrosum  (Shi Gao) | 12 g |
| Radix Paeoniae Rubra  (Chi Shao) | 6 g |

| | |
|---|---|
| Fructus Forsythiae (Lian Qiao) | 6 g |
| Flos Carthami (Hong Hua) | 3 g |
| Table salt (Shi Yan) | 6 g |
| Flos Lonicerae (Jin Yin Hua) | 6 g |

The original records require that raw Gypsum Fibrosum should be used. All the above ingredients were boiled for rinsing the mouth.

### Comments

This prescription was modified on the basis of the previous one with priority being given to clearing toxic heat.

## XI.6. MOUTHWASH REMEDY II

Mouthwash Remedy II (Shu Kou Fang Er) was carefully prepared by the imperial physician Tong Chenhai around seven to nine o'clock in the evening on the 27th day of the third month of the lunar calendar, with no information given concerning the year.

### Ingredients

| | |
|---|---|
| Berba Menthae (Bo He) | 3 g |
| Flos Lonicerae (Jin Yin Hua) | 4.5 g |
| Gypsum Fibrosum (Shi Gao) | 9 g |
| Radix Paeoniae Rubra (Chi Shao) | 6 g |
| Fructus Forsythiae (Lian Qiao) | 4.5 g |
| Resina Murrhae (Mo Yao) | 3 g |
| Pericarpium Zanthoxyli (Chuan Jiao) | 1.8 g |
| Table salt (Shi Yan) | 6 g |

The original records prescribe that green Fructsu Forsythiae and the leaves of Herba Menthae should be used.

### Comments

This prescription chiefly consists of ingredients that have the effect of relieving toxic heat, plus those for clearing gastric heat, subduing fire, activating blood circulation and removing obstruction from channels and collaterals. The paradox is that Pericarpium Zanthoxyli, pungent and warming, was added into it. This is an example of combining cold and heat properties in clinical practice. According to *Medicinal Plants* (*Yao Xing Ben Cao*), Fructus Forsythiae can "alleviate toothache," so its use in the remedy should be helpful.

## XI.7. MOUTHWASH REMEDY III

Mouthwash Remedy III (Shu Kou Fang San) was carefully prepared by the imperial physician Tong Chenhai around seven to nine o'clock in the evening on the second day of the sixth month of the lunar calendar, with no information given as to the year.

### Ingredients

| | |
|---|---|
| Herba Schizonepetae (Jing Jie Sui) | 3 g |
| Herba Menthae (Bo He) | 3 g |

| | |
|---|---|
| Bombyx Batryticatus  (Jiang Can) | 4.5 g |
| Fructus Forsythiae  (Lian Qiao) | 6 g |
| Radix Paeoniae Rubra  (Chi Shao) | 6 g |
| Flos Lonicerae  (Jin Yin Hua) | 4.5 g |
| Gypsum Fibrosum  (Shi Gao) | 9 g |
| Table salt  (Shi Yan) | 12 g |

The original recipe calls for raw Gypsum Fibrosum to be processed into powder before use. The above ingredients were well boiled for oral rinsing when convenient.

### Comments

Herba Schizonepetae, pungent and warming, eliminates wind and relieves superficial symptoms and signs. It also has an ascending property, thus eliminating wind from the facial and head regions. Herba Menthae, pungent and cooling, eliminates wind-heat. Because of its cooling and dispersing property, Herba Menthae also helps eliminate wind-heat that attacks the head region. These two ingredients, one cold and the other hot in property, mutually assist in playing their therapeutic actions. Gypsum Fibrosum, mainly cold in property, is a major ingredient for eliminating gastric heat. Table salt also relieves toxic heat. Bombyx Batryticatus eliminates wind and softens masses. According to *Compendium of Materia Medica* (*Ben Cao Gang Mu*), it relieves toothache caused by invasion of wind-heat. It is a medicinal ingredient in TCM that can also be used for rubbing against the teeth to ease toothache.

## XI.8. MOUTHWASH REMEDY IV

Mouthwash Remedy IV (Shu Kou Fang Si) was carefully prepared by the imperial physician Tong Chenhai for Emperor Guangxu on the ninth day of the sixth month of the lunar calendar, with no information given concerning the year.

### Ingredients

| | |
|---|---|
| Flos Lonicerae  (Jin Yin Hua) | 6 g |
| Radix Paeoniae Rubra  (Chi Shao) | 6 g |
| Herba Menthae  (Bo He) | 3 g |
| Bombyx Batryticatus  (Jiang Can) | 2.4 g |
| Gypsum Fibrosum  (Shi Gao) | 1.2 g |
| Pollen Typhae  (Pu Huang) | 3 g |
| Radix seu Rhizoma Rhei·  (Da Huang) | 2.1 g |
| Table salt  (Shi Yan) | 12 g |

The original records say that raw Gypsum Fibrosum, and Pollen Typhae in powder form should be used. The above ingredients were boiled for oral rinsing.

### Comments

There is no doubt that this prescription has the action of clearing stomach fire. Radix seu Rhizoma Rhei, bitter and cold, clears fire and cools blood. It also has the effect of relieving swelling, stopping pain and relieving toxic heat. According to *Supplement to Prescriptions for Emergency Cases* (*Bu Que Zhou Hou Fang*), Radix seu Rhizoma Rhei pounded into pieces together with millet wine in paste form applied to swollen areas may treat boils with burning pain. According to *Peaceful Holy Benevolent Prescriptions* (*Tai Ping Shen Hui Fang*), "Rubbing the inside of the mouth with equal proportions of powdered Radix seu Rhizoma Rhei and dried Alum, and spitting out the saliva" may help patients with oral ulcer. Modern test-tube studies show that Radix seu Rhizoma Rhei has an anti-bacteria effect against some gram-positive and gram-negative bacteria. The effective anti-bacteria element is a derivative substance from anthraquinone. Its main function is to restrict bacteria growth. Radix seu Rhizoma Rhei Decoction (Da Huang Tang) also has the effect of restraining the growth of fungi. The use of Radix seu Rhizoma Rhei should therefore be effective in treating the Emperor's oral ulcer.

## XI.9.  MOUTHWASH REMEDY V

Mouthwash Remedy V (Shou Kou Fang Wu) was carefully prepared for Emperor Guangxu by the imperial physician Tong Chenhai on the 15th day of the sixth month of the lunar calendar, with no information given as to the year.

*Ingredients*

| | |
|---|---|
| Gypsum Fibrosum  (Shi Gao) | 6 g |
| Radix Paeoniae Rubra  (Chi Shao) | 4.5 g |
| Bombyx Batryticatus  (Jiang Can) | 3 g |
| Fructus Forsythiae  (Lian Qiao) | 4.5 g |
| Flos Lonicerae  (Jing Yin Hua) | 3 g |
| Resina Murrhae  (Mo Yao) | 3 g |
| Table salt  (Shi Yan) | 6 g |

The original recipe says that raw Gypsum Fibrosum should be prepared in powder form before use. The above ingredients were boiled for oral rinsing.

### Comments

The main actions of the prescription are to clear stomach fire, eliminate wind, relieve toxic heat, activate blood circulation and remove obstruction from channels and collaterals.

## XI.10.  MOUTHWASH REMEDY VI

Mouthwash Remedy VI (Shu Kou Fang Liu) was carefully prepared by the imperial physician Tong Chenhai for Emperor Guangxu around seven to nine o'clock in the evening on the 26th day of the 10th month of the lunar calendar, with no information given as to the year.

*Ingredients*

| | |
|---|---|
| Pollen Typhae  (Pu Huang) | 3 g |
| Gypsum Fibrosum  (Shi Gao) | 9 g |
| Radix Paeoniae Rubra  (Chi Shao) | 6 g |
| Flos Lonicerae  (Jin Yin Hua) | 3 g |
| Radix seu Rhizoma Rhei  (Da Huang) | 3 g |
| Pericarpium Zanthoxyli  (Chuan Jiao) | 3 g |
| Herba Menthae  (Bo He) | 2.1 g |
| Table salt  (Shi Yan) | 3 g |

The original record says that raw Pollen Typhae and Gypsum Fibrosum should be used. The Pollen Typhae should be packed, and table salt prepared very fine before use. The above ingredients were boiled for oral rinsing.

**Comments**

This prescription combining both dispersing and clearing principles acts to clear stomach fire, relieve accumulation of heat in the intestines, promote blood circulation, and eliminate wind-heat. The chapter "An Approach to Real Principles" in *Plain Questions* ("Zhi Zheng Yao Da Lun," *Su Wen*), says, "Apply heat-property ingredients in the treatment of cold conditions and vice versa for heat conditions." The mouth and teeth conditions of Emperor Guangxu were mainly caused by heat accumulation. This was the reason why many ingredients in the prescription were cool or cold in property. What cannot be ignored is that chronic illness must have led to cold retention in the stomach. Warming ingredients were thus used to assist in achieving good therapeutic effects.

Oral rinsing is a type of external therapy in TCM. In this prescription, ingredients of cold and heat property were used almost in balance. Most may be directly applied for external therapy. Due to their therapeutic effect in relieving swelling and toxic heat, they were effective in dealing with oral conditions.

Also, it is quite possible that the Emperor was suffering from oral illness at the time this prescription was made.

## XI.11.  HERBAL MOUTHWASH REMEDY I

Herbal Mouthwash Remedy I (Shu Yao Fang Yi) was prepared for Emperor Guangxu on the 23rd day of the seventh month of the lunar calendar, with no information concerning the year or the name of the imperial physician who prepared the remedy.

**Ingredients**

| | |
|---|---|
| Gypsum Fibrosum  (Shi Gao) | 6 g |
| Herba Menthae  (Bo He) | 3 g |
| Pericarpium Zanthoxyli  (Chuan Jiao) | 3 g |
| Lignum Cercis Chinensis  (Zi Jing Pi) | 6 g |
| Radix Angelicae Pubscentis  (Du Huo) | 6 g |
| Table salt  (Shi Yan) | 12 g |

The original recipe calls for raw Gypsum Fibrosum to be used. The above ingredients were boiled in water for oral rinsing at any time.

**Comments**

In this prescription, Gypsum Fibrosum, sweet and cold, was used to clear heat from the stomach channel. Pericarpium Zanthoxyli, pungent and strongly warm, may eliminate cold and stop pain. These two ingredients, one being cold and the other warm in property, were prescribed together. Lignum Cercis Chinensis promotes blood circulation and relieves swelling. According to *Classified Materia Medica* (*Fen Lei Cao Yao Xing*) Lignum Cercis Chinensis can be applied to treat patients for "sore throat and toothache." Radix Angelicae Pubscentis, pungent, bitter and slightly warm, can eliminate wind and dampness and stop pain. *Prescrip-*

*tions for Emergencies* (*Zhou Hou Bei Ji Fang*) says, "Radix Angelicae Pubscentis decocted with millet wine for rinsing may stop toothache and control swollen gums caused by wind-heat invasion." The combination of Lignum Cercis Chinensis and Radix Angelicae Pubscentis is also significant. The former activates blood circulation and relieves toxicity while the latter may disperse wind and stop pain. Their combined use also serves to integrate cooling and warming properties in one prescription. Herba Menthae, pungent and cooling, disperses wind in the upper part of the body. Table salt clears heat, relieves toxicity and enters into the kidney. The formulation of ingredients in this prescription is of profound significance. Ingredients of both cold and hot properties were used at the same time in consideration of both excess and deficiency of the Emperor's physical state. The remedy can be used over a long period of time, and because the original record says "for oral rinsing at any time."

## XI.12. HERBAL MOUTHWASH REMEDY II

Herbal Mouthwash Remedy II (Shu Yao Fang Er) was carefully prepared for Emperor Guangxu by the imperial physician Tong Chenhai around five to seven o'clock on the third day of the sixth month of the lunar calendar, with no information given as to the year.

*Ingredients*

| | |
|---|---|
| Herba Menthae  (Bo He) | 3 g |
| Bombyx Batryticatus  (Jiang Can) | 4.5 g |
| Fructus Forsythiae  (Lian Qiao) | 6 g |
| Radix Paeoniae Rubra  (Chi Shao) | 9 g |
| Gypsum Fibrosum  (Shi Gao) | 9 g |
| Resina Murrhae  (Mo Yao) | 6 g |
| Cortex Moudan Radicis  (Mu Dan Pi) | 6 g |
| Table salt  (Shi Yan) | 12 g |

The original scripts require that the leaves of Herba Menthae and raw Gypsum Fibrosum in powder form should be used. The above ingredients were well boiled for oral rinsing p.r.n.

*Comments*

The main actions of this prescription were to clear wind-heat and relieve toxic heat. At that time it was applied for oral ulcer, swollen gums and sore throat.

## XI.13. HERBAL MOUTHWASH REMEDY III

Herbal Mouthwash Remedy III (Shu Yao Fang San) was carefully prepared for Emperor Guangxu by the imperial physician Fan Yimei around five to seven o'clock on the eighth day of the eighth month of the lunar calendar, with no information given concerning the year.

*Ingredients*

| | |
|---|---|
| Gypsum Fibrosum  (Shi Gao) | 9 g |
| Radix Scutellariae  (Huang Qin) | 4.5 g |
| Caulis Lonicerae  (Ren Dong Teng) | 3 g |

| Cortex Moudan Radicis (Dan Pi) | 3 g |
| Herba Menthae (Bo He) | 1.8 g |
| Pericarpium Zanthoxyli (Chuan Jiao) | 1.5 g |

The Gypsum Fibrosum should be prepared in powder form raw, and the Radix Soutellariae roasted with millet wine before use, according to the original records. All the ingredients were well boiled in water for oral rinsing p.r.n.

*Comments*

The main therapeutic purpose of this prescription was to clear fire and heat from the lung and stomach channels. It acts to eliminate wind, clear heat and cool blood. It was basically applied in this case for relieving swelling and stopping pain.

## XI.14. HERBAL MOUTHWASH REMEDY IV

Herbal Mouthwash Remedy IV (Shu Yao Fang Si) was carefully prepared for Emperor Guangxu by the imperial physician Tong Chenhai around five to seven o'clock on the 26th day of the 11th month of the lunar calendar, with no information given as to the year.

*Ingredients*

| Bombyx Batryticatus (Jiang Can) | 4.5 g |
| Fructus Forsythiae (Lian Qiao) | 6 g |
| Resina Olibani (Ru Xiang) | 6 g |
| Flos Lonicerae (Jin Yin Hua) | 6 g |
| Rhizoma Corydalis (Yuan Hu Suo) | 6 g |
| Gypsum Fibrosum (Shi Gao) | 12 g |
| Natrii Sulfas Exsiccatus (Xuan Ming Fen) | 3 g |

The original records require that roasted Bombyx Batryticatus, raw Gypsum Fibrosum in powder form and prepared Rhizoma Corydalis should be used. The above ingredients were well boiled for rinsing at any time.

*Comments*

The composition of this prescription is similar to some of the previous ones. The only difference is that it includes Rhizoma Corydalis. According to *Collective Comments on Materia Medica* (*Ben Cao Hui Yan*), "Rhizoma Corydalis, if intended for the purpose of activating blood, must be prepared with wine." The Rhizoma Corydalis in this prescription mainly plays the role of activating circulation and stopping pain. *The Orthodoxy of Materia Medica* (*Ben Cao Zheng Yi*) claims that Rhizoma Corydalis is applicable to all kinds of disorders due to poor mechanism of *qi* and blood, either internally or externally, in upper or lower parts of the body.

In recent years, professionals in various places have been using Rhizoma Corydalis extract to make 0.2% Rhizoma Corydalis base injection for local anesthesia in certain minor surgical operations, where its pain-relieving effect is remarkable.

## XI.15. HERBAL MOUTHWASH REMEDY V

Herbal Mouthwash Remedy V (Shu Yao Fang Wu) was carefully prepared

for Emperor Guangxu by the imperial physician Tong Chenhai on the 27th day of
the 11th month of the lunar calendar, with no information given concerning the
year.

### Ingredients

| | |
|---|---|
| Flos Mume Pill for Tongue Ulcer (Mei Hua Dian She Dan) | 6 pills |
| Borneoleum Syntheticum and Borax Powder (Bing Peng San) | 0.9 g |
| Flos Lonicerae (Jin Yin Hua) | 6 g |
| Gypsum Fibrosum (Shi Gao) | 12 g |
| Pollen Typhae (Pu Huang) | 3 g |
| Resina Olibani (Ru Xiang) | 6 g |
| Pericarpium Zanthoxyli (Chuan Jiao) | 4.5 g |
| Table salt (Shi Yan) | 4.5 g |

The original recipe calls for six pieces of Flos Mume Powder for Tongue
Ulcer (Mei Hua Dian She Dan) to be ground into powder and packed into a small
bag for use. Borneoleum Syntheticum and Borax Powder and raw Pollen Typhae
should both be packed before use. Resina Olibani and raw Gypsum Fibrosum
should be prepared in powder form before use. The above ingredients were boiled
for oral rinsing.

### Comments

Apart from ingredients that have the effect of clearing heat, eliminating wind
and relieving toxicity, this prescription also contains Flos Mume Pill for Tongue
Ulcer (Mei Hua Dian She Dan) and Borneoleum Syntheticum and Borax Powder
(Bing Peng San). Both are traditional patent medicines. The former includes
Resina Murrhae, Borax, Resina Olibani, Resina Draconis, Borneoleum Syntheticum, Cinnabari, and Calculus Bovis. The latter consists mainly of Borneoleum
Syntheticum, Cinnabari, Natrii Sulfas Exsiccatus, and Borax. Flos Mume Pill for
Tongue Ulcer was first recorded in *Complete Collection of Patterns and Treatments
in External Medicine* (*Wai Ke Zheng Zhi Quan Sheng Ji*). This patent pill has the
action of clearing toxic heat and stopping pain. It is applied in the treatment of
furuncles, boils, sore throat, acute tonsillitis, and painful and swollen gums. The
original remedy does not include Flos Mume. When the imperial physicians
prepared such prescriptions, they intended to include Flos Mume, especially by
adding white Flos Mume that was known as Lu'emei, according to *Supplement to
Compendium of Materia Medica* (*Ben Cao Gang Mu Shi Yi*). Being bland and
astringent, it has the action of soothing the liver, pracifying the stomach and
resolving phlegm. *Origins of Materia Medica* (*Ben Cao Yuan Shi*) says, "White Flos
Mume clears heat from the head and eyes, promotes lung *qi*, and eliminates
phlegm-heat in the lung." For the treatment of ulcer on the lip, *Red Water and
Profound Pearl Collection* (*Chi Shui Xuan Zhu*) says to "stick a flower petal of white
Flos Mume to the boil; the bleeding will soon be stopped provided the boil is
already broken." Borneolum Syntheticum and Borax Powder (Bing Peng San) was
first mentioned in *True Lineage of External Medicine* (*Wai Ke Zheng Zong*). It was
traditionally spread over affected areas for toothache and sore throat.

# XII. PRESCRIPTIONS FOR ORAL ULCER

## XII.1. REMEDY FOR CLEARING GASTRIC HEAT AND ULCER

The date and the imperial physician who made this Remedy for Clearing Gastric Heat and Ulcer (Qing Wei Xiao Mi San) remain unknown.

*Ingredients*

| | |
|---|---:|
| Natrii Sulfas Exsiccatus (Xuan Ming Fen) | 3 g |
| Indigo Naturalis (Qing Dai) | 0.6 g |
| Moschus (She Xiang) | 0.15 g |
| Borneolum Syntheticum (Bing Pian) | 0.9 g |
| Pollen Typhae (Pu Huang) | 0.9 g |
| Resina Olibani (Ru Xiang) | 0.9 g |
| Herba Violae (Zi Hua Di Ding) | 6 g |

The original recipe says Pollen Typhae should be used raw. The above ingredients were ground into fine powder and sifted through a silk net, after which it was ready for spreading over the affected area. The powder soon dissolves in the saliva.

*Comments*

Oral ulcer known as Koumi in TCM was first recorded in *Yellow Emperor's Internal Medicine* (*Huang Di Nei Jing*). "On *Qi* Obstruction" in *Plain Questions* ("Qi Bi Lun," *Su Wen*) says, "The urinary bladder shifts heat to the small intestine and causes obstruction, giving rise to ulcer in the oral cavity." Factors such as stomach fire or deficiency fire, or dampness retention in the spleen turning into dormant heat that forms upward damp-heat along the spleen channel will eventually cause ulcer in the whole oral cavity. The therapeutic principle is mainly to eliminate heat from the stomach and sedate stomach fire, strengthen the spleen and eliminate dampness. External therapy actually plays a significant role in the treatment of oral ulcer. In this prescription, Indigo Naturalis, salty and cold, may eliminate toxic heat. Its external use can help in cases of ulcer with oozing fluid. It was used also in combination with Pollen Typhae for bleeding or epistaxis caused by excessive heat. Moschus, pungent and warm, often applied externally in boils and carbuncles, activates blood, disperses masses and prevents ulcer. Borneolum Syntheticum, slightly cold and applied externally, has the effect of eliminating heat and stopping pain. It is considered as a common ingredient for oral conditions. The purpose of using Natrii Sulfas Exsiccatus in this prescription was to clear heat and calm fire, especially when used externally.

## XII.2. STOMACH HEAT-CLEARING POWDER

The date and the imperial physician who formulated the prescription was not recorded.

*Ingredients*

| | |
|---|---:|
| Human urine sediment (Ren Zhong Bai) | 9 g |
| Indigo Naturalis (Qing Dai) | 4.5 g |
| Radix Angelicae Dahuricae (Bai Zhi) | 4.5 g |

| | |
|---|---|
| Radix Paeoniae Lactiflorae  (Bai Shao) | 4.5 g |
| Gypsum Fibrosum  (Shi Gao) | 6 g |
| Borneolum Syntheticum  (Bing Pian) | 3 g |
| Calculis Bovis  (Niu Huang) | 1.5 g |
| Moschus  (She Xiang) | 0.3 g |

The original records require that raw Gypsum Fibrosum should be used. The above ingredients were ground into fine powder and sifted through a silk net for external application to the affected areas.

### Comments

In this prescription, prepared human urine sediment eliminates toxic heat, resolves blood stasis and stops bleeding. It is applied externally in oral and tongue ulcer, and sore throat. The external use of Calculis Bovis also helps eliminate toxic heat in the treatment of pain and swelling of the mouth. These two ingredients plus Borneolum Syntheticum, Moschus and Indigo Naturalis are very effective in sedating fire, relieving toxic heat and alleviating swelling. Badix Paeoniae Lactiflorae promotes blood circulation. Radix Angelicae Dahuricae eliminates wind. Raw Gypsum Fibrosum, applied externally, treats patients for furuncles with swelling and oozing fluid, while its internal use can clear stomach fire and hence the name Stomach Heat-clearing Powder. The prescription is also significant in that it approaches the disease from its root cause.

## XIII.  ODONTOPATHY PRESCRIPTIONS

### XIII.1. MOUTHWASH REMEDY FOR TEETH

The time and name of the the imperial physician who formulated Mouthwash Remedy for Teeth (Shu Ya Fang) were not recorded.

### Ingredients

| | |
|---|---|
| Flos Lonicerae  (Jin Yin Hua) | 9 g |
| Cortex Lycci Radicis  (Di Gu Pi) | 6 g |
| Gypsum Fibrosum  (Shi Gao) | 18 g |
| Table salt  (Shi Yan) | 9 g |
| Cortex Phellodendri  (Huang Bai) | 3 g |
| Herba Menthae  (Bo He) | 3 g |
| Pericarpium Zanthoxyli  (Chuan Jiao) | 1.2 g |

### Comments

According to the health records of the late Qing Dynasty, Emperor Guangxu has "toothache on the left side" for many years. It was accompanied by "blisters in the throat and palate." Judging from this assumption, he suffered from periodontitis or periapical abscess. Note: Multiple factors such as wind-heat, or wind-cold, or deficiency of the liver and kidney or tooth cavities may give rise to toothache. Because of the different causative factors, the clinical manifestations of toothache may vary, and therapeutic principles should alter accordingly.

In this prescription, the Cortex Lycii Radicis clears heat and cools blood. The

Cortex Phellodendri sedates fire and toxic heat and the Flos Lonicerae eliminates toxic heat. The table salt, entering into the kidney, relieves toxic heat and fortifies the teeth. The Pericarpium Zanthoxyli, pungent and warm, stops toothache and kills bacteria. *Medicinal Plants* (*Yao Xing Ben Cao*) claims, "Pericarpium Zanthoxyli eases toothache." In this prescription, the Pericarpium Zanthoxyli was used to counter-balance the cold property ingredients. It was also an example of combining ingredients of both hot and cold properties. Analysis of the ingredients indicates that the tooth conditions complained of by Emperor Guangxu were mainly caused by wind-heat invasion.

## XIII.2. MOUTHWASH REMEDY FOR CLEARING STOMACH HEAT

Mouthwash Remedy for Clearing Stomach Heat (Qing Wei Shu Ya Fang) was carefully prepared by the imperial physician Zhao Wenkui for Emperor Guangxu on the 16th day of the sixth month of the lunar calendar, with no information given as to the year.

*Ingredients*

| | |
|---|---|
| Gypsum Fibrosum  (Shi Gao) | 12 g |
| Flos Carthami  (Hong Hua) | 6 g |
| Radix Rubiae  (Qian Cao) | 6 g |
| Resina Murrhae  (Mo Yao) | 3 g |
| Pollen Typhae  (Pu Huang) | 4.5 g |
| Table salt  (Shi Yan) | 9 g |
| Herba Taraxaci  (Pu Gong Ying) | 3 g |

The original records say that both the Gypsum Fibrosum and Pollen Typhae should be packed in bags raw. The ingredients were boiled for oral rinsing.

*Comments*

In this prescription, the Gypsum Fibrosum and Pollen Typhae eliminate heat from both the stomach and lung, and relieve toxic heat and swelling. The Resina Murrhae relieves swelling and alleviate pain. The Radix Rubiae and Pollen Typhae activate blood circulation and relieve swelling. The Flos Carthami activates blood and stops pain and the table salt relieves toxicity. The combination of these ingredients had the effect of clearing stomach fire, relieving toxic heat, resolving blood stasis, and relieving swelling. The prescription was specifically made for Emperor Guangxu's gum swelling and toothache.

## XIII.3. MOUTHWASH REMEDY FOR CLEARING STOMACH HEAT AND RELIEVING TOOTHACHE

The date and the imperial physician who formulated Mouthwash Remedy for Clearing Stomach Heat and Relieving Toothache (Qing Wei Zhi Tong Shu Chi Fang) remain unknown.

*Ingredients*

| | |
|---|---|
| Herba Menthae  (Bo He) | 4.5 g |
| Gypsum Fibrosum  (Shi Gao) | 9 g |
| Herba Eclipta  (Han Lian Cao) | 6 g |

Cortex Lycci Radicis  (Di Gu Pi)                                         6 g
Radix Puerariae  (Ge Gen)                                               6 g
Radix Glycyrrhizae  (Gan Cao)                                         0.9 g

The original recipe requires that the Radix Glycyrrhizae and Gypsum Fibrosum should be used raw. The above ingredients were well decocted before the
residue was separated out. The decoction was stored for rinsing the mouth three
to five times daily.

### Comments

The actions of this prescription are explained in its nomenclature. Gypsum
Fibrosum, sweet and cold, clears stomach fire. Herba Menthae eliminates wind and
heat. Radix Glycyrrhizae relieves toxicity. Herba Eclipta cools blood and stops
bleeding. Radix Puerariae relieves symptoms and signs in the superficial syndrome.
It also has the effect of elevating clear Yang and sending stomach *qi* upward. The
use of Radix Puerariae on the one hand helps disperse the pathogenic factors; on
the other it produces fluid and guides the herbal effect to the respective channels.

# XIV. OTOPATHY PRESCRIPTIONS

## XIV.1. PRESCRIPTION FOR DEAFNESS

The date and the imperial physician who prepared Prescription for Deafness
(Zhi Er Long Fang) remain unknown.

### Ingredients

Radix Rehmanniae  (Sheng Di Huang)                               12 g
Radix Paeoniae Lactiflorae  (Bai Shao)                             6 g
Radix Achyranthis Bidentatae  (Huai Niu Xi)                      6 g
Rhizoma Anemarrhebae  (Zhi Mu)                                   6 g
Pericarpium Citri Reticulatae  (Chen Pi)                          3 g
Fructus Aurantii  (Zhi Ke)                                        6 g
Rhizoma Alimatis  (Ze Xie)                                        3 g
Radix Ledebouriellae  (Fang Feng)                              4.5 g
Cortex Clycine Max  (Hei Dou Pi)                                 6 g

The original recipe requires that both the Radix Achyranthis Bidentatae and
Rhizoma Anemarrhebae should be roasted with salt water, and the Fructus
Aurantii roasted with wheat flour. Six grams of raw Magnetitum should also be
roasted and prepared in fine powder for use.

Factors leading to the onset of deafness can be either excess of fire or
deficiency of kidney water. Several doses of this remedy will relieve deafness
remarkably.

### Comments

There are many causes of deafness. In addition to congenital and traumatic
factors, a number of internal diseases may also give rise to deafness. As far as the
mechanism is concerned, the onset of deafness is inseparable from either excess or
deficiency. The deficient conditions are often caused by deficiency of the liver and

kidney, while excessive ones mostly result from accumulation of phlegm and fire internally. Emperor Guangxu's deafness due to constitutional deficiency and over consumption of kidney essence was the so-called "essence collapsing-type deafness" according to the chapter "On Collapsing of *Qi*" in *Miraculous Pivot* ("Jue Qi Pian," *Lin Shu*). Obviously, so many frustrations due to unachieved aspirations, low mood, liver *qi* stagnation, and so forth in time resulting in accumulation of dormant fire that unsymptomatically over-consumed liver Yin could also worsen his deafness. The etiology of the deafness suffered by Emperor Guangxu should be the deficiency or at least the disharmony between the liver and kidney. This selection of ingredients therefore agreed with his actual condition.

The Radix Rehmanniae, Cortex Moudan Radicis, Rhizoma Anemarrhebae and Cortex Phellodendri nourish Yin and sedate fire. The Radix Alismatis eliminates dampness from the urine. The Radix Ledebouriellae eliminates wind and dampness. Radix Paeoniae Lactiflorae and Radix Achyranthis Bidentatae soothe the liver and the Pericarpium Citri Reticulatae and Fructus Aurantil strengthen the spleen. The Cortex Clycine Max nourishes blood and clears wind. The use of Magnetitum is quite significant here, as it enters two channels, and can be applied in the treatment of deafness caused by upward disturbance of floating Yang resulting from Yin deficiency of the liver and kidney.

## XIV.2. PRESCRIPTION FOR DEAFNESS WITH OBSTRUCTION

The date and the imperial physician who formulated Prescription for Deafness with Obstruction (Zhi Er Long Bi Fang) remain unknown.

*Ingredients*
  Radix Glycyrrhizae  (Gan Cao)
  Radix Rehamnniae  (Sheng Di Huang)

The original recipe calls for three equal portions of each ingredient to be processed into fine powder. The powder was then made into the shape of a date kernel and covered with rouge before inserting it into the ear orifice.

*Comments*

Radix Glycyrrhizae, possessing the action of relieving toxic heat, is effective for boils and furuncles when it is applied externally. Radix Rehamnniae entering into the liver and kidney channels can eliminate heat, cool blood and produce fluid. Rouge has the effect of relieving blockage of *qi* in the ear due to its fragrance.

## XIV.3. PRESCRIPTION FOR EAR OBSTRUCTION

The date and the imperial physician who made Prescription for Ear Obstruction (Zhi Er Men Fang) remain unknown.

*Ingredients*

| | |
|---|---|
| Herba Asari  (Xi Xin) | 0.1 g |
| Rhizoma Acori Graminei  (Shi Chang Pu) | 0.1 g |
| Caulis Akebiae  (Mu Tong) | 0.1 g |
| Moschus  (She Xiang) | 0.01 g |

The above ingredients were processed into fine powder and wrapped in cotton before inserting into the ear. The blockage of *qi* in the ear is promptly cleared.

### Comments

Both the Moschus and Rhizoma Acori Graminei in this prescription are fragrant ingredients for clearing *qi* obstruction. The Herba Arari, pungent and warm, clears obstruction in the channels. The Caulis Adebiae may reach the nine orifices. All of the above ingredients have the effect of opening the various orifices. Their combined use here can be effective.

## XIV.4. PRESCRIPTION FOR PROMOTING HEARING

Prescription for Promoting Hearing (Li Qiao Tong Er Fang) was carefully prepared by the imperial physician Guo Rong for Emperor Guangxu on the first day of the fourth month of the lunar calendar, with no information given as to the year.

### Ingredients

| | |
|---|---|
| Caulis Akebiae  (Mu Tong) | 3 g |
| Scorpio  (Quan Xie) | 1.5 g |
| Radix Polygalae  (Yan Zhi) | 0.2 g |
| Moschus  (She Xiang) | 0.015 g |

According to the original records, the Scorpio should be detoxicated before use. The above ingredients were processed into powder and made into wax-coated rolls three centimetres long. These were wrapped in brocade and a roll was inserted into the ear.

### Comments

The fragrant Moschus opens the orifice. Caulis Akebiae is known to open into the nine orifices. Radix Polygalae also opens into the orifice. The combined use of these ingredients can promote hearing.

## XIV.5.  External Remedy for Treating Deafness

The date and the imperial physician who formulated External Remedy for Treating Deafness (Zhi Er Long Wai Yong Fang) for Emperor Guangxu remain unknown.

### Ingredients

| | |
|---|---|
| Rhizoma Acori Graminei  (Shi Chang Pu) | 3 g |
| Caulis Akebiae  (Mu Tong) | 3 g |
| Scorpio  (Quan Xie) | 1.5 g |
| Radix Polygalae  (Yan Zhi) | 1.5 g |
| Moschus  (She Xiang) | 0.3 g |

The above ingredients were processed into fine powder which was mixed with three grams of melted wax. While still quite warm, this mixture was made into pills the size of date kernels. These pills were preserved in chinaware so that their original flavour was maintained. They were wrapped in cotton and made into fine rolls three centimetres long for insertion into the ear orifice, the rolls being replaced every three days. Hearing was thus promoted.

**Comments**

This prescription was formed on the basis of the previous one by adding Rhizoma Acori Graminei for it is also fragrant for opening the ear. The preservation method introduced here, "preserve them in chinaware so as to maintain the original flavour," is significant. This is because fragrant substances may be volatile.

## XIV.6.  EXTERNAL LOZENGE FOR PROMOTING HEARING

The date and the imperial physician who formulated the prescription External Lozenge for Promoting Hearing (Li Qi Cong Er Fang) remain unknown.

**Ingredients**

| | |
|---|---|
| Periostracum Cicadae  (Chan Tui) | 3 g |
| Herba Asari  (Xi Xin) | 2.4 g |
| Green tea  (Qing Cha) | 2.4 g |
| Folium Nelumbinis  (He Ye) | 2.4 g |
| Moschus  (She Xiang) | 0.3 g |

The above ingredients were processed into fine powder and mixed with fresh crushed onion and made into very small sticks which were wrapped in brocade and put into the ear orifice.

**Comments**

The Periostracum Cicadae in this prescription disperses wind-heat. The Herba Asari with its warming effect removes obstruction from the ear. The Folium Nelumbinis helps clear Yang to ascend. Green tea clears the head and brightens the vision. These ingredients are helped by the fragrant Moschus to promote hearing.

## XIV.7.  HERBAL TEA FOR CLEARING LIVER HEAT AND PROMOTING HEARING

Herbal Tea for Clearing Liver Heat and Promoting Hearing was carefully prepared by the imperial physician Zhang Zhongyuan for Emperor Guangxu on the 15th day of the fourth month of the lunar calendar.

**Ingredients**

| | |
|---|---|
| Flos Chrysanthemi  (Ju Hua) | 6 g |
| Rhizoma Acori Graminei  (Shi Chang Pu) | 4.5 g |
| Radix Polygalae  (Yuan Zhi) | 2.4 g |
| Radix Paeoniae Lactiflorae  (Bai Shao) | 9 g |

The original recipe requires raw Radix Paeoniae Lactiflorae collected in Hangzhou to be used. The above ingredients were prepared to be used as Chinese tea.

**Comments**

This prescription was proposed as a tea replacement for healing. The Flos Chrysanthemi clears heat from the liver. The Rhizoma Acori Graminei and Radix

Polygalae, fragrant opening ingredients, calm the mind. It also deals with the root cause of a disease.

## XIV.8.  EXTERNAL LOZENGE FOR TINNITUS

The date and the imperial physician who made External Lozenge for Tinnitus (Zhi Er Ming Fang) remain unknown.

### Ingredient
Radix Rehmanniae  (Di Huang)

The original processing method was for raw Radix Rehmanniae to be sliced and packed in paper. These were decocted using mild heat. When ready, they were inserted into the ear orifice as a kind of external therapy.

### Comments
The Radix Rehmanniae enters the kidney channel to cool the blood and produce body fluid. As most cases of tinnitus are due to kidney deficiency, this is also an approach to deal with the root cause of the disease.

## XIV.9.  EXTERNAL LOZENGE FOR DEFICIENCY TINNITUS

The date and the imperial physician who made External Lozenge for Deficiency Tinnitus (Zhi Er Xu Ming Fang) remain unknown.

### Ingredients
| | |
|---|---|
| Moschus  (She Xiang) | 0.3 g |
| Scorpio  (Quan Xie) | 14 |
| Folium Nelumbinis  (He Ye) | 14 |
| Herba Menthae  (Bo He) | 3 g |

The original recipe requires fresh Folium Nelumbinis to be used. The Scorpio and Moschus were first wrapped in lotus leaves and baked on tile, then ground into fine powder, mixed with water and the wet powder also made into small sticks which were inserted into the ear for healing purpose.

### Comments
In this prescription, the Herba Menthae, pungent and cooling, has the effect of eliminating wind from the superficial portion of the body. Moschus, fragrant, opens into the orifice. Scorpio may soothe the liver and search for wind in the body. The processing introduced here is very special. It was possible that Herba Menthae leaves were used for their fragrant effect. Note: The original records suggest this prescription was made up by Emperor Guangxu himself.

## XIV.10.  EXTERNAL REMEDY FOR DEAFNESS AND TINNITUS

The date and the imperial physician who made External Remedy for Deafness and Tinnitus (Zhi Er Ming Er Long Fang) remain unknown.

### Ingredients
Semen Zanthaxylum  (Jiao Mu)
Rhizoma Acori Graminei  (Shi Chang Pu)

Magnetitum  (Ci Shi)

The above ingredients were processed into fine powder and mixed with Ganlis Perillae and yellow wax to make very small sticks each six centimetres long. These sticks were wrapped in brocade for external application at ear orifice and changed daily.

*Comments*

The Semen Zanthaxylum, pungent warming, opens into the ear, while Rhizoma Acori Graminei also has a fragrant opening effect. Magnetitum, entering the kidney, may soothe the liver and reduce hyperactivity of liver Yang. This remedy also serves as an example of simultaneously dealing with both the liver and kidney.

## XIV.11.  REMEDY FOR TREATING EAR OBSTRUCTION

The date of preparation of Remedy for Treating Ear Obstruction (Zhi Er Du Fang) remains unknown.

*Ingredients*
Herba Asari  (Xi Xin)
Rhizoma Acori Graminei  (Shi Chang Pu)

The above two ingredients were processed into fine powder and mixed with shredded tobacco for water-pipe smoking. Whether it was effective in dealing with ear *qi* obstruction or not is still a question.

*Comments*

It seems that this prescription was formulated by Emperor Guangxu himself as it is in his handwriting. Fragrant and pungent warming ingredients were mixed for removing *qi* obstruction in the ear. External application could be effective, though it is doubtful whether the water-pipe smoking method would be useful.

## XIV.12.  PRESCRIPTION FOR EARACHE AND DEAFNESS

The date and the imperial physician who formulated Prescription for Earache and Deafness (Zhi Er Tong Er Long Fang) remain unknown.

*Ingredients*
Radix Euphorbiae Kansui  (Gan Sui)
Radix Aconiti Kusneziffii  (Cao Wu)

The original recipe calls for three portions of each ingredient to be processed into fine powder and made in the shape of date seeds wrapped in brocade for ear inserting at night.

*Comments*

This prescription possesses the actions of relieving swelling and mass, eliminating wind and stopping pain. According to *Collection of Highly Recommended Prescriptions* (*Bai Yi Xuan Fang*), Radix Euphorbiae Kansui powder mixed with water to be spread over the affected area may be applied for all sorts of boils. Radix Aconiti Kusneziffii, drastically pungent and warm, may eliminate wind, clear dampness and stop pain.

Analysis of the handwritten manuscripts suggests that this prescription might have been formulated by Emperor Guangxu himself, as he was that eager to rid himself of his ear problem.

## XIV.13. PRESCRIPTION FOR EAR OBSTRUCTION AND DEAFNESS

The date and the imperial physician who formulated Prescription for Ear Obstruction and Deafness (Zhi Qi Bi Er Long Fang) were not recorded.

### Ingredients

| | |
|---|---|
| Radix Glycyrrhizae (Gan Cao) | 1.5 g |
| Radix Euphorbiae Kansui (Gan Sui) | 1.5 g |
| Moschus (She Xiang) | 0.3 g |

The above ingredients were processed into fine powder and filled into the tube of green Chinese onion. Inserting the tube into the ear was believed to be able to clear *qi* obstruction promptly.

### Comments

In this prescription, the fragrant Moschus was applied to remove the obstruction of *qi* in the ear. Radix Glycyrrhizae and Radix Euphorbiae Kansui counteract according to the 18 counter-actings. In recent years, however, studies and efforts have been made in various parts of China to combine these two ingredients in the same remedy but with no dramatic results. Some scholars believe that the two can be used at the same time. Some experiments show that the two could be safely applied in combination. They also show that it would cause no problem if the dosage of Radix Glycyrrhizae was equal or less than that of Radix Euphorbiae Kansui. Radix Glycyrrhizae may even at times help detoxicate Radix Euphorbiae Kansui. Side-effects could occur should the dosage of Radix Glycyrrhizae surpass that of Radix Euphorbiae Kansui, i.e., the toxicity of Radix Euphorbiae Kansui would increase following a positive ratio with the dosage of Radix Glycyrrhizae. Still, the effect of the combined use of the two at the same time requires further studies and observation.

## XIV.14. SIMPLE RECIPE FOR DEAFNESS

The date and the imperial physician who formulated Simple Recipe for Deafness (Zhi Er Long Dan Fang) remain unknown.

### Ingredient

Scorpio (Quan Xie)

According to the original records the Scorpio was detoxicated and ground, then mixed with water for ear drops. The ear *qi* obstruction was removed when the water sound was heard in the ear.

### Comments

Scorpio has the effect of searching for winds, releasing spasm and soothing the liver. This simple remedy was based on the principle of clearing the *qi* obstruction in the ear.

## XIV.15. EXTERNAL REMEDY FOR EAR OBSTRUCTION

External Remedy for Ear Obstruction (Er Bi Wai Zhi Fang) was carefully prepared by the imperial physician Zhong Xun on the 16th day of the fifth month of the lunar calendar in 1908.

*Ingredients*

| | |
|---|---|
| Rhizoma Corydalis  (Yuan Hu Suo) | 3 g |
| Squama Manitis  (Chuan Shan Jia) | 3 g |
| Scorpio  (Quan Xie) | 1 |
| Lumbricus  (Qiu Yin) | 3 |
| Fuligo  (Bai Cao Shuang) | 6 g |
| Borneolum Syntheticum  (Bing Pian) | 1.5 g |

The original recipe requires the Squama Manitis to be roasted and the Scorpio detoxicated before use. Three fresh earthworms or four dried worms without skin should be used. The Fuligo should be mixed with lard.

The above ingredients were ground into fine powder and mixed with onion juice for making small sticks which were inserted into the ear for healing purpose, and were changed daily.

*Comments*

This prescription possesses the actions of eliminating wind, removing obstruction, activating blood circulation, and regulating *qi*. The earthworms clear heat and invigorate the collaterals. Scorpio searches for wind. Squama Manitis activates blood. Rhizoma Corydalis regulates *qi*, while the fragrant Borneolum Syntheticum opens the ear orifice. Fuligo stops bleeding.

## XIV.16. PRESCRIPTION FOR PROMOTING HEARING AND EAR *QI*

Pescription for Promoting Hearing and Ear *Qi* (Li Qiao Cong Er Fang) was carefully prepared by the imperial physician Li Decang on the sixth day of the second month of the lunar calendar, with no information given as to the year.

*Ingredients*

| | |
|---|---|
| Squama Manitis  (Chuan Shan Jia) | 6 g |
| Periostracum Cicadae  (Chan Tui) | 6 g |
| Rhizoma Acori Graminei  (Shi Chang Pu) | 6 g |
| Flos Momordica Cochinchinensis  (Mu Bi Hua) | 6 g |
| Semen Ricini  (Bi Ma Ren) | 4.5 g |
| Scorpio  (Quan Xie) | 4 |
| Fel Cyperinus Carpio  (Li Yu Dan) | 4 |
| Moschus  (She Xiang) | 3 g |

The original prescription says that raw Squama Manitis, Periostracum Cicadae without feet and detoxicated dried Scorpio should be used. The oil from the Semen Ricini should be separated out before use. The Fel Cyperinus Carpio and Moschus should be added last.

The above ingredients were processed into fine powder and mixed with Moschus and Fel Cyperinus Carpio, and further mixed with melted yellow wax. This was made into small sticks while still slightly warm. These sticks, about 3 centimetres long, would fit people of all ages. They should be wrapped in brocade and inserted into the ear orifice to remove *qi* obstruction.

### Comments

In this prescription, the Squama Manitis activates blood in the channels and collaterals. Scorpio and Periostracum Cicadae eliminate wind and stop pain. Moschus and Rhizoma Acori Graminel open into the ear orifice due to their fragrant aromas. Fel Cyperinus Carpio eliminates heat and calms fire. Semen Ricini moistens and promotes bowel movement. Flos Momordica Cochinchinensis eliminates heat and soothes the liver. The combination of ingredients in this prescription was very well thought out, and sufferers from similar problems may try it out.

# XV.  PRESCRIPTIONS FOR TREATING COUGH

## XV.1. DECOCTION FOR CLEARING PULMONARY HEAT

Decoction for Clearing Pulmonary Heat (Shu Jie Qing Fei Yin) was carefully prepared by the imperial physician Li Dechang for Emperor Guangxu on the 21st day of the 12th month of the lunar calendar, with no information given as to the year.

### Ingredients

| | |
|---|---|
| Herba Schizonepetae  (Jing Jie) | 2.4 g |
| Radix Peucedani  (Qian Hu) | 3 g |
| Ganlis Perillae  (Su Gen) | 1.2 g |
| Folium Perillae  (Su Ye) | 1.2 g |
| Cortex Mori Radicis  (Sang Bai Pi) | 3 g |
| Semen Armenicacae  (Xing Ren) | 4.5 g |
| Radix Platycodi  (Jie Gen) | 3 g |
| Massa Fermentata Medicinalis  (Shen Qu) | 4.5 g |
| Radix Glycyrrhizae  (Gan Cao) | 1.5 g |
| Radix Ophiopogonis  (Mai Men Dong) | 6 g |

The original recipe calls for the Cortex Mori Radicis processed with honey and powdered Semen Armenicacae to be used. The kernel of the Radix Ophiopogonis should be removed before use. Two pieces of ginger should be added.

### Comments

Most of the ingredients in this prescription are pungent and dispersing, to help the lungs perform their dispersing and descending functions. The main function of the decoction was to eliminate pathogenic factors from the lung. This prescription was probably used in the early years of Emperor Guangxu's era.

## XV.2. PRESCRIPTION FOR VARIOUS TYPES OF COUGH

The eunuch Fan Changchun conveyed the imperial edict to prepare Prescription for Various Types of Cough (Zhi Ke Fang) on the 20th day of the first month of the lunar calendar. The year in which it was made remains unknown.

*Ingredients*

| | |
|---|---|
| Radix Platycodi  (Jie Gen) | 240 g |
| Herba Schizonepetae  (Jing Jie) | 240 g |
| Radix Asteris  (Zi Wan) | 240 g |
| Radix Stemonae  (Bai Bu) | 240 g |
| Rhizoma Cynanchi Stauntonii  (Bai Qian) | 240 g |

According to the original records, the Radix Platycodi and Herba Schizone-petae should be roasted before use. The Radix Asteris, Radix Stemonae and Rhizoma Cynanchi Stauntonii should be steamed on rice bofore being roasted for future use.

The above ingredients were ground into fine powder, three grams of which were taken each time with boiled water. Ginger tea should be used instead of boiled water if the invasion of exogenous pathogenic wind-cold has just taken place.

*Comments*

This prescription aims at eliminating wind and resolving phlegm. It originated from *Medical Revelations* (*Yi Xue Xin Wu*) though without Pericarpium Citri Reticulatae. It has the actions of stopping cough, resolving phlegm and alleviating superficial symptoms and signs of the lung, while Herba Schizonepetae actually relieves the superficial symptoms and signs. Rhizoma Cynanchi Stauntonii and Radix Platycodi resolve phlegm. Radix Asteris and Radix Stemonae disperse the lungs and stop cough. In the early stage of invasion of exogenous pathogenic invasion, ginger tea was suggested because its pungent warming effect helps relieve superficial symptoms and signs. It should be mentioned that this remedy, being dry in nature, should not be prescribed for chronic cough due to Yin deficiency. It was believed to be one of the prescriptions used by Emperor Guangxu in his early years.

## XV.3. HERBAL SYRUP FOR EASING COUGH AND CLEARING HEAT

Herbal Syrup for Easting Cough and Clearing Heat (Qing Sou Zhi Ke Yi Huo Hua Yin Gao) was carefully prepared for Emperor Guangxu by the imperial physician Zhuang Shouhe on the 14th day of the 10th month of the lunar calendar, with no mention of the year.

*Ingredients*

| | |
|---|---|
| Ganlis Perillae  (Su Geng) | 1.5 g |
| Semen Perillae  (Su Zi) | 1.5 g |
| Radix Peucedani  (Qian Hu) | 9 g |
| Pericarpium Citri Reticulatae Rubra  (Ju Hong) | 6 g |
| Radix Trichosanthis  (Tian Hua Fen) | 9 g |
| Folium Mori  (Sang Ye) | 9 g |
| Flos Chrysanthemi  (Gan Ju) | 9 g |
| Radix Ophiopogonis  (Mai Men Dong) | 9 g |
| Poria  (Fu Ling) | 9 g |
| Fructus Oryzae Germinature  (Gu Ya) | 9 g |
| Massa Fermentata Medicinalis  (Shen Qu) | 9 g |

| Caulis Bambusae in Taeniam (Zhu Ru) | 6 g |
| Radix Glycyrrhizae (Gan Cao) | 3 g |

According to the original records, frosted Folium Mori, raw Radix Gyloyrrhizae, and Massa Fermentata Medicinalis and Fructus Oryzae Germinature, the latter both roasted, should be used.

The above ingredients were first well boiled, the residue separated out and the remaining liquid further concentrated. Processed honey was added to make a syrup with the concentrated liquid. Two spoonfuls of the syrup were taken together with boiled water each time.

### Comments

In this prescription, the Ganlis Perillae and Radix Peucedani disperse the lungs and stop cough. Radix Trichosanthis and Radix Ophiopogonis produce fluid, stop thirst and nourish body Yin. Folium Mori and Flos Chrysanthemi eliminate wind-heat. Two-old-drug Decoction (Er Chen Tang) consisting of Rhizoma Pinelliae, Pericarpium Citri Reticulatae Rubra, Poria and Radix Glycyrrhizae, here resolves phlegmatic fluid and dampness. Rhizoma Pinelliae was not included here because the imperial physician intended to prevent its causing pungent drying. Caulis Bambusae in Taeniam clears phlegm and stops nausea. Fructus Oryzae Germinature and Massa Fermentata Medicinalis strengthen the spleen to eliminate dampness. This prescription, using both dispersing and nourishing ingredients for eliminating pathogenic factors while not neglecting reinforcing the anti-pathogenic *qi*, may therefore be used over a long period of time.

## XV.4. PEAR SYRUP WITH BAMBOO LIQUID

Pear Syrup with Bamboo Liquid (Jia Zhu Li Li Gao) was recorded on the 26th day of the second month of the lunar calendar, with no mention of the year or the imperial physician who formulated it.

### Ingredients

| Pear (Huang Li) | 100 |
| Folium Phyllostachyos (Zhu Ye) | 100 |
| Rhizoma Phragmitis (Lu Gen) | 30 |
| Pericarpium Citri Reticulatae Rubra (Ju Hong) | 20 |
| Bulbus Eleocharis Tuberosae (Bi Qi) | 50 |

The original recipe calls for fresh Folium Phyllostachyos and Rhizoma Phragmitis to be used. Pericarpium Citri Reticulatae Rubra, the orange skin from oranges grown on an old tree, should be used. Bulbus Eleocharis Tuberosae juice was used rather than the Bulbus Eleocharis Tuberosae itself.

### Comments

In this prescription, the pear and Bulbus Eleocharis Tuberosae nourish Yin, produce fluid, moisten the lungs and stop cough. Folium Phyllostachyos, Rhizoma Phragmitis and Pericarpium Citri Reticulaltae Rubra were also added to clear heat and resolve phlegm. Prepared as syrup, it was suitable for chronic cough due to Yin deficiency. Steamed bamboo liquid might produce similar effect.

# XVI. PRESCRIPTIONS FOR TREATING CARDIAC CONDITIONS

## XVI.1. PILL FOR NOURISHING THE HEART AND STRENGTHENING THE SPLEEN

Pill for Nourishing the Heart and Strengthening the Spleen (Yang Xin Jian Pi Wan) was recorded for Emperor Guangxu on the 24th day of the fifth month of the lunar calendar, with no mention of the year or the imperial physician who formulated it.

### Ingredients

| | |
|---|---|
| Radix Codonopsis Pilosulae (Dang Shen) | 9 g |
| Rhizoma Atractylodis Macrocephalae (Bai Zhu) | 9 g |
| Poria (Fu Shen) | 15 g |
| Semen Ziziphi Spinosae (Suan Zao Ren) | 12 g |
| Radix Polygalae (Yuan Zhi) | 3 g |
| Radix Angelicae Sinensis (Dang Gui) | 9 g |
| Radix Paeoniae Lactiflorae (Bai Shao) | 9 g |
| Cortex Eucommiae (Du Zhong) | 12 g |
| Pericarpium Citri Reticulatae (Chen Pi) | 6 g |
| Semen Coicis (Yi Yi Ren) | 15 g |
| Fructus Amomi (Sha Ren) | 4.5 g |
| Fructus Tribuli Terrestris (Bai Ji Li) | 9 g |
| Semen Nelumbinis (Lian Zi Rou) | 12 g |
| Fructus Oryzae Germinature (Gu Ya) | 9 g |
| Rhizoma Dio (Shan Yao) | 12 g |
| Radix Glycyrrhizae Praeparatae (Zhi Gan Cao) | 4.5 g |

The original recipe calls for both the Radix Angelicae Sinensis and Rhizoma Atractylodis Macrocephalae to be roasted with earth before use. The Semen Ziziphi Spinosae should be roasted until burnt yellow before use. The Cortex Eucommiae Semen Coicis, Fructus Amomi, Radix Paeoniae Lactiflorae, Fructus Oryzae Germinature and Rhizoma Dio should be roasted. The kernels of the Semen Nelumbinis and Radix Polygalae should be used. The Radix Glycyrrhizae should be processed before use.

The above ingredients were processed into fine powder and mixed with date soup and Massa Fermentata Medicinalis paste to make the Cinnabari-coated pills the size of Chinese mung beans. Three grams of the pills were taken each time with boiled water. The same prescription was repeated on the 23rd day of the ninth month of the lunar calendar.

### Comments

This prescription, formed on the basis of modifying Spleen-governing Blood Decoction (Gui Pi Tang) and Ginseng Powder with Poria and Bighead Atractylodis (Shen Ling Bai Zhu San), has the action of nourishing the heart and strengthening the spleen. Since Emperor Guangxu had constitutional Yin deficiency, Radix Astragali seu Hedysari from Spleen-governing Blood Decoction

(Gui Pi Tang) was omitted in order to prevent an over strong effect in ascending Yang and reinforcing *qi*. Radix Auchlandiae was also omitted because its fragrant pungent property might overconsume body Yin. Arillus Longan was also omitted as being too greasy. The primary aim of this prescription was to nourish the heart. Ginseng Powder with Poria and Bighead Atractylodis is basically meant to pacify the stomach and eliminate dampness. In that part of the prescription, Fructus Tribuli Terrestris, Radix Paeoniae Lactiflorae and Cortex Eucommiae were used instead of Semen Dolichoris and Radix Platycodi because the imperial physician who formulated this prescription also took the liver and kidney into consideration. This prescription bears the characteristics of a comprehensive option of ingredients, neither too warm nor too cold. It should therefore have been one of the prescriptions presented to Emperor Guangxu in his later years.

## XVI.2. CINNABARI-NELUMBINIS POWDER

Cinnabari-Nelumbinis Powder (Zhu Sha Lian Xin San) was presented to Emporer Guangxu, with no time or name of the imperial physician who formulated it given.

### Ingredients
| | |
|---|---|
| Plumula Nelumbinis  (Lian Zi Xin) | 6 g |
| Cinnabari  (Zhu Sha) | 0.3 g |

The above ingredients were ground into fine powder and packed into 10 small bags.

### Comments
In this prescription, the Plumula Nelumbinis, bitter and cold, enters into the heart channel and clears heart fire. According to *Compendium of Materia Medica* (*Ben Cao Gang Mu*), Plumula Nelumbinis has the effect of clearing heart fire. Cinnabari, entering into the heart channel, may clear heart fire and tranquilize the heart and mind. According to *The Original Classics* (*Ben Jing*), Cinnabari calms the soul. Contemporary studies also demonstrate its tranquilizing effect. The combination of these two ingredients has the effect of clearing heart fire and calming the mind. Emperor Guangxu often took the medicine. Very important is that the dosage of Cinnabari should be kept at a minimum, for it contains such minerals as mercuric sulfide, and frequent over-dosing could be harmful.

## XVI.3. HERBAL TEA FOR CALMING THE MIND

The date and the imperial physician who concocted Herbal Tea for Calming the Mind (An Shen Dai Cha Yin) remain unknown.

### Ingredients
| | |
|---|---|
| Dens Draconis  (Long Chi) | 3 g |
| Rhizoma Acori Graminei  (Shi Chang Pu) | 3 g |

The original records require the Dens Draconis to be fired. The two ingredients were prepared to be taken as Chinese tea.

*Comments*

In this prescription, the Rhizoma Acori Graminei, entering the spleen and heart channels, has the effect of tranquilizing the mind. *The Original Classics (Ben Jing)* claims, "Rhizoma Acori Gramine opens into the heart and nourishes the five Zang organs." Modern studies show that its decoction has the effect of tranquilizing animals. Dens Draconis, entering the heart and liver channels, may tranquilize frightened patients and calm the mind, reduce hyperactive liver Yang, and lessen palpitation and convulsions. The combined use of the two was to calm the heart and mind. According to the health records of Emperor Guangxu around 1905 he "often laughed impulsively for nothing," and "murmured to himself. This prescription was perhaps presented for the above conditions." It was made as a tea replacement in an attempt to achieve a gradual therapeutic process.

## XVI.4. TREASURE-GATHERING PILL

The year and the imperial physician who formulated the prescription for Treasure-gathering Pill (Ju Bao Dan) remain unknown. The pill was suggested for all heart or stomach pains.

*Ingredients*

| | |
|---|---|
| Resina Murrhae (Mo Yao) | 15 g |
| Resina Olibani (Ru Xiang) | 15 g |
| Unidentified | |
| Unidentified | |
| Cinnabari (Zhu Sha) | 15 g |
| Succinum (Hu Po) | 15 g |
| Radix Auchlandiae (Mu Xiang) | 30 g |
| Radix Angelicae Sinensis (Dang Gui) | 30 g |
| Rhizoma Cyperi (Xiang Fu) | 30 g |
| Moschus (She Xiang) | 3 g |
| Lignum Dalbergiae Odoriferae (Jiang Xiang) | 15 g |
| Benzoinum (An Xi Xiang) | 15 g |

The original records require that the oily substance from the Resina Murrhae and Resina Olibani should be separated out before use. The above ingredients were ground into fine powder together with six grams of Radix Glycyrrhizae, to be made into pills or syrup. The weight of each pill was three grams, and the dosage was one pill each time, taken with millet wine or boiled water. The prescription was repeated and made another package for the use of the Emperor.

*Comments*

The ingredients in this prescription have the effect of removing obstruction from the channels and collaterals by means of fragrant warming, activating blood circulation and resolving blood stasis. The intention of the imperial physician who made this prescription was to treat the heart and stomach at the same time. "Blood circulation will be stagnant when it encounters cold." "Where there is no obstruction, there is no pain." The fragrant, pungent warming ingredients in this prescription help remove obstruction from the channels and collaterals, activate blood and resolve blood stasis so that the blood circulates normally and the pain is relieved spontaneously. This prescription may also be suggested for angina pectoris. However, attention should be paid to avoiding the strong effect of fragrant, pungent warming ingredients in over-consuming the body Yin. However, too strong an effect of resolving blood stasis may cause bleeding. This was why Radix Glycyrrhizae was used here to harmonize the ingredients; it was made in syrup form to avoid too drastic an effect. Records concerning the use of this prescription by Emperor Guangxu are quite rare. It was probably a prescription presented for his personal use in his early years.

There was another remedy of the same name recorded in the collection of the imperial hospital prescriptions, though the ingredients were quite different from this one.

## XVI.5. SPIRIT-REGAINING PILL

The year and the imperial physician who formulated Spirit-regaining Pill (Gui Shen Dan) remain unknown.

### Ingredients

| | |
|---|---|
| Cinnabari (Zhu Sha) | 60 g |
| Medulla Junci Effusi (Deng Xin Cao) | 90 g |

According to the original records, two boar hearts were cut for containing the above two ingredients, after which the cuts were sutured with fine thread and both were placed in an earthenware utensil for cooking. That done the boar hearts and Medulla Junci Effusi were cast away and the processed Cinnabari was left to be ground into fine powder. Sixty grams of Radix Poria powder were added and all were mixed with millet wine to make pills the size of Chinese parasol-tree seeds. The initial dosage of nine to 15 pills was gradually increased to 25 pills, taken with Radix Ophiopogonis soup. In severe cases the pills were taken with soup made from Resina Olibani and Radix Ginseng.

### Comments

Cinnabari, heavy, cold and slightly toxic, enters the heart channel. Its cold property can be applied to clear heat while its heavy property is a tranquilizer. Cinnabari has the actions of calming the mind and tranquilizing frightened patients; it also prevents ulceration. The internal use of Cinnabari may ease palpitation, anxiety, insomnia and mental disorder. Its external use can be applied for boils and carbuncles as well as oral ulcers. Medula Junci Effusi may clear heart fire, while Radix Poria nourishes the heart and calms the mind. The combined use of these ingredients helps give a stronger effect in nourishing the heart and calming the mind. After Guangxu was made emperor, hard work, fear and worry over-consumed his energy and spirit. It was therefore appropriate for imperial physicians to present him with such nourishing prescriptions.

In the theory of TCM the heart houses the mind. The production of heart blood will be sufficient when heart $qi$ is well reinforced, and the mind will subsequently be calmed. Hence the name Spirit-regaining Pill.

In addition to the above-mentioned conditions, this prescription was recommended for mental disorder and epilepsy. The boar heart was used in line with the opinion in TCM to reinforce a Zang organ by using an animal Zang organ. Even today some people still use boar heart filled with Cinnabari for the treatment of epilepsy. When the powdered Cinnabari thus prepared was taken with Radix Ophiopogonis soup, it was more suitable for the epileptic with heart-Yin deficiency. Taken with soup made from Resina Olibani and Radix Ginseng, it is more suitable for the *qi*-deficiency type of epilepsy, a difference to be noticed in practice.

# XVII.  PRESCRIPTIONS FOR TREATING SPLEEN AND STOMACH CONDITIONS

## XVII.1.  MODIFIED ANCIENT FIVE-JUICE DRINK

Modified Ancient Five-juice Drink (Jia Jian Gu Fang Wu Zhi Yin) was carefully prepared by the imperial physician Zhao Wenkui on the 23rd day of the first month of the lunar calendar, with no mention of the year.

*Ingredients*

| | |
|---|---:|
| Fructus Citrus Cochinchinensis  (Mi Gan) | 2 |
| Nodus Nelumbinis Rhizomatis  (Xian Ou) | 120 g |
| Bulbus Eleocharis Tuberosae  (Bi *Qi*) | 20 |
| Fructus Canarit  (Qing Guo) | 20 |
| Rhizoma Zingiberis Recens  (Sheng Jiang) | 1 slice |

The original recipe calls for the Fructus Citrus Cochinchinensis, Nodus Nelumbinis Rhizomatis and Rhizoma Zingiberis Recens to be peeled before use, and the bits of the Fructus Citrus Cochinchinensis and Fructus Canarit to also be discarded. The above ingredients were mashed and wrapped in a piece of cloth to squeeze out the juice for oral use at any time.

*Comments*

Fructus Citrus Cochinchinensis, Fructus Canarit and Bulbus Eleocharis Tuberosae, entering the lung and stomach channels, have the effect of promoting lung *qi*, clearing the throat, producing fluid and relieving toxication. Rhizoma Zingiberis Recens, entering the spleen channel, may stimulate the appetite, warm the channels and stop nausea. Nodus Nelumbinis Rhizomatis, entering the heart, stomach and spleen channels, may also clear heat and produce fluid. According to *A Complete Record of Holy Benevolence* (*Shen Ji Zong Lu*) there was a type of powder called Lotus and Ginger Powder (Jiang'ou San) which was indicated in the vomiting and severe thirst of cholera. The prescription may be applied for sore throat, congestion of the eye, severe thirst, cough, poor appetite and nausea. According to historical data, Zhao Wenkui served as an imperial physician in the late Qing Dynasty. Also, according to the health records of Emperor Guangxu in 1908, he had "blisters on the left palate, and bloody discharge when he brushed his teeth. From time to time, he could feel blisters on the left palate, slight pain on the right side, and a foreign body sensation when he swallowed food." Similar records such as "poor appetite, belching and discomfort in the stomach," and "thirst with desire to drink" were also found dated around that time. Judging from these sources of information, it is estimated that this prescription was presented for Emperor Guangxu to use when he was seriously ill. Although it is a sort of tonic, it also serves therapeutic purposes.

## XVII.2. GINSENG-PORIA AND ATRACTYLODIS MACROCEPHALAE PILL

Ginseng-Poria and Atractylodis Macrocephalae Pill (Shen Ling Bai Zhu Wan), presented to Emporer Guangxu on the ninth day of the first month of the lunar calendar, was carefully prepared by the imperial physicians Zhang Zhongyuan and Zhong Xun in reply to the questions: Can I use this prescription? If so, how shall I take it? The answer: Divide the pill into 10 packs of six grams each.

Your Excellency, Ginseng-Poria and Atractylodis Macrocephalae Pill (Shen Ling Bai Zhu Wan), consisting of mild ingredients, is indicated in diarrhea due to spleen deficiency, poor appetite and retention of cold-damp.

### Comments

According to copies of prescriptions in the imperial hospital, the composition of Ginseng-Poria and Atractylodis Macrocephalae Pill was the same as Ginseng-Poria and Atractylodis Macrocephalae Powder (Shen Ling Bai Zhu San) as recorded in *A Collection of Prescriptions with Notes (Yi Fang Ji Jie)*. Notes in the imperial hospital claimed that the pill was applicable for all kinds of conditions due to deficiency of the spleen and stomach, and that it could be used regularly. "Strong functions of the spleen and stomach drive away all diseases. On the other hand, should the function of the spleen and stomach be out of harmony, ailments will flood into one's body."

As Emperor Guangxu had constitutional deficiency of the spleen and stomach, this prescription was often presented to him. Though it failed to help the emperor solve his problem completely, it did apparently give some relief. It was possibly related to his liver *qi* stagnation over-riding the spleen and lack of physical activity. This prescription is even today often recommended in clinical practice of TCM.

Note that in the prescription's notes, "Can I use this prescription? If so, how shall I take it? Divide...." should have been written by Emperor Guangxu himself. According to the reply presented by the imperial physician to the Emperor, it should be used without any doubt.

## XVII.3. DECOCTION FOR PACIFYING THE STOMACH AND STRENGTHENING THE SPLEEN

Decoction for Pacifying the Stomach and Strengthening the Spleen (Yi *Qi* Ping Wei Jian Pi Yin) was presented to Emperor Guangxu on the third day of the.

sixth month of the lunar calendar, with no information given as to the year or the imperial physician who made it.

### Ingredients

| | |
|---|---|
| Radix Panacis Quequifloii  (Xi Yang Shen) | 9 g |
| Rhizoma Atractylodis Macrocephalae  (Bai Zhu) | 6 g |
| Rhizoma Dio  (Shan Yao) | 12 g |
| Semen Dolichoris  (Bian Dou) | 12 g |
| Radix Poria  (Fu Shen) | 12 g |
| Radix Polygalae  (Yuan Zhi) | 4.5 g |
| Radix Paeoniae Lactiflorae  (Bai Shao) | 9 g |
| Fructus Gardeniae  (Shan Zhi Zi) | 6 g |
| Periostracum Cicadae  (Chan Tui) | 6 g |
| Cortex Magnoliae Officinalis  (Hou Po) | 3 g |
| Pericarpium Citri Reticulatae  (Chen Pi) | 4.5 g |
| Radix Glycyrrhizae  (Gan Cao) | 3 g |

The original records direct that Cinnabari-coated Radix Poria, roasted Fructus Gardeniae and powdered Radix Panacis Quequifloii should be used in the prescription, with the addition of half of a fresh lotus leaf.

### Comments

The ingredients in this prescription were mainly based on Stomach-pacifying Powder (Ping Wei San), implying at the same time the therapeutic features of Ginseng-Poria and Atractylodis Macrocephalae Pill (Shen Ling Bai Zhu Wan). It was formulated to strengthen spleen *qi* and pacify the stomach. Cinnabari-coated Poria, Radix Polygalae and Radix Paeoniae Lactiflorae were added to calm the heart and mind. This prescription was used in mid summer, a hot and humid season. Periostracum Cicadae, Fructus Gardeniae and Herba Menthae were therefore used to clear heat and relieve restlessness. This prescription was formed rather cautiously and in full compliance with principles.

## XVII.4. DECOCTION FOR NOURISHING YIN AND REINFORCING SPLEEN *QI*

Decoction for Nourishing Yin and Reinforcing Spleen *Qi* (Yi Qi Zi Yin Jian Pi Yin) was presented to Emperor Guangxu on the sixth day of the sixth month of the lunar calendar, with no information given as to the year or the imperial physician who made it.

### Ingredients

| | |
|---|---|
| Radix Panacis Quiquefloii  (Xi Yang Shen) | 9 g |
| Rhizoma Atractylodis Macrocephalae  (Bai Zhu) | 9 g |
| Rhizoma Dio  (Shan Yao) | 12 g |
| Semen Dolichoris  (Bian Dou) | 12 g |
| Radix Poria  (Fu Shen) | 12 g |
| Radix Polygalae  (Yuan Zhi) | 4.5 g |
| Radix Paeoniae Lactiflorae  (Bai Shao) | 9 g |
| Radix Trichosanthis  (Tian Hua Fen) | 9 g |
| Periostracum Cicadae  (Chan Tui) | 6 g |

| | |
|---|---|
| Pericarpium Citri Reticulatae  (Chen Pi) | 6 g |
| Cortex Eucommiae  (Du Zhong) | 12 g |
| Fructus Chaenomelis  (Mu Gua) | 12 g |

The original recipe requires that the Radix Panacis Quiquefloii should be processed into powder before use. The Rhizoma Atractylodis Macrocephalae should be roasted in earth. The Rhizoma Dio, Semen Dolichoris, Radix Paeoniae Lactiflorae and Cortex Eucommiae should also be roasted before use, while the Radix Poria should be coated with Cinnabari. Thirty grams of fresh lotus leaves and nine grams of fried Fruotus Oryzae Germinature should also be included.

### Comments

This prescription was modified on the basis of Decoction for Pacifying the Stomach and Strengthening the Spleen (XVII. 3). Referring to the original prescription, Cortex Magnoliae Officinalis and Fructus Gardeniae were omitted because the former was fragrant and dry while the latter was bitter and cold. Radix Trichosanthis was added in order to help produce fluid and quench thirst. Fructus Chaenomelis and Cortex Eucommiae were ingredients for reinforcing the kidney, activating blood and stopping pain. The inclusion of these ingredients may indicate that Emperor Guangxu suffered from lumbar soreness and pain in the knees.

According to *Notes on Daily Life* written by the Emperor himself in 1907, such phrases as "The pain in my lumbar region, commencing from the 11th month of the lunar calendar the year before last up until now has lasted for nearly two years. I should be active in seeking a prompt approach in dealing with it. Otherwise, I am afraid it may become a problem." It is clear that around 1907 his lumbar pain was already quite severe. The prescription, however, appears to take lumbar pain only as a secondary problem, and may date from around 1907.

## XVII.5. SYRUP FOR STRENGTHENING THE SPLEEN TO ELIMINATE DAMP-HEAT

Syrup for Strengthening the Spleen to Eliminate Damp-Heat (Qing Re Li Pi Chu Shi Gao) was carefully prepared by the imperial physician Yang Angui for Emperor Guangxu on the 13th day of the ninth month of the lunar calendar in 1882.

### Ingredients

| | |
|---|---|
| Poria  (Fu Ling) | 15 g |
| Pericarpium Citri Reticulatae  (Chen Pi) | 12 g |
| Rhizoma Atractylodis Macrocephalae  (Bai Zhu) | 12 g |
| Semen Coicis  (Yi Yi Ren) | 15 g |
| Rhizoma Dio  (Shan Yao) | 9 g |
| Herba Dendrobii  (Shi Hu) | 15 g |
| Radix Ophiopogonis  (Mai Dong) | 15 g |
| Massa Fermentata Medicinalis  (Shen Qu) | 6 g |
| Fructus Oryzae Germinature  (Gu Ya) | 6 g |
| Fructus Hordei Germinatus  (Mai Ya) | 6 g |

| Semen Dolichoris  (Bian Dou) | 15 g |
| Herba Artemisiae Capillaris  (Yin Chen Hao) | 12 g |
| Flos Chrysanthemi  (Ju Hua) | 9 g |
| Radix Glycyrrhizae  (Gan Cao) | 6 g |

The original records state that the Semen Coicis, Rhizoma Dio and Semen Dolichoris should be roasted before use, while the Radix Glycyrrhizae should be used raw. The above ingredients were well decocted before removing the residue. Refined honey was then added to make a syrup. Six grams of the syrup was taken each time with boiled water.

### Comments

This prescription was aimed at strengthening the spleen by means of eliminating dampness and heat from urinary tract. In 1882 the young Emperor Guangxu started using herbal decoctions frequently, indicating how poor his body constitution was.

## XVII.6. MODIFIED SYRUP FOR STRENGTHENING THE SPLEEN TO ELIMINATE DAMP-HEAT

Modified Syrup for Strengthening the Spleen to Eliminate Damp-Heat (Jia Jian Li Pi Qing Re Chu Shi Gao) was carefully prepared by the imperial physicians Zhuang Shouhe and Tong Wenbin on the 20th day of the sixth month of the lunar calendar in 1902.

### Ingredients

| Radix Codonopsis Pilosulae  (Dang Shen) | 6 g |
| Rhizoma Atractylodis Macrocephalae  (Bai Zhu) | 9 g |
| Poria  (Fu Ling) | 9 g |
| Fructus Amomi  (Sha Ren) | 3 g |
| Pericarpium Citri Reticulatae  (Chen Pi) | 4.5 g |
| Massa Fermentata Medicinalis  (Shen Qu) | 9 g |
| Herba Dendrobi  (Shi Hu) | 9 g |
| Semen Dolichoris  (Bian Dou) | 9 g |
| Radix Paeoniae Lactiflorae  (Bai Shao) | 4.5 g |
| Kitchen-range earth  (Zao Xin Tu) | 9 g |
| Semen Coicis  (Yi Yi Ren) | 9 g |
| Vital Energy-reinforcing Powder  (Yi Yuan San) | 6 g |

The original records state that the Rhizoma Atractylodis Macrocephalae, Massa Fermentata Medicinalis, Radix Paeoniae Lactiflorae and Semen Coicis should be roasted before use.

The above ingredients were well boiled and the residue was discarded. The concentrated liquid was mixed with the year-long preserved honey to make a syrup. Six grams of the syrup, infused in boiled water, were taken each time. On the fourth day of the sixth month of the lunar calendar, early summer, the prescription was repeated, omitting Radix Ophiopogonis and adding nine grams of Semen Dolichoris. On the 20th day of the sixth month of the lunar calendar, the mid-summer season, the prescription was altered by omitting Radix Angelicae

Sinensis and kitchen-range earth (9 g).

## Comments

This prescription was formed on the basis of Five Ingredients Miraculous Powder (Wu Wei Yi Gong San) plus ingredients that have the effect of strengthening the spleen by clearing damp-heat from the urinary tract. It was a mild remedy to produce slow and stable effect. The use of kitchen-range earth was largely related to its effect in warming the Middle Jiao, drying out dampness and stopping nausea. The Radix Paeoniae Laotiflorae was added to strengthen the effect in nourishing the liver and spleen. In the early summer season, Radix Ophiopogonis was omitted while Semen Dolichoris was added. In mid-summer, Radix Angelicae Sinensis was omitted while kitchen-range earth was added. The records show that the original prescription did contain Radix Ophiopogonis and Radix Angelicae Sinensis. The imperial physicians Zhuang Shouhe and Tong Wenbin considered long-term use of the prescription when they began preparing it. The purpose of changing the ingredients in accordance with the season was because in summer, damp-heat was oppressive, and in early summer the greasy Radix Ophiopogonis was removed from the prescription while Semen Dolichoris with the effect of eliminating dampness was added. In mid-summer, Radix Angelicae Sinensis was omitted while kitchen-range earth was added to increase its effect in drying out dampness. This comprehensive application of herbal remedies according to seasonal changes is no doubt a peculiarity of the imperial physicians, a point to be remembered.

## XVII.7. SYRUP FOR REINFORCING THE SPLEEN AND STOMACH AND ELIMINATING DAMPNESS

Syrup for Reinforcing the Spleen and Stomach and Eliminating Dampness (Li Pi Yang Wei Chu Shi Gao) was carefully prepared by the imperial physicians Fan Shaoxiang, Zhong Ling and Quan Shun in the second month of the lunar calendar in 1884.

### Ingredients

| | |
|---|---|
| Radix Codonopsis Pilosulae  (Dang Shen) | 6 g |
| Rhizoma Actratylodis Macrocephalae  (Bai Zhu) | 9 g |
| Poria  (Fu Ling) | 9 g |
| Semen Nelumbinis  (Lian Rou) | 9 g |
| Semen Dolichoris  (Bian Dou) | 9 g |
| Herba Agastachis  (Huo Xiang Gen) | 4.5 g |
| Massa Fermentata Medicinalis  (Shen Qu) | 6 g |
| Fructus Hordei Germinatus  (Mai Ya) | 9 g |
| Pericarpium Citri Reticulatae  (Chen Pi) | 4.5 g |
| Fructus Amomi  (Sha Ren) | 3 g |
| Radix Glycyrrhizae  (Gan Cao) | 2.4 g |

According to the original scripts, the Rhizoma Atractylodis Macrocephalae, Semen Dolichoris and Fructus Hordei Germinature should be baked before use, while the Fructus Amomi should be processed into powder.

The above ingredients were well decocted and the residue removed. The remaining liquid was further concentrated and refined honey added to make a syrup. Six grams of the syrup infused in boiled water was taken each time.

On the 23rd day of the second month of the lunar calendar, in mid spring, the mild prescription was studied critically and then followed without changing any of the ingredients.

### Comments

This prescription was modified on the basis of Ginseng-Poria and Atractylodis Macrocephalae Powder (Shen Ling Bai Zhu Wan). Radix Platycodi in the original remedy was omitted, but Massa Fermentata Medicinalis and Fructus Hordei Germinature were added in order to strengthen its effect in regulating the function of the spleen. Rhizoma Dio was replaced by Herba Agastachis because imperial physicians were afraid that Rhizoma Dio would be too greasy for the Emperor. The pharmaceutical properties of this prescription were rather mild with neither preponderance of heat nor of cold. This was done in view of the fact that Emperor Guangxu had deficiency of the spleen and stomach, plus indigestion, and so often needed to have his spleen and stomach condition treated.

## XVII.8. SYRUP FOR REGULATING THE SPLEEN AND STOMACH AND ELIMINATING DAMPNESS

Syrup for Regulating the Spleen and Stomach and Eliminating Dampness (Li Pi He Wei Chu Shi Gao) was carefully prepared by the imperial physicians Tong Wenbin and Quan Shun on the fourth day of the second month of the lunar calendar in 1885.

### Ingredients

| | |
|---|---|
| Radix Codonopsis Pilosulae (Dang Shen) | 4.5 g |
| Rhizoma Atractylodis Macrocephalae (Bai Shu) | 4.5 g |
| Poria (Fu Ling) | 9 g |
| Semen Coicis (Yi Yi Ren) | 9 g |
| Semen Nelumbinis (Lian Rou) | 9 g |
| Fructus Oryzae Germinature (Gu Ya) | 6 g |
| Pericarpium Citri Reticulatae (Chen Pi) | 3 g |
| Rhizoma Cyperi (Xiang Fu) | 3 g |
| Radix Angelicae Sinensis (Dang Gui) | 6 g |
| Fructus Lycii (Gou Qi Zi) | 6 g |
| Radix Paeoniae Lactiflorae (Bai Shao) | 4.5 g |
| Radix Rehmanniae (Sheng Di Huang) | 6 g |

According to the original records, raw Rhizoma Atractylodis Macrocephalae, roasted Fructus Oryzae Germinature, processed Rhizoma Cyperi, roasted Radix Paeoniae Laotiflorae, and Radix Angelicae Sinensis roasted with earth should be used.

The above ingredients were well decocted before the herbal residue was discarded. The remaining liquid was further concentrated before refined honey was added to make a syrup. Six grams of the syrup infused with boiled water were taken each time.

On the 19th day of the first month of the lunar calendar, the date marking Jingzhe, the time in spring to waken the hibernating animals, the same prescription was again critically studied. The prescription was appropriate and the ingredients were mild, so no further modification was required.

### Comments

Although the main therapeutic purpose of the prescription was to regulate the spleen and pacify the stomach, it was in fact a formulation of the Eight Treasures Decoction (Ba Zhen Tang). Only Radix Glycyrrhizae was omitted because of dampness retention in the Middle Jiao. Rhizoma Ligustici Chuanxiong, pungent and warming, was also omitted on account of Emperor Guangxu's Yin deficient constitution, and Rhizoma Ligustici Chuanxiong may over-consume Yin in the body. Fructus Lycii was added to nourish the liver and kidney. This was an approach significant in dealing with the root cause of the disease. The mild Rhizoma Cyperi may also consume Yin because of its dry and bitter properties, yet it was included in the prescription probably because of the Emperor's emotional disturbances. Its use could help relieve his stagnation of liver *qi*.

Judging the whole prescription again shows that it accorded with both reinforcing and activating principles. Its effect was gradual so it could be taken over a long period of time. This is also the reason why imperial physicians claimed repeatedly that the ingredients were mild and could be applied continuously according to changes in season.

## XVII.9. SYRUP FOR REGULATING THE LIVER AND SPLEEN AND ELIMINATING DAMPNESS

Syrup for Regulating the Liver and Spleen and Eliminating Dampness (Li Pi He Gan Hua Shi Gao) was sent to the imperial hospital for preparation, though the date and imperial physician who prescribed it remain unknown.

### Ingredients

| | |
|---|---|
| Radix Panacis Quiquefloii  (Xi Yang Shen) | 9 g |
| Rhizoma Actratylodis Macrocephalae  (Bai Zhu) | 6 g |
| Radix Paeoniae Lactiflorae  (Bai Shao) | 15 g |
| Radix Schrophulariae  (Xuan Shen) | 15 g |
| Pericarpium Citri Reticulatae Rubra  (Ju Hong) | 9 g |
| Polyporus Umbellatus  (Zhu Ling) | 15 g |
| Rhizoma Alimatis  (Zhe Xie) | 9 g |
| Poria  (Fu Ling) | 15 g |
| Flos Inulae  (Xuan Fu Hua) | 9 g |
| Fructus Aurantii  (Zhi Ke) | 9 g |
| Bulbus Fritillariae Cirhosae  (Chuan Bei) | 9 g |
| Pericarpium Trichosanthis  (Gua Lou Pi) | 9 g |
| Semen Cuscutae  (Tu Si Zi) | 15 g |
| Rhizoma Polygonati Odorati  (Yu Zhu) | 9 g |
| Flos Chrysanthemi  (Ju Hua) | 9 g |
| Cortex Mori Radicis  (Sang Bai Pi) | 9 g |

| | |
|---|---|
| Semen Raphani  (Lai Fu Zi) | 9 g |
| Caulis Bamusae in Taeniam  (Zhu Ru) | 9 g |
| Endothelium Corneum Gigeriae Galli  (Ji Nei Jin) | 12 g |
| Massa Fermentata Medicinalis  (Shen Qu) | 9 g |
| Fructus Hordei Germinatus  (Mai Ya) | 9 g |
| Fructus Crataegi (Shan Zha) | 9 g |

The original records say that both the Radix Panacis Quiquefloii and Bulbus Fritillariae Cirhosae should be powdered before use, while the Flos Inulae should be packed before placing in the decoction. The Fructus Aurantii should be roasted and the Semen Raphani should be powdered before use.

The above ingredients were well decocted and the herbal residue discarded. The remaining liquid was further concentrated and then 150-g refined honey added to make a syrup. Three spoonfuls of the syrup infused with boiled water were taken each time.

### Comments

The main action of this prescription is to regulate the function of the spleen and resolve dampness. Therapeutically, it follows the Five Ingredients Powder to help regulate the function of the spleen. Cortex Cinnamomi was omitted to increase the action of eliminating dampness from the urine. Fructus Hordei Germinatus, Fructus Crataegi, Massa Fermentata Medicinalis, Semen Raphani, Fructus Aurantii and Endothelium Corneum Gigeriae Galli help strengthen the spleen and pacify the stomach. Cortex Mori Radicis and Pericarpium Trichosanthis clear the lung so that the function of the lung, also known as the upper source of water, is reinforced. Bulbus Fritillariae Cirhosae is used here to clear the sputum and stop cough. Radix Paeoniae Lactiflorae, Flos Chrysanthemi, Radix Schrophulariae and Semen Cuscutae regulate both the liver and kidney. Rhizoma Atractylodis Macrocephalae and Caulis Bambusae in Taeniam relieve the dryness and stop nausea. Flos Inulae reduces abnormal ascending of *qi*, pacifies the stomach and clears the sputum. This prescription, if followed over a long period of time, will benefit such conditions as deficiency of the liver and kidney, and retention of dampness due to spleen deficiency. Unfortunately, the disease conditions of Emperor Guangxu were so changeable that his chronic illnesses were difficult to treat despite the careful working out of therapeutic principles and the implementation of treatments.

## XVII.10.  REINFORCED THREE ELIXIRS DECOCTION

Reinforced Three Elixirs Decoction (Jia Wei San Xian Yin) was presented to the Emperor on the seventh day of the sixth month of the lunar calendar, with no information given as to the year and the imperial physician who made it.

### Ingredients

| | |
|---|---|
| Fructus Crataegi  (Shan Zha) | 6 g |
| Fructus Hordei Germinatus  (Mai Ya) | 6 g |
| Massa Fermentata Medicinalis  (Shen Qu) | 6 g |
| Caulis Bamusae in Taeniam  (Zhu Ru) | 6 g |
| Semen Coicis  (Tu Si Zi) | 9 g |

The original script says that prepared Semen Coicis cake was used.

**Comments**

This decoction can be used as Chinese tea replacement. Fructus Crataegi, Fructus Hordei Germinatus and Massa Fermentata Medicinalis promote digestion and pacify the spleen and stomach. Caulis Bambusae in Taeniam clears deficiency heat and stops nausea. The cake made from Semen Coicis nourishes the liver and kidney, reducing pain in the lumbar region. This prescription was applied mainly to deal with hiccups due to food retention. It was also used to treat the Emperor for his lumbar pain. It is believed that it was the prescription used in Emperor Guangxu's last few years.

## XVII.11. PRESCRIPTION FOR PACIFYING THE STOMACH AND PRODUCING FLUID

No information is available as to the date and the imperial physician who formulated the Prescription for Pacifying the Stomach and Producing Fluid (Sheng Jing He Wei Fang).

**Ingredients**

| | |
|---|---|
| Pear  (Da Li) | 3 |
| Nodus Nelumbinis Rhizomatis  (Xian Ou) | 1 |
| Ramulus Nelumbinis  (He Gen) | 1 |
| Pericarpium Citri Reticulatae Rubra  (Ju Luo) | 3 g |
| Radix Glycyrrhizae  (Gan Cao) | 2.4 g |
| Radix Zingiberis Recens  (Sheng Jiang) | 3 |
| Plumula Nelumbinis  (Lian Zi Xin) | 10 |
| Radix Scrophulariae  (Xuan Shen) | 6 g |

According to the original recipe, the pears, lotus root (Xian Ou) and fresh Ginger (Sheng Jiang) should be crushed for their juice only.

**Comments**

This prescription has the actions of clearing heat, stopping cough, producing fluid and pacifying the stomach. The Radix Scrophulariae nourishes Yin, sedates fire and relieves restlessness. It was applied mainly to nourish the kidney. According to *Explanation of Prescription Actions* (*Yao Pin Hua Yi*), "The effect of Radix Scrophulariae in nourishing the kidney is as good as Rhizoma Anemarrhenae." Radix Glyoyrrhizae pacifies the Middle Jiao, relieves spasmodic pain and moistens the lung. *A Collection of Comments on Materia Medica* (*Ben Cao Hui Yan*) claims Radix Glycyrrhizae to be "the ingredient for overcoming deficiency and relieving toxicity." Plumula Nelumbinis, Ramulus Nelumbinis and Nodus Nelumbinis all belong to plants of the family Nymphaeaceae. They are different parts of lotus, namely the seeds, stem and root, having the actions of clearing summer heat, strengthening the stomach and relieving restlessness. Radix Zingiberis Recens stops nausea and eliminates cold. The great medical scientist Sun Simiao (581-682) described it as a "sacred ingredient for nausea and vomiting." Pears can produce fluid and correct the dryness. Pericarpium Citri Reticulatae can remove obstruction from channels and resolve phlegm.

These ingredients were all prescribed according to the precise condition of Emperor Guangxu at that time.

# XVIII. PRESCRIPTIONS FOR CONSTIPATION AND DIARRHEA

## XVIII.1. CONSTIPATION REMEDY

Constipation Remedy (Bian Bi Fang) was presented for imperial use on the 21st day of the 11th month of the lunar calendar, with no information given as to the year and the imperial physician who formulated it.

### Ingredients

| | |
|---|---|
| Semen Armenicacae  (Xin Ren) | 9 g |
| Semen Pini Nodi  (Song Zi Ren) | 9 g |
| Fructus Cannabis  (Huo Ma Ren) | 9 g |
| Semen Biota  (Bai Zi Ren) | 9 g |

The above ingredients were pounded into pieces and brewed in boiling water to be taken as tea.

### Comments

All the ingredients in this prescription, having the effect of moistening the intestines and moving the bowels, are indicated in constipation due to Yin deficiency or lack of fluid in aged patients. The so-called Bada Xinren, according to *Compendium of Materia Medica* (Ben Cao Gang Mu), was called Badan Xinren. Both mean the ordinary sort of Semen Armenicacae. It belongs to the Rosaceae family and refers only to the kernels of Badan Xinren. *A Profound Explanation to Materia Medica* (*Ben Cao Tong Xuan*) says: "Badan Xinren may moisten the intestines and resolve phlegm." Emperor Guangxu had a Yin-deficient body constitution. Many of his health records mention his constipation, and this prescription must have been empirical and effective.

## XVIII.2. DIARRHEA PRESCRIPTION

Diarrhea Prescription (Zhi Fu Xie Fang) was presented for imperial use on the eighth day of the ninth month of the lunar calendar, with no information given as to the year and the imperial physician who formulated it.

### Ingredients

| | |
|---|---|
| Rhizoma Alismatis  (Ze Xie) | 9 g |
| Rhizoma Atractylodis Macrocephalae  (Bai Zhu) | 9 g |
| Fructus Evodiae (Wu Zhu Yu) | 3 g |
| Pericarpium Citri Reticulatae Rubra  (Ju Luo) | 9 g |
| Caulis Bamusae in Taeniam  (Zhu Ru) | 6 g |
| Polyporus Umbellatus  (Zhu Ling) | 9 g |
| Radix Paeoniae Lactiflorae  (Bai Shao) | 15 g |
| Rhizoma Coptidis  (Huang Lian) | 2.1 g |

The original scripts require that the Rhizoma Atractylodis Macrocephalae should be roasted in earth and the Rhizoma Coptidis ground into powder before use.

**Comments**

This prescription was formed on the basis of Five Accumulations Pill (Wu Ji Wan) and simplified Five Ingredients Powder with Poria (Wu Ling San), plus Pericarpium Citri Reticulatae Rubra and Caulis Bambusae in Taeniam. It is estimated to have been made especially for nausea, vomiting and loose stools suffered by Emperor Guangxu. Ingredients from Five Accumulations Pill in the prescription were applied to deal with damp-heat diarrhea, while the Polyporus Umbellatus, Rhizoma Alismatis and Rhizoma Atractylodis Macrocephalae strengthen the spleen in eliminating dampness. Pericarpium Citri Reticulatae Rubra and Caulis Bambusae in Taeniam pacify the Middle Jiao and stop nausea.

# XIX.  PRESCRIPTION FOR URINARY BLADDER CONDITIONS

## XIX.1.  FIVE INGREDIENTS POWDER WITH PORIA

Five Ingredients Powder with Poria (Wu Ling San) was prepared on the eighth day of the intercalary fourth month of the lunar calendar in 1887 by the imperial physicians Zhang Zhongyuan and Zhong Xun.

**Ingredients**

| | |
|---|---:|
| Poria  (Fu Ling) | 24 g |
| Rhizoma Atractylodis Macrocephalae  (Bai Zhu) | 12 g |
| Rhizoma Alismatis  (Ze Xie) | 18 g |
| Polyporus Umbellatus  (Zhu Ling) | 18 g |
| Cortex Cinnamomi  (Rou Gui) | 2.4 g |

According to the original records, roasted Atractylodis Macrocephalae and peeled Cortex Cinnamomi with purple oil should be used. The above ingredients were ground into fine powder, three grams of which were infused with the decoction from the Three Elixirs Decoction (San Xian Tang) for internal use.

**Comments**

This prescription, taken from *Treatise on Febrile Diseases* (*Shang Han Lun*), has actions in strengthening the spleen, eliminating dampness, and promoting the *qi* mechanism in discharging water. Specifically, Poria, Polyporus Umbellatus and Rhizoma Alismatis were applied to promote the function of the urinary bladder in transforming *qi* and smoothing the water passage so that the dampness could be eliminated through the urinary tract. Rhizoma Atractylodis Macrocephalae strengthens the spleen and eliminates dampness. Cortex Cinnamomi was used instead of Ramulus Cinnamomi to strengthen its effect of promoting the source of fire. During the era of Emperor Guangxu, the intercalary fourth month of the lunar calendar took place in 1887 and 1906. Judging from the physical condition of the Emperor, this prescription should be the one used for him in 1906.

# XX.  PRESCRIPTIONS FOR SEMINAL EMISSION

## XX.1.  PILL FOR REINFORCING AND WARMING KIDNEY ESSENCE

Pill for Reinforcing and Warming Kidney Essence (Zi Yin Yi Shen Xuan Jing Wan) was recommended for Emperor Guangxu to take regularly so as to achieve a slow effect starting from the 15th day of the 11th month of the lunar calendar. The year and the imperial physician who formulated the prescription remain unknown.

*Ingredients*

| | |
|---|---:|
| Radix Rehmanniae  (Sheng Di Huang) | 30 g |
| Fructus Corni  (Shan Zhu Yu) | 12 g |
| Cortex Eucommiae  (Du Zhong) | 18 g |
| Fructus Tribuli Terrestris  (Bai Ji Li) | 18 g |
| Poria  (Fu Ling) | 18 g |
| Rhizoma Dio  (Shan Yao) | 18 g |
| Fructus Psoraleae  (Bu Gu Zhi) | 12 g |
| Semen Allii  (Jiu Cai Zi) | 12 g |
| Radix Angelicae Sinensis  (Dang Gui) | 18 g |
| Radix Paeoniae Lactiflorae  (Bai Shao) | 12 g |
| Rhizoma Cibotii  (Jin Mao Gou) | 12 g |
| Fructus Alpiniae Oxyphylla  (Yi Zhi Ren) | 9 g |
| Radix Achyranthis Bidentatae  (Niu Xi) | 12 g |
| Fructus Nelumbinis  (Shi Lian Xin) | 15 g |
| Glycine Max  (Lu Dou Pi) | 18 g |
| Fructus Amomi  (Sha Ren) | 4.5 g |

According to the original records, the Rhizoma Dio, Semen Allii and Radix Paeoniae Lactiflorae should be roasted before use. The hairy coating from the Rhizoma Cibotii should be discarded during processing.

The above ingredients were ground into fine powder and made with date jam into pills the size of Chinese mung beans. Six grams of the pills were taken morning and evening with salt water.

*Comments*

Many prescriptions for nourishing the kidney Yin are available from different sources. This prescription mainly reinforces the kidney and warms sperm. Emperor Guangxu had seminal emission for years, accompanied by scrotum eczema and spermacrasia. His weak body would not accept drastic nourishing. As deficient Yin and Yang were not supposed to be warmed instantly, a mild prescription was used to achieve the effect of reinforcing both Yin and Yang gradually.

# XX.2. MODIFIED PILL FOR REINFORCING AND WARMING KIDNEY ESSENCE

Modified Pill for Reinforcing and Warming Kidney Essence (Jia Jian Zi Yin Yi Shen Xuan Jing Wan) was prepared by the imperial physicians Zhuang Shouhe and Quan Shun on the 13th day of the 12th month of the lunar calendar. The year in which it was made remains unknown.

*Ingredients*

| | |
|---|---|
| Radix Rehmanniae  (Sheng Di Huang) | 30 g |
| Fructus Corni  (Shan Zhu Yu) | 12 g |
| Rhizoma Dio  (Shan Yao) | 18 g |
| Cortex Eucommiae  (Du Zhong) | 18 g |
| Fructus Tribuli Terrestris  (Bai Ji Li) | 18 g |
| Poria  (Fu Ling) | 15 g |
| Fructus Psoraleae  (Bu Gu Zhi) | 12 g |
| Radix Polygalae  (Yuan Zhi) | 6 g |
| Radix Angelicae Sinensis  (Dang Gui) | 18 g |
| Radix Paeoniae Lactiflorae  (Bai Shao) | 12 g |
| Rhizoma Cibotii  (Jing Mao Gou) | 12 g |
| Fructus Alpiniae Oxyphylla  (Yi Zhi Ren) | 9 g |
| Radix Achyranthis Bidentatae  (Niu Xi) | 12 g |
| Fructus Nelumbinis  (Shi Lian Xin) | 15 g |
| Pericarpium Citri Reticulatae  (Chen Pi) | 6 g |
| Glycine Max  (Lu Dou Pi) | 18 g |

According to the original recipe, roasted Rhizoma Dio and Radix Paeoniae Lactiflorae, Cortex Eucommiae roasted in salt water, and prepared Rhizoma Cibotii should be used.

The above ingredients were ground into fine powder and made with date jam into pills the size of Chinese mung beans. Six grams of the pills were taken with salt water morning and evening.

*Comments*

This pill was also based on Pill for Reinforcing and Warming Kidney Essence (Zi Yin Yi Shen Xuan Jing Wan) with slight modifications. Since Emperor Guangxu had a body constitution typical of flaring up of deficient fire, he was not supposed to have Semen Allii in his prescription for too long a time because it would further assist the flaring up of fire, and was therefore omitted. Nor was Semen Armenicacae, pungent and warm, appropriate for Emperor Guangxu for the same reason. The prescription was also aimed at nourishing the Yin of the heart, stopping cough and resolving phlegm. So, Radix Polygalae was definitely to be used. Pericarpium Citri Reticulatae would be the best choice for regulating the spleen *qi* and pacifying the stomach, resolving phlegm and stopping cough. According to the health record of Emperor Guangxu on the 13th day of the 12th month of the lunar calendar, statements such as "hyperactivity of fire and deficiency of water made him unable to receive tonifying decoctions" were found. His own notes on his physical condition contained such information as "occasional premature ejaculation and damp-cold sensation in the lower part of the body," "poor appetite, restlessness and sweating." It was possible that this prescription was used for the Emperor at that period of time.

## XX.3.  KIDNEY ESSENCE REINFORCING PILL I

The prescription for Kidney Essence Reinforcing Pill I (Yi Shen Gu Jing Wan Yi) was prepared by the imperial physicians Zhuang Shouhe, Yang Jihe and Zhang Zhongyuan on the third day of the seventh month of the lunar calendar. The year in which it was made remains unknown.

### Ingredients

| | |
|---|---|
| Plastrum Testudinis  (Gui Ban) | 18 g |
| Conchae Ostreae  (Mu Li) | 12 g |
| Colla Cornu Cervi  (Lu Jiao Jiao) | 9 g |
| Gecko  (Ge Jie) | 1 pair |
| Radix Rehmanniae Praeparatae  (Shu Di Huang) | 9 g |
| Radix Paeoniae Lactiflorae  (Bai Shao) | 6 g |
| Fructus Alpiniae Oxyphylla  (Yi Zhi Ren) | 6 g |
| Semen Cuscutae  (Tu Si Zi) | 12 g |
| Poria  (Fu Ling) | 9 g |
| Rhizoma Dio  (Shan Yao) | 6 g |
| Fructus Corni  (Shan Zhu Yu) | 6 g |
| Cortex Moudan Radicis  (Mu Dan Pi) | 9 g |
| Fructus Schisandrae  (Wu Wei Zi) | 3 g |
| Fructus Rosae Laevigata  (Jin Yin Zi) | 6 g |
| Fructus Nelumbinis  (Shi Lian Zi) | 9 g |
| Rhizoma Alismatis  (Ze Xie) | 6 g |

The original records state that processed Plastrum Testudinis, raw Conchae Ostreae and Colla Cornu Cervi roasted with Gecko powder should be used. Gecko tail and Semen Cuscutae cake should also be used. Dry Radix Paeoniae Lactiflorae, Rhizoma Dio and Fructus Alpiniae Oxyphylla roasted with salt water should be used.

The above ingredients were ground into fine powder and made with malt sugar into pills the size of Chinese mung beans. Six grams of the pills were taken with boiled water morning and evening.

### Comments

This is a comprehensive prescription consisting of the Two Immortals of Plastrum Testudinis and Colla Cornu Cervi (Gui Lu Er Xian Jiao), Six Ingredients Rehmanniae Pill with Fructus Schisandrae (Qi Wei Du Qi Wan) and Poria-Semen Cuscutae Powder (Fu Tu Dan) together with other kidney-tonifying and sperm fortifying ingredients. It was aimed at reinforcing both Yin and Yang of the kidney, nourishing the liver and regulating the qi of the spleen. Malt sugar was used as the pill binder for its sweet flavour and bland property. According to Prescriptions Worth a Thousand Gold (Qian Jin Yao Fang), malt sugar has the effect of driving away the deficient cold and reinforcing qi. Materia Medica on Diet Therapy (Shi Xing Ben Cao) also says, "Malt sugar may strengthen the spleen and stomach and pacify the Middle Jiao." The ingredients in this prescription are actually greasy. Malt sugar was used to strengthen the spleen, thus making the construction of the remedy quite ideal.

## XX.4. KIDNEY ESSENCE REINFORCING PILL II

The prescription for Kidney Essence Reinforcing Pill II (Yi Shen Gu Jing Wan Er) was prepared by the imperial physicians Zhang Zhongyuan and Quan Shun on the 22nd day of the 11th month of the lunar calendar. The year in which it was made remains unknown.

*Ingredients*

| | |
|---|---|
| Radix Rehmanniae Praeparatae  (Shu Di Huang) | 240 g |
| Fructus Corni  (Shan Zhu Yu) | 120 g |
| Rhizoma Dio  (Shan Yao) | 120 g |
| Cortex Moudan Radicis  (Mu Dan Pi) | 120 g |
| Poria  (Fu Ling) | 120 g |
| Os Draconis  (Long Gu) | 9 g |
| Radix Nelumbinis  (Lian Xu) | 30 g |
| Semen Euryales  (Qian Shi) | 60 g |
| Colla Corii Asini  (Xian Jiao) | 120 g |

The original recipe requires the Os Draconis to be ground into powder in water and the Semen Euryales roasted before use.

The preparation of this kind of pill was fairly complicated. Prepared Conchae Ostreae Powder (Mu Li San) was used to roast the Colla Corii Asini until particles were formed. Then the Conchae Ostreae was discarded. The remaining part was mixed with the above ingredients to be ground into fine powder and made into honey pills the size of Chinese mung beans. The pills were taken twice daily morning and evening. Twelve grams of the pills were taken each time orally with Herba Pyrolae soup.

*Comments*

This prescription was actually the Rehmanniae Pill with Six Ingredients (Liu Wei Di Huang Wan) but without Rhizoma Alismatis and Golden Lock Pill for Keeping Kidney Essence (Jin Suo Gu Jing Wan) using Colla Corii Asini but without Fructus Tribuli Terrestris. Rhizoma Alismatis was omitted to prevent its strong effect in eliminating dampness from affecting the body Yin. Adding Colla Corii Asini and omitting Fructus Tribuli Terrestris was to strengthen the effect of the prescription in reinforcing Yin. Using Herba Pyrolae soup to take the pill was to strengthen the effect of reinforcing the kidney and fortifying the kidney essence.

## XX.5. PRESCRIPTION FOR CHRONIC NOCTURNAL EMISSION

Prescription for Chronic Nocturnal Emission (Jiu Huan Meng Yi Fang) was recorded without the date or names of the imperial physicians who made it.

*Ingredients*

| | |
|---|---|
| Fructus Tribuli Terrestris  (Bai Ji Li) | 240 g |
| Radix Dipsaci  (Chuan Xu Duan) | 60 g |

| | |
|---|---|
| Semen Cuscutae  (Tu Si Zi) | 90 g |
| Fructus Corni  (Shan Zhu Yu) | 120 g |
| Semen Euryales  (Qian Shi) | 120 g |
| Radix Nelumbinis  (Lian Xu) | 120 g |
| Fructus Fubi  (Fu Peng Zi) | 60 g |
| Fructus Lycii  (Gou Qi Zi) | 60 g |

The original records state that raw Fructus Cornu, Semen Euryales, Radix Nelumbinis, Fructus Fubi and Fructus Lycii should be used. The Fructus Dipsaci should be prepared with millet wine, while a half dose of Fructus Tribuli Terrestris was made into powder and the other half was made into syrup.

The above ingredients were ground into fine powder and made with Fructus Tribuli Terrestris syrup and refined honey into pills the size of Chinese mung beans. Fifteen grams of the pills were taken with salt water on an empty stomach.

### Comments

This prescription was formed on the basis of the Excellent Immortal Pill (Cui Xian Wan) from copies of the prescription in the Qing Dynasty imperial hospital. Os Draconis and Fructus Rosae Laevigata were omitted but Radix Nelumbinis was added into the present prescription, which was aimed solely at reinforcing the kidney essence, promoting blood circulation, strengthening the lumbus and knees, stopping seminal emission, rejuvenating the facial complexion and halting night sweating. Suitable for the condition of Emperor Guangxu, it was often presented for his use.

## XX.6. SEMINAL EMISSION PRESCRIPTION

Seminal Emission Prescription (Zhi Yi Jing Fang) was recorded without the date or the names of imperial physicians who formulated it.

### Ingredients

| | |
|---|---|
| Radix Rehmanniae Praeparatae  (Shu Di Huang) | 9 g |
| Rhizoma Alismatis  (Ze Xie) | 9 g |
| Cortex Moudan Radicis  (Mu Dan Pi) | 2.4 g |
| Poria  (Fu Ling) | 3 g |
| Rhizoma Dio  (Shan Yao) | 3 g |
| Semen Ziziphi Spinosae  (Suan Zao Ren) | 3 g |
| Semen Euryales  (Qian Shi) | 3 g |
| Semen Cuscutae  (Tu Si Zi) | 3 g |
| Cortex Eucommiae  (Du Zhong) | 3 g |
| Radix Morindae Officinalis  (Ba Ji Tian) | 3 g |
| Pig fat  (Zhu You) | 3 g |

The original records require that the Semen Euryales should be ground into powder before use. The above ingredients were made into a decoction to be taken while still warm for achieving optimum effect.

### Comments

This prescription was formed on the basis of Radix Rehmanniae Pill with Six Ingredients (Liu Wei Di Huang Wan) plus certain ingredients with the effect of warming the kidney and consolidating the kidney essence. Radix Morindae Officinalis in combination with Semen Cusoutae produced remarkable effect in strengthening the kidney and consolidating the kidney essence. Cortex Eucommiae in combination with Semen Euryales strengthens the action of the prescription in reinforcing the spleen and the kidney. The original text claimed that it had excellent effect, probably an over-statement. However, long-term use of the remedy would no doubt be helpful. The ingredients in this prescription were handwritten by Emperor Guangxu himself. The so-called excellent effect may have been the personal experience of the Emperor, or so it would seem.

## XX.7. PRESCRIPTION FOR PREMATURE EJACULATION AND NOCTURNAL EMISSION

Prescription for Premature Ejaculation and Nocturnal Emission (Zhi Jing Hua Meng Yi Fang) was recorded without the date or the name of the imperial physician who made it.

### Ingredients

| | |
|---|---|
| Fructus Rosae Laevigata  (Jin Yin Zi) | 15 g |
| Semen Euryales  (Qian Shi) | 15 g |
| Plumula Nelumbinis  (Lian Zi Xin) | 15 g |
| Os Draconis  (Long Gu) | 15 g |

According to the original records, the Os Draconis should be fired before use. The above ingredients were ground into fine powder and made with rice gruel into pills the size of Chinese mung beans. Seventy grams of the pills were taken each time with salt and millet wine mixture.

### Comments

Several factors contribute to seminal emission. Generally speaking, it is mainly related to the following three: flaring up of deficient fire, accumulation of internal damp-heat, and deficient kidney failing to retain the essence. The main purpose of this prescription was to strengthen the kidney. It was formed on the basis of Land and Water Immortal Pill (Shui Lu Er Xian Dan) recorded in the *Collection of Hong's Proved Prescriptions* (*Hong Shi Ji Yan Fang*). It is indicated in seminal emission, frequency of urination and cloudy urine. Plumula Nelumbinis consolidates the kidney essence and clears heart fire. Os Draconis prepared on fire also helps retain the essence. Should the kidney *qi* be reinforced and the gate for essence be locked, nocturnal emission may cease spontaneously. This prescription was also handwritten by Emperor Guangxu himself.

## XX.8. PROVED PRESCRIPTION FOR SEMINAL EMISSION

Proved Prescription for Seminal Emission (Zhi Yi Jing Yan Fang) was recorded without the date or the name of the imperial physician who formulated it.

### Ingredients

| | |
|---|---|
| Radix Ginseng (Ren Shen) | 60 g |
| Radix Astragali seu Hedysari  (Huang Qi) | 60 g |

| | |
|---|---:|
| Poria (Fu Ling) | 60 g |
| Cortex Eucommiae (Du Zhong) | 60 g |
| Semen Euryales (Qian Shi) | 60 g |
| Radix Polygalae (Yuan Zhi) | 60 g |
| Radix Poria (Fu Shen) | 30 g |
| Rhizoma Dio (Shan Yao) | 240 g |
| Radix Platycodi (Jie Geng) | 12 g |
| Radix Auchlandiae (Mu Xiang) | 6 g |
| Cinnabaris (Chen Sha) | 6 g |
| Moschus (Dang Men Zi) | 1 g |

The above ingredients were ground into fine powder and made with refined honey into pills the size of Chinese mung beans. Six grams of the pills were taken together with rice gruel.

### Comments

This prescription was formed on the basis of Excellent Fragrant Powder (Miao Xiang San) as recorded in *Imperial Grace Formulary of the Tai Ping Era* (*Tai Ping Hui Min He Ji Ju Fang*). It was modified by omitting Radix Glycyrrhizae from the original, while adding Cortex Eucommiae and Semen Euryales. It was indicated in heart *qi* deficiency, palpitation, fright, dizziness and vertigo, seminal emission and night sweating. In order to strengthen the effect of the remedy, Cortex Eucommiae was used to reinforce the kidney and consolidate the kidney essence. Semen Euryales was added to help clear heart fire and retain kidney essence. Most of the prescriptions presented to Emperor Guangxu for his seminal emission were aimed at reinforcing the kidney and retaining kidney essence. Yet this prescription was primarily to reinforce heart *qi*, starting from regaining harmony between the heart and kidney. Reinforcing the kidney and retaining kidney essence, and taking both the heart and kidney into consideration may be regarded as the chief characteristics of this prescription.

## XX.9. SINGLE INGREDIENT DECOCTION FOR RETAINING KIDNEY ESSENCE

Single Ingredient Decoction for Retaining Kidney Essence (Yi Wei Mi Jing Tang) was carefully prepared by the imperial physician Yang Jihe on the 10th day of the fifth month of the lunar calendar, with no information given as to the year.

### Ingredient

| | |
|---|---:|
| Semen Juglandis film (Fen Xin Mu) | 15 g |

The original records say the woody film from the Semen Juglandis should be washed before use. It was decocted with one and half teacups of water until half a cup of decoction was left. This was taken before sleep.

### Comments

Semen Juglandis belongs to the family Juglandaceae. Its wooden film, also known as walnut coating, has the effect of consolidating kidney essence, being popularly applied as the principal ingredient in the treatment of seminal emission. The reason why it has been used for treating seminal emission is its effect of consolidating kidney essence. Emperor Guangxu therefore often took it. Today, people tend to use it for dealing with neurasthenia as well as seminal emission. Its therapeutic effect is beyond doubt.

## XX.10. LIGNUM AQUILARIAE RESINATUM PILL WITH MAGNETITUM

The prescription for Lignum Aquilariae Resinatum Pill with Magnetitum (Chen Xiang Ci Shi Wan) was prepared by the imperial physicians Zhang Zhong-yuan, Quan Shun and Zhong Xun on the 29th day of the ninth month of the lunar calendar, with no information given as to the year.

### Ingredients

| | |
|---|---|
| Lignum Aquilariae Resinatum  (Chen Xiang) | 30 g |
| Fructus Viticis  (Man Jing Zi) | 30 g |
| Halite  (Qing Yan) | 30 g |
| Flos Chrysanthemi  (Ju Hua) | 30 g |
| Radix Morindae Officinalis  (Ba Ji Tian) | 30 g |
| Semen Trigonella  (Hu Lu Ba) | 30 g |
| Rhizoma Dio  (Shan Yao) | 30 g |
| Pericarpium Zanthoxyli  (Chuan Jiao) | 30 g |
| Magnetitum  (Ci Shi) | 30 g |
| Fructus Corni  (Shan Zhu Yu) | 30 g |
| Radix Aconiti Praeparata  (Fu Zi) | 30 g |
| Actinolitum  (Yang Qi Shi) | 30 g |

The original records say that both the Magnetitum and Actinolitum should be first fired with vinegar and then ground into powder in water before use. All the ingredients were ground into fine powder before mixing with millet wine-cooked wheat paste for processing into pills the size of Chinese parasol-tree seeds. Fifty pills were taken with salty soup on an empty stomach. The dosage was later increased to 70 pills.

### Comments

This prescription has the effect of warming the kidney Yang and is mainly applied for such conditions as the kidney Yang deficiency, cold retention in the sperm palace, damp scrotum, impotence and premature ejaculation. The prescription chiefly consists of ingredients that have the function of warming the kidney and strengthening Yang *qi*, plus ingredients also for retaining and receiving the vital *qi*. The nomenclature of the remedy Lignum Aquilariae Resinatum Pill with Magnetitum has the following rationales: Lignum Aquilariae Resinatum "is warm in property but never dry, promotes *qi* but not to the state of sedating *qi*"; and Magnetitum "can work into the kidney and appease Yin so that the dragon fire resulting from Yin deficiency does not ascend." The above quotes are from *Essence of Materia Medica* (*Ben Cao Qiu Zhen*). The combination of the two ingredients may remarkably strengthen the effect of the prescription in warming the kidney and promoting the kidney in receiving *qi*.

# XXI.  LIVER CONDITION PRESCRIPTIONS

## XXI.1.  PILL FOR SOOTHING THE LIVER AND SOFTENING MASSES

Pill for Soothing the Liver and Softening Masses (Tiao Gan Shu Jin Ruan Jian Wan) was prepared by the imperial physician Tong Chenhai for Emperor Guangxu on the 15th day of the ninth month of the lunar calendar, with no information given as to the year.

### Ingredients

| | |
|---|---|
| Radix Rehmanniae  (Sheng Di Huang) | 18 g |
| Radix Paeoniae Rubra  (Chi Shao) | 12 g |
| Rhizoma Cyperi  (Xiang Fu) | 12 g |
| Pericarpium Citri Reticulatae Viride  (Qing Pi) | 12 g |
| Radix Curcumae  (Chuan Yu Jin) | 18 g |
| Rhizoma Corydalis  (Yuan Hu Suo) | 12 g |
| Resina Murrhea  (Mo Yao) | 9 g |
| Sargassum  (Hai Zao) | 9 g |
| Spica Prunellae  (Xia Ku Cao) | 15 g |
| Herba Menthae  (Bo He) | 6 g |
| Flos Chrysanthemi  (Ju Hua) | 9 g |

According to the original records, the Pericarpium Citri Reticulatae Viride and Radix Curcumae should be ground into powder, while the Rhizoma Cyperi and Rhizoma Corydalis should be processed, both before use.

The above ingredients were ground into fine powder and made into water-bound pills the size of Chinese mung beans, 4.5 grams of which were taken each time with boiled water.

### Comments

This prescription has the actions of nourishing the kidney, soothing the liver, regulating *qi*, activating blood, relieving *qi* stagnation and softening masses. Tong Chenhai, who served as an imperial physician in the late Qing Dynasty, was carefully working out this prescription when Emperor Guangxu was already seriously ill. His condition was characterized by deficiency of kidney water, stagnation of liver *qi* and hypofunction of both the spleen and stomach. Judging from the ingredients and actions of this prescription, the Emperor probably had such clinical manifestations as lumbar soreness, premature ejaculation, wandering pain in both hypochondriac regions, belching, hiccups and a full sensation in the epigastric region. These symptoms and signs were those contained in Emperor Guangxu's health records around 1884.

## XXI.2. DECOCTION FOR REGULATING THE LIVER AND REINFORCING THE KIDNEY

Decoction for Regulating the Liver and Reinforcing the Kidney (He Gan Yi Shen Yin) was carefully prepared by the imperial physician Zhong Xun for Emperor Guangxu on the seventh day of the fourth month of the lunar calendar, with no information given as to the year.

*Ingredients*

| | |
|---|---|
| Rhizoma Acori Graminei (Shi Chang Pu) | 3 g |
| Fructus Chaenomelis (Mu Gua) | 6 g |
| Fructus Liquidambaris (Lu Lu Tong) | 5 |
| Radix Auchlandiae (Mu Xiang) | 1.5 g |
| Massa Fermentata Medicinalis (Shen Qu) | 3 g |
| Fructus Hordei Germinatus (Mai Ya) | 3 g |
| Fructus Crataegi (Shan Zha) | 3 g |
| Flos Chrysanthemi (Ju Hua) | 3 g |
| Semen Cuscutae (Tu Si Zi) | 9 g |
| Radix Paeoniae Lactiflorae (Bai Shao) | 6 g |
| Medulla Junci Effusi (Deng Xin Cao) | 1 |

According to the original recipe, the Fructus Chaenomelis should be roasted with salt water, while the Fructus Liquidambaris should be ground into powder before use. The above ingredients were made into decoction for oral administration while still warm.

*Comments*

The Radix Paeoniae Lactiflorae, Radix Auchlandiae and Flos Chrysanthemi in the prescription were used for regulating liver *qi*. Semen Cuscutae reinforces the kidney and fortifies the kidney essence. Rhizoma Acori Graminei calms the heart and tranquilizes the mind. Fructus Liquidambaris and Fructus Chaenomelis remove obstruction from channels. Massa Fermentata Medicinalis, Fructus Crataegi and Fructus Hordei Germinatus reinforce the spleen and strengthen the stomach. Medulla Junci Effusi promotes water discharge and clears heat from the heart. As the actions of this prescription are mild, it was applied in an attempt to achieve a gradual effect.

# XXII. PRESCRIPTIONS FOR MUSCLE AND TENDON PAIN

## XXII.1. PRESCRIPTION FOR LUMBAGO AND BACK PAIN

Prescription for Lumbago and Back Pain (Zhi Jian Bei Jin Gu Teng Tong Fang) was prepared and submitted on the 11th day of the 11th month of the lunar calendar, with no mention of the year.

*Ingredients*

| | |
|---|---|
| Flos Sophora Immaturus (Huai Hua Zi) | 15 g |
| Juglandis (Hei Tao) | 15 g |
| Semen Sesame (Zhi Ma) | 15 g |
| Folium Camelliae Sinensis (Cha Ye) | 15 g |

The above ingredients were immersed in five bowls of water and decocted to half the volume. The decoction was then taken while still warm.

*Comments*

This prescription embodies both clearing and reinforcing principles. Among them, the Semen Sesame, having the action of nourishing the liver and the kidney, is usually applied in the treatment of such conditions as liver and kidney deficiency, wind type Bi-syndrome and paralysis. According to *Supplement to Chinese Materia Medica (Ben Cao Shi Yi)*, the use of 15 grams of Semen Sesame decocted with millet wine was suggested for the treatment of paralysis. Juglandis also reinforces the kidney and consolidates the kidney essence. It can be applied for lumbar pain and weakness in the lower limbs due to kidney deficiency. Flos Sophora Immaturus is good for cooling blood and clearing heat. Modern studies prove that it also contains anti-bacterial substance, effective in resisting staphylococous and bacillus coli. Folium Camelliae Sinensis, the Chinese tea, may help clear toxic heat from the head and eyes. The tannic acid in Chinese tea acts as the vitamin P that is helpful in capillary wall metabolism.

## XXII.2. PRESCRIPTION FOR SPINAL AND NECK PAIN

Prescription for Spinal and Neck Pain (Zhi Xiang Jie Ji Bei Tong Fang) was prepared on the 23rd day of the fifth month of the lunar calendar for the purpose of helping relieve Emperor Guangxu's pain in the cervical and thoracic portions of the spinal column.

*Ingredients*

| | |
|---|---|
| Rhizoma seu Radix Notopterygii (Qiang Huo) | 6 g |
| Radix Angelicae Pubescentis (Du Huo) | 4.5 g |
| Rhizoma Ligustici (Hao Ben) | 4.5 g |
| Fructus Viticis (Man Jing Zi) | 6 g |
| Radix Ledebouriellae (Fang Feng) | 6 g |
| Rhizoma Ligustici Chuanxiong (Chuan Xiong) | 6 g |
| Ramulus Uncariae cum Uncis (Gou Teng) | 4.5 g |
| Rhizoma Curcumae Longae (Jiang Huang) | 6 g |
| Radix Glycyrrhizae (Gan Cao) | 2.4 g |

The above ingredients were made into decoction to be taken while still warm.

*Comments*

This prescription was formed on the basis of Radix Notopterygii Decoction for Resolving Dampness (Qiang Huo Shen Shi Tang) as recorded in *Imperial Grace Formulary of the Tai Ping Era (Tai Ping Hui Min He Ji Ju Fang)*, plus Ramulus Uncariae cum Uncis and Rhizoma Curcumae Longae. It was indicated in pain of the neck and nape, and also pain in the back and lumbar regions due to the invasion of dampness in the superficial portion of the body. Many wind-dispersing ingredients were contained in the prescription. It was thus formulated according to the principle that "wind can drive away dampness" in *The Yellow Emperor's Internal Medicine (Huang Di Nei Jing)*. The Rhizoma seu Radix Notopterygii, Radix Angelicae Pubescentis, Radix Ledebouriellae, Rhizoma Ligustici and Fructus Viticis were used to eliminate wind and dampness. The Rhizoma Ligustici Chuanxiong and Rhizoma Curcumae Longae were applied to activate blood and remove obstruction from channels and collaterals. Ramulus Uncariae cum Uncis activates collateral circulation and guides the herbal effect to work in the expected areas. The Radix Glycyrrhizae harmonizes all of the ingredients while helping the dispersing action of the pungent warming ingredients. It should be noted that from 1907 Emperor Guangxu experienced fairly serious pain in the hip and lumbar region while his health was continuing to fall and therefore this prescription was not suitable for him though it may have been in the early stage of his illness.

## XXII.3.  HERBAL BATH REMEDY FOR SOOTHING TENDONS AND RELIEVING PAIN

Herbal Bath Remedy for Soothing Tendons and Relieving Pain (Shu Jing Zhi Tong Xi Yao Fang) was carefully prepared for Emperor Guangxu by the imperial physician Fan Yimei, with no information given as to the year.

*Ingredients*

| | |
|---|---|
| Radix Angelicae Sinensis  (Dang Gui) | 9 g |
| Radix Paeoniae Rubra  (Chi Shao) | 6 g |
| Cortex Moudan Radicis  (Mu Dan Pi) | 6 g |
| Radix Ledebouriellae  (Fang Feng) | 6 g |
| Radix Stephaniae Tetrandurae  (Han Fang Ji) | 9 g |
| Radix Gentianae Macrophyllae  (Qin Jiao) | 6 g |
| Fructus Chaenomelis  (Mu Gua) | 6 g |

The original recipe states that the Radix Angelicae Sinensis should be prepared with millet wine before use. All ingredients were well boiled for herbal bathing.

*Comments*

This prescription has the effect of activating blood and stopping pain. It is especially effective, however, in soothing the tendons. Compared with the immediate previous prescription, such blood-moving ingredients as Resina Olibani, Resina Murrhae and Flos Carthami were omitted. The moistening ingredients Radix Gentianae Macrophyllae and Fructus Chaenomelis among wind-eliminating ones were used to nourish the liver and soothe the tendons. The treatment suggested for eliminating wind and that for circulating blood should be considered as different therapeutic strategies.

## XXII.4.  HERBAL BATH REMEDY FOR SOOTHING TENDONS AND ACTIVATING BLOOD

Herbal Bath Remedy for Soothing Tendons and Activating Blood (Shu Jing Huo Luo Xi Yao Fang) was carefully prepared by the imperial physician Fan Yimei for Emperor Guangxu on the fifth day of the fifth month of the lunar calendar, with no mention of the year.

*Ingredients*

| | |
|---|---|
| Radix Angelicae Pubescentis  (Du Huo) | 6 g |
| Radix Gentianae Macrophyllae  (Qin Jiao) | 9 g |

| | |
|---|---|
| Radix Stephaniae Tetrandrae  (Fang Ji) | 9 g |
| Fructus Chaenomelis  (Mu Gua) | 9 g |
| Radix Paeoniae Lactiflorae  (Chi Shao) | 9 g |
| Cortex Moudan Radicis  (Mu Dan Pi) | 6 g |
| Ramulus Mori  (Sang Zhi) | 9 g |
| Radix Auchlandiae  (Mu Xiang) | 3 g |

The original directions were for the **Radix Auchlandiae** to be ground into fine powder before use. The above ingredients were well boiled in water for herbal bathing of affected areas of the body.

### Comments

This prescription has the action of eliminating wind and dampness. Most of the ingredients were for clearing wind. Theoretically, it was carried out in line with the principal philosophy from *Plain Questions* (*Su Wen*) that "wind communicates with the liver," and "liver manufactures blood." A treatment suggested for eliminating wind also means to treat the blood by means of circulation. Tendons acquire normal blood nutrition only when obstruction from channels and collaterals are removed. Like previous prescriptions, this suited the physical condition of Emperor Guangxu which was characterized by painful tendons and muscles, and pain and soreness in the hip and lumbar region, though it was further modified with various ingredients.

## XXII.5. HERBAL BATH REMEDY FOR RESOLVING BLOOD STASIS AND RELIEVING PAIN

Herbal Bath Remedy for Resolving Blood Stasis and Relieving Pain (Huo Yu Zhi Tong Xi Yao Fang) was carefully prepared by the imperial physician Fan Yimei for Emperor Guangxu between 4:00 and 6:00 p.m. on the 20th day of the fifth month of the lunar calendar. The year was not given.

### Ingredients

| | |
|---|---|
| Radix Angelicae Sinensis  (Dang Gui) | 9 g |
| Radix Paeoniae Lactiflorae  (Chi Shao) | 6 g |
| Cortex Moudan Radicis  (Mu Dan Pi) | 4.5 g |
| Radix Ledebouriellae  (Fang Feng) | 4.5 g |
| Flos Carthami  (Hong Hua) | 3 g |
| Radix Auchlandiae  (Mu Xiang) | 1.8 g |

The original scripts require that both the Radis Angelicae Sinensis and Flos Carthami should be prepared with millet wine, while the Radix Auchlandiae should be prepared as powder. The above ingredients were well boiled in water for local hot compress or wash.

### Comments

This prescription was similar to the previous ones. Local hot compress and wash over the affected areas helps work the herbal effect deeper into the body. It also fits the principle that "blood circulates faster when encountering heat." Pain was relieved when blood stasis was removed.

## XXII.6. HERBAL BATH REMEDY FOR NOURISHING TENDONS AND ACTIVATING COLLATERALS

Herbal Bath Remedy for Nourishing Tendons and Activating Collaterals (Rong Jing Huo Luo Xi Yao Fang) was carefully prepared for Emperor Guangxu by the imperial physician Zhao Wenkui on the 24th day of the third month of the lunar calendar. The year was not given.

*Ingredients*

| | |
|---|---|
| Fructus Chaenomelis (Mu Gua) | 9 g |
| Ramulus Pini Nodi (Song Jie) | 9 g |
| Radix Paeoniae Lactiflorae (Chi Shao) | 12 g |
| Herba Speranskia Tuberculata (Tou Gu Cao) | 6 g |
| Caulis Sinomenii (Qing Feng Teng) | 9 g |
| Resina Olibani (Ru Xiang) | 6 g |
| Resina Murrhae (Mo Yao) | 6 g |
| Flos Carthami (Hong Hua) | 6 g |
| Radix Angelicae Sinensis (Dang Gui) | 12 g |
| Caulis Aristolochia Debilis (Tian Xian Teng) | 9 g |

The above ingredients were boiled in water and 100 grams of liquor were added for local wash.

*Comments*

This prescription followed the therapeutic principle of nourishing blood, soothing the liver, activating blood and removing obstruction from channels and collaterals, not contradicting the disease condition of Emperor Guangxu at that time. Caulis Sinomenii has been a common ingredient for relieving pain due to Bi-syndrome resulting from wind or dampness invasion. Caulis Aristolochia Debilis, also known as Qing Mu Xiang in Chinese, may promote qi circulation and also stop pain. Experiments show that it has the function of obstructing the sympathetic nerve. Clinically, it has been used to lower blood pressure and cure eclampsia gravidarum. It was also recorded in ancient TCM literature that the stems of Fructus Chaenomelis Viride were used for Bi-syndrome pain due to wind-damp invasion. It is used in this prescription for its actions of promoting qi circulation, activating blood and so stopping pain. Zhao Wenkui served as president of the Imperial Hospital in the late Qing Dynasty during the later years of Emperor Guangxu, whose lingering and serious illness was beyond help despite Zhao's efforts in constantly modifying the prescriptions. Even marvellous remedies could have offered little help.

## XXII.7. HERBAL BATH REMEDY FOR RELIEVING WIND-DAMP

Herbal Bath Remedy for Relieving Wind-Damp (Qu Feng Shi Xi Yao Fang) was recorded without indicating the date or the imperial physician who prepared it.

*Ingredients*

| | |
|---|---|
| Flos Carthami (Hong Hua) | 9 g |

| | |
|---|---|
| Rhizoma seu Radix Notopterygii  (Qiang Huo) | 15 g |
| Herba Speranskia Tuberculata  (Tou Gu Cao) | 15 g |
| Fructus Chaenomelis  (Mu Gua) | 18 g |
| Radix Stephaniae Tetrandrae  (Fang Ji) | 15 g |
| Ramulus Mori  (Sang Zhi) | 18 g |

The above ingredients were mashed together and packed for use as the external wash remedy.

### Comments

This was a prescription aimed at eliminating wind and dampness. Rhizoma seu Radix Notopterygii disperses wandering wind from the Taiyang channel, for wind may aggravate dampness invading the body. Fructus Chaenomelis, Radix Stephaniae Tetrandrae and Ramulus Mori remove dampness from the channels and collaterals. Herba Speranskia Tuberculatae in combination with Flos Carthami was used to activate blood and stop pain. However, its combination with Radix Stephaniae Tetrandrae and Rhizoma seu Notopterygii was to eliminate wind and dampness. These ingredients were boiled in water for herbal washing when it was suitably warm, its therapeutic effect in curing pain due to wind-damp invasion being good.

## XXII.8.  HERBAL BATH REMEDY I

Herbal Bath Remedy I (Xi Yao Fang Yi) was carefully prepared by the imperial physician Fan Yimei between 8:00 and 10:00 p.m. on the sixth day of the sixth month of the lunar calendar, with no year given.

### Ingredients

| | |
|---|---|
| Fructus Chaenomelis  (Mu Gua) | 9 g |
| Radix Gentianae Macrophyllae  (Qin Jiao) | 6 g |
| Radix Ledebouriellae  (Fang Feng) | 6 g |
| Radix Stephaniae Tetrandrae  (Fang Ji) | 6 g |
| Herba Lycopodii  (Shen Jing Cao) | 6 g |
| Radix Angelicae Dahuricae  (Bai Zhi) | 6 g |

The above ingredients were well boiled in water for herbal washing.

### Comments

This was a prescription that had the effect of eliminating wind, clearing dampness and soothing the tendons. According to *Standards for Syndrome Differentiation and Treatments* (*Zheng Zhi Zhun Sheng*), both Radix Ledebouriellae and Radix Stephaniae Tetrandrae were used together in the powdery remedy called Radix Stephaniae Tetrandrae Powder (Fang Ji San). It was recorded as having good effect in the treatment of pain due to wind-damp invasion, and also the stubborn Bi-syndrome affecting hands and feet.

## XXII.9.  HERBAL BATH REMEDY II

Herbal Bath Remedy II (Xi Yao Fang Er) was carefully prepared by the imperial physician Fan Yimei. No date was provided in the original records.

*Ingredients*

| | |
|---|---|
| Fructus Chaenomelis  (Mu Gua) | 9 g |
| Cortex Eucommiae  (Du Zhong) | 9 g |
| Radix Achyranthis Bidentatae  (Niu Xi) | 9 g |
| Radix Gentiane Macrophyllae  (Qin Jiao) | 9 g |
| Radix Stephaniae Tetrandrae  (Han Fang Ji) | 9 g |
| Ramulus Uncariae cum Uncis  (Gou Teng) | 6 g |
| Rhizoma Atractylodis Macrocephalae  (Bai Zhu) | 9 g |
| Ramulus Mori  (Sang Zhi) | 12 g |

The original recipe requires the Cortex Eucommiae to be roasted before use, and raw Rhizoma Atractylodis Macrocephalae should be used. The above ingredients were well boiled in water and 100 grams of alcohol added for local wash.

*Comments*

In this prescription, Fructus Chaenomelis, Cortex Eucommiae and Radix Achyranthis Bidentatae, ingredients for nourishing the liver and reinforcing the kidney, were mixed with those for eliminating wind and dampness. It should be one of the remedies for dealing with pain in the lumbar region and legs for Emperor Guangxu. Strong alcohol was added to promote blood circulation. It was therefore effective for pain due to cold retention and qi stagnation.

# XXIII.  LUMBAR PAIN PRESCRIPTIONS

## XXIII.1. PRESCRIPTION FOR SPLEEN DAMPNESS-RELATED LUMBAR PAIN

Information concerning the date and imperial physician who made the Prescription for Spleen Dampness-related Lumbar Pain (Zhi Pi Shi Yao Tong) was not appear in the original records.

*Ingredients*

| | |
|---|---|
| Rhizoma Atractylodis Macrocephalae  (Bai Zhu) | 60 g |
| Semen Coicis  (Yi Yi Ren) | 30 g |

Three bowls of water were used for decocting the ingredients, the decoction being simmered until only one bowl of liquid was left. This was drunk in one breath. It was believed to be effective for lumbar pain due to retention of dampness in the spleen.

*Comments*

The Radix Atractylodis Macrocephalae, with sweet flavour and warming property, has the actions of strengthening the spleen, drying out dampness and pacifying Middle Jiao. It was applied for general lassitude, painful joints, poor appetite and loose stools due to spleen qi deficiency and retention of dampness in the body. *The Original Classics* (*Ben Jing*) claims that "Radix Atractylodis Macrocephalae is indicated in Bi-syndrome due to invasion of wind, cold and dampness." Semen Coicis, entering the spleen, kidney and lung channels, has the effect of strengthening the spleen, nourishing the lung and clearing damp-heat. It was used to treat loose stools and Bi-syndrome due to dampness invasion. Again, *The Original Classics* claims that "Semen Coicis treats patients for tendon spasm as well as Bi-syndrome due to invasion of wind and dampness." According to *Materia Medica on Diet Therapy* (*Shi Liao Ben Cao*), "Semen Coicis can clear both the dry and damp types of beriberi." The combination of Rhizoma Atractylodis Macrocephalae and Semen Coicis actually enhances the effect of both strengthening the spleen and eliminating dampness. Eliminating lingering dampness enables normal circulation of qi and blood in the channels and collaterals, while lumbar pain stops when qi and blood are in harmony. *The Revised Materia Medica* (*Ben Cao Xin Bian*) says, "Semen Coicis is best at eliminating water from the body without damaging the real body Yin. It would be most appropriate to suggest it for retention of dampness in the lower part of the body. Using 30 to 60 grams of Semen Coicis as principal ingredient assisted by ingredients for strengthening the spleen and eliminating dampness for conditions caused by damp-water, it would be rare for prompt therapeutic effect not to occur." However, there were also opinions against the combined use of Semen Coicis and Rhizoma Atractylodis Macrocephalae. The book entitled *Supplementary Proof to Materia Medica* (*Ben Jing Shu Zheng*) states: "Obviously, Semen Coicis and Rhizoma Atractylodis Macrocephalae are not opposing ingredients.... Rhizoma Atractylodis Macrocephalae gives instant effect while Semen Coicis produces a slow one. Combination of the two might cause a difficult situation where prompt therapeutic effect is expected and vice versa. Nevertheless, in case where a slow effect is expected, the partial instant effect might also give rise to excessive dryness."

## XXIII.2. LUMBAGO PRESCRIPTION

Information concerning the date and the imperial physician who formulated Lumbago Prescription (Zhi Yao Tong Fang) was not contained in the original records.

### Ingredient

Semen Crataegi  (Shan Zha He)

The original records require Semen Crataegi to be roasted on tiles so as to preserve its medicinal properties. Roasted Semen Crataegi was ground into fine powder to be taken p.o. 3 grams each time in a course of 10 individual doses. In the treatment of lumbar pain, it was taken with old millet wine.

### Comments

Semen Crataegi, seed of hawthorn fruits of the family Dioscoreaceae, can be used to treat patients for food retention and hernia. According to *Magic Formulae of the Sea* (*Hai Shang Fang*), it can be used in difficult labour. TCM medical classics rarely contain any records of its use for lumbar pain. But Radix Crataegi can be applied for joint pain. The actual effect of this prescription in the treatment of lumbar pain therefore needs further verification.

## XXIII.3.  HOT-PACK REMEDY FOR LUMBAR PAIN

No information concerning the date or imperial physician who formulated Hot-pack Remedy for Lumbar Pain (Zhi Yao Tong Tang Fang) was available in the original records.

### Ingredients

| | |
|---|---|
| Concha Ostreae  (Mu Li) | 15 g |
| Radix Achyranthis Bidentatae  (Chuan Niu Xi) | 9 g |
| Radix Angelicae Pubescentis  (Du Huo) | 4.5 g |

The above three ingredients were ground into fine powder which was baked with salt water and 10 green onion roots. The product was wrapped in a piece of fine cloth for local hot compress. The Conchae Ostreae was to be used raw.

### Comments

This remedy was suggested for external application only. Conchae Ostreae helps constrain Yin and sedate hyperactive Yang. *The Original Classics* (*Ben Jing*) claims that it was good for "strengthening joints." Radix Achyranthis Bidentatae, having the effect of nourishing the liver and kidney, and strengthening the tendons, was applied here to deal with lumbar pain. According to *The Orthodox of Materia Medica* (*Ben Cao Zheng Yi*), "the application of Radix Achyranthis Bidentatae on the back and arm.... for the purpose of removing obstruction from channels and collaterals and promoting motor functions of joints could give remarkable effects." Radix Angelicae Pubescenti has the effect of eliminating wind and dampness, dispersing cold and stopping pain. It was claimed also in the book *The Orthodox Materia Medica* that "Radix Angelicae Pubescentis was the right medicine for eliminating wind and removing obstruction from channels and collaterals," and "was specially applied for treating painful conditions of lumbar region, knees and calf. Onion roots have the action of promoting Yang *qi* and eliminating cold." *Explanation of Prescription Actions* (*Yao Pin Hua Yi*) says that onion roots remove obstruction from joints. The above two books prove that this prescription has the action of removing obstruction from channels and collaterals, eliminating cold and promoting motor functions of joints.

## XXIII.4.  MASSAGE FOR LUMBAR PAIN

The prescription for Massage for Lumbar Pain (Zhi Yao Tong Cha Xi Fang) was carefully prepared by the imperial physician Shi Huan on the 28th day of the seventh month of the lunar calendar in 1908.

### Ingredients

| | |
|---|---|
| Pericarpium Zanthoxyli  (Chuan Jiao) | 15 g |
| Radix Angelicae Pubescenti  (Du Huo) | 9 g |
| Herba Asari  (Xi Xin) | 3 g |
| Radix Aconiti  (Chuan Wu) | 7.5 g |
| Droppings  (Wan Can Sha) | 15 g |

| | |
|---|---|
| Resina Olibani  (Ru Xiang) | 9 g |
| Caulis Abekiae  (Mu Tong) | 9 g |
| Resina Murrhae  (Mo Yao) | 9 g |

The above eight ingredients were first mashed into fine pieces and decocted, the decoction being mixed with strong alcohol for external use on the affected area.

## Comments

This remedy, meant for local rubbing and washing, has the action of eliminating wind-cold, removing dampness and obstruction from channels and collaterals, activating blood and easing pain. Strong alcohol was applied for its effect of activating blood and removing obstruction from channels and collaterals. As Radix Aconiti is toxic, this remedy should not be applied on lesions where skin is broken.

## XXIII.5.  BI-SYNDROME HERBAL WASH REMEDY

Bi-syndrome Herbal Wash Remedy (Xi Yao Fang) was carefully prepared for the use of Emperor Guangxu by the imperial physician Ren Xigen on the 13th day of the sixth month of the lunar calendar, while the year was not mentioned.

### Ingredients

| | |
|---|---|
| Flos Carthami  (Hong Hua) | 6 g |
| Semen Persicae  (Tao Ren) | 6 g |
| Radix Angelicae Sinensis  (Dang Gui Wei) | 3 g |
| Radix Ledebouriellae  (Fang Feng) | 3 g |
| Ramulus Cinnamomi  (Gui Zhi) | 4.5 g |
| Flos Chrysanthemi  (Ju Hua) | 6 g |
| Flos Lonicerae  (Jin Yin Hua) | 4.5 g |
| Radix Glycyrrhizae  (Gan Cao Shao) | 2.4 g |

The above ingredients were decocted for bathing.

## Comments

This remedy was prepared for treating Emperor Guangxu's painful joints. Ingredients applied here have the effect of eliminating toxic heat, activating blood and resolving blood stasis. The underlying mechanism of the remedy was that "there would be no pain if the obstruction in the channels was removed." According to Emperor Guangxu's case history, his painful joints, also known as Bi-syndrome in TCM, often involved his lumbar region and legs.

## XXIII.6.  HERBAL WASH REMEDY FOR ACTIVATING BLOOD AND EASING PAIN

The date and the imperial physician who prepared this remedy remain unknown.

### Ingredients

| | |
|---|---|
| Rhizoma seu Radix Notopterygii  (Qiang Huo) | 6 g |

Rhizoma Drynariae  (Gu Sui Bu)                                    6 g
Resina Olibani  (Ru Xiang)                                       9 g
Radix Notoginseng  (San Qi)                                      6 g
Radix Angelicae Sinensis  (Dang Gui)                             6 g
Radix Scrophulariae  (Xu Duan)                                   6 g
Resina Murrhae  (Mo Yao)                                         9 g
Radix Achyranthis Bidentatae  (Niu Xi)                           6 g
Flos Carthami  (Hong Hua)                                        6 g
Semen Strychni  (Ma Qian Zi)                                     6 g
Resina Draconis  (Xue Jie)                                       6 g
Radix Stephaniae Tetrandrae  (Fang Ji)                           6 g
Radix Ledebouriellae  (Fang Feng)                                9 g
Herba Speranskia Tuberculata  (Tou Gu Cao)                       6 g
Rhizoma Angelicae Dahuricae  (Bai Zhi)                           6 g
Radix Glycyrrhizae  (Gan Cao)                                    6 g
Radix Allii Fistulosi  (Lao Cong Xu)                             6 g
Halitum  (Shi Yan)                                              30 g
Alcohol  (Shao Jiu)                                            250 g

The above ingredients were ground into fine powder, omitting Semen Strychni but adding nine grams of Ganlis Perillae. Strong alcohol was mixed with the other ingredients and all were placed in a bag for herbal compress and washing daily. The prepared powder should be packed into two cloth bags. It would be appropriate to steam the bags before applying them to the affected area of the body.

### Comments

All ingredients in this remedy activate blood. They offer very strong effect in resolving phlegm, removing obstruction from channels and collaterals and easing pain, while ingredients tonifying the kidney were added to the remedy. The health condition of Emperor Guangxu would suggest that this remedy was applied to deal with pain in his lumbar and hip regions, but this condition failed to improve despite repeated efforts in using herbal ingredients of such properties as cold, heat, warm and cool. This remedy approached the condition by working through the blood system, with reference to the ancient prescription the Eight Li Powder (Ba Li San). Also, it was applied according to the underlying mechanism of "treating the clinical manifestations in the acute stage of the condition." Over-dosage of Semen Strychni will poison the patient along with its strong effect in activating blood and removing obstruction from the channels and collaterals. According to modern pharmaceutical studies, Ganlis Perillae prepared in decoction may reduce the excitement of the central nerve system caused by Semen Strychni base and cocaine. This was why imperial physicians conventionally reduced Semen Strychni and added Ganlis Perillae when basing on the ancient prescription. This also serves to demonstrate the valuable clinical experience of imperial physicians in the Qing Dynasty. Packing the ingredients in cloth bags and steaming them before use was believed to reduce the toxicity of the ingredients in the remedy.

# XXIV. PRESCRIPTIONS FOR CONDITIONS OF THE FOUR LIMBS

## XXIV.1. Hand Wash Remedy for Nourishing Tendons

Hand Wash Remedy for Nourishing Tendons (Xi Shou Rong Jin Fang) was carefully prepared by the imperial physician Zhao Wenkui, without indicating date and time.

### Ingredients

| | |
|---|---|
| Ramulus Cinnamomi  (Gui Zhi) | 6 g |
| Radix Paeoniae Rubra  (Chi Shao) | 6 g |
| Resina Murrhae  (Mo Yao) | 4.5 g |
| Resina Olibani  (Ru Xiang) | 3 g |
| Fructus Chaenomelis  (Mu Gua) | 9 g |
| Radix Gentianae Macrophyllae  (Qin Jiao) | 6 g |
| Semen Luffae  (Si Gua) | 3 g |
| *Jia Zhu* | 6 g |
| Caulis Aristolochia Debilis  (Tian Xian Teng) | 9 g |

The above ingredients were decocted in water for external wash only.

### Comments

Ingredients in this prescription, having the actions of removing obstruction from channels and collaterals, resolving stasis, eliminating cold and stopping pain, are effective in dealing with Bi-syndrome due to invasion of wind, cold and dampness. The fine stems of Ramulus Cinnamomi were used in combination with Semen Luffae and Caulis Aristolochia Debilis to clear obstruction from the channels because they were believed to be effective by working in the arms. Both Resina Murrhae and Resina Olibani were used to sedate pain. The theory of TCM holds that the liver dominates the tendons. Soothing and nourishing the liver may in fact help to nourish the tendons. Therefore, Radix Paeoniae Rubra, Fructus Chaenomelis and *Jia Zhu* were used to sedate liver Yang, nourish the liver and regulate liver *qi*. The actual formation of this prescription is fairly comprehensive and systematic. This external remedy should be applied warm to obtain optional therapeutic results in activating blood and soothing tendons.

## XXIV.2. LEG WASH REMEDY FOR NOURISHING TENDONS AND EASING PAIN

Leg Wash Remedy for Nourishing Tendons and Easing Pain (Rong Jing Nian Tong Xi Yao Fang) was carefully prepared by the imperial physician Zhao Wenkui for Emperor Guangxu on the 28th day of the 11th month of the lunar calendar, with no information given as to the year.

### Ingredients

| | |
|---|---|
| Fructus Chaenomelis  (Mu Gua) | 12 g |
| Radix Paeoniae Rubra  (Chi Shao) | 9 g |
| Retinervus Citri Fructus  (Ju Luo) | 9 g |

| | |
|---|---|
| Resina Olibani  (Ru Xiang) | 9 g |
| Radix Angelicae Sinensis  (Dang Gui) | 12 g |
| Resina Murrhae  (Mo Yao) | 6 g |
| Flos Carthami  (Hong Hua) | 6 g |
| Radix Ledebouriellae  (Fang Feng) | 9 g |
| Herba Speranskia Tuberculata  (Tou Gu Cao) | 9 g |

The above ingredients were first decocted, then 200 grams of strong alcohol were added for external washing p.r.n.

### Comments

A sharp contrast to the previous prescription is that the former was applied for pain in the arms while the latter was used for pain in the legs. The selection of ingredients were different, though the therapeutic principles were similar, i.e. nourishing the tendons and easing pain. The former included the fine stems of Ramulus Cinnamomi that has an upward moving tendency to work into the arms. The latter included heavier doses of ingredients that have the effect of relieving blood stasis, thus driving the ingredients to work more in eliminating pain in the legs. Strong alcohol was mixed here to promote the effect of activating blood circulation.It was therefore believed that the effect of activating blood circulation, resolving blood stasis, nourishing tendons and easing pain would be very remarkable.

## XXIV.3.  LEG WASH REMEDY

Leg Wash Remedy (Xi Tui Fang) was carefully prepared by the imperial physician Yang Shifen for Emperor Guangxu on the second day of the 11th month of the lunar calendar. The year in which it was prepared remains unknown.

### Ingredients

| | |
|---|---|
| Radix Angelicae Sinensis  (Dang Gui) | 9 g |
| Fructus Chaenomelis  (Mu Gua) | 9 g |
| Radix Glycyrrhizae  (Gan Cao) | 3 g |
| Radix Paeoniae Lactiflorae  (Bai Shao) | 6 g |
| Retinervus Citri Fructus  (Ju Luo) | 9 g |
| Resina Olibani  (Ru Xiang) | 9 g |
| Caulis Sinomenii  (Qing Feng Teng) | 9 g |
| Cortex Dictamni Radicis  (Bai Xian Pi) | 9 g |

The original recipe requires the Radix Angelicae Sinensis and Radix Paeoniae Lactiflorae to be prepared in wine before use.

### Comments

In this prescription the Cortex Dictamni Radicis can also be applied in treating patients for carbuncles and furuncles and tinea in addition to its application here for eliminating wind and dampness.

## XXIV.4.  LEG WASH REMEDY PLUS

Leg Wash Remedy Plus (Xi Tui Fang You) was carefully prepared by the imperial physician Yang Shifen for Emperor Guangxu between 22:00 and 24:00

hours on the seventh day of the 12th month of the lunar calendar. The year in which it was made remains unknown.

### Ingredients

| | |
|---|---|
| Radix Angelicae Sinensis  (Dang Gui) | 9 g |
| Chaulis Sinomenii  (Qing Feng Teng) | 9 g |
| Fructus Chaenomelis  (Mu Gua) | 9 g |
| Radix Paeoniae Rubra  (Chi Shao) | 9 g |
| Herba Sperranskia Tuberculata  (Tou Gu Cao) | 9 g |
| Radix Ledebouriellae  (Fang Feng) | 4.5 g |

According to the original records, the Radix Angelicae Sinensis should be prepared in wine and the Radix Paeoniae Rubra should be baked in wine before use. The above ingredients were boiled for external wash and compress.

### Comments

The pain Emperor Guangxu complained of in the arms, legs and back was caused by invasion of wind and dampness in the channels and collaterals due to deficiency of *qi* and blood. Therefore, in addition to using ingredients of eliminating wind and dampness, and removing obstructions from channels and collaterals, such ingredients as Radix Angelicae Sinensis and Radix Paeoniae Rubra for nourishing the nutrient system and blood were also combined in the prescription. The ingredients in this prescription were carefully worked out even if it was only for external use. It was not merely mixing a few ingredients with the effect of eliminating wind and dampness.

## XXIV.5. PRESCRIPTION FOR COLD BI OF LEG

Prescription for Cold Bi of Leg (Zhi Han Tui Fang) was prepared for Emperor Guangxu for leg pain due to invasion of exogenous pathogenic cold. Neither the date nor the imperial physician who made it was provided in the original records.

### Ingredients

| | |
|---|---|
| Radix Angelicae Sinensis  (Dang Gui) | 60 g |
| Arillus Longan  (Gui Yan Rou) | 90 g |
| Radix Rehmanniae Praeparatae  (Shu Di) | 60 g |
| Radix Stephaniae Tetrandrae  (Fang Ji) | 30 g |
| Radix Rubiae  (Qian Cao) | 6 g |
| Radix Ledebouriellae  (Fang Feng) | 18 g |
| Rhizoma Homalomenae  (Nian Jian) | 60 g |
| Radix Achyranthis Bidentatae  (Niu Xi) | 24 g |
| Ramulus Cinnamomi  (Gui Zhi) | 24 g |
| Rhizoma Dioscoreae Septemlobae  (Bi Xie) | 21 g |
| Unidentified | 30 g |
| Cortex Eucommiae  (Du Zhong) | 21 g |
| Scolopendra  (Wu Gong) | 3 pcs |
| Os Tigris  (Hu Gu) | 60 g |
| Rock sugar  (Bing Tang) | 120 g |
| Alcohol  (Gan Jiu) | 2880 g |

## Comments

Ingredients in this prescription were prescribed for treating pain in the legs due to cold invasion, though the remedy was not composed merely of warming-property ingredients but rather, mainly consisted of ingredients having actions of reinforcing both the liver and kidney. The secondary ingredients were those for eliminating cold and dampness. According to the health records of Emperor Guangxu, he had been suffering from renal disease for a long time. When the imperial physicians worked out a prescription to deal with his leg pain, they were focusing on reinforcing the liver and kidney in an attempt to treat the root cause of the condition. Such an application of herbs agrees with the statements. "The lower portion of the body is dominated by earth *qi*," and "The liver dominates tendons and the kidney dominates bones," as recorded in *Yellow Emperor's Internal Medicine* (*Huang Di Nei Jing*). Yet, three pieces of Scolopendra were used to search for any remaining wind in the body. It is also apparent that the imperial physicians tended to include insects in the prescription even if their patient was the Emperor. They selected the ingredients according to the necessity of the condition, not for whom they were providing the medicine.

# XXV. ARTICULAR PAIN REMEDIES

## XXV.1. PRESCRIPTION FOR JOINT PAIN

Prescription for Joint Pain (Zhi Gu Jie Tong Fang) was prepared for Emperor Guangxu on the eighth day of the 12th month of the lunar calendar. Neither the year nor the physician who made it were noted in the original records.

### Ingredients

| | |
|---|---|
| Resina Olibani  (Ru Xiang) | 30 g |
| Resina Murrhae  (Mo Yao) | 30 g |
| Colla Cori Asini  (Pi Jiao) | 60 g |
| Rhizoma Zingiberis Recens  (Sheng Jiang) | 80 g |

According to the original scripts, the Rhizoma Zingiberis Recens was mashed into fine pieces and its juice obtained by means of pressing. The Rhizoma Zingiberis Recens juice was used to cook with Colla Cori Asini. This was followed by mixing the powdery ingredients inside to make a medicinal paste to be spread onto pieces of clean cloth and plastered onto the affected area. This was followed by ironing the plaster with a heated cloth shoe sole. No metal was used in ironing. Should juice from Rhizoma Zingiberis Recens be unavailable, juice from onions or garlic could be applied instead.

## Comments

The combination of Resina Olibani and Resina Murrhae has the action of activating blood circulation and stopping pain. One is believed to be an ingredient working on blood among those normally working on *qi* while the other ingredient working on *qi* was among those normally working on blood. Colla Cori Asini was applied here to make the prepared ingredients into a paste for the convenience of plastering. The random selection of any of the three kinds of juice was to increase the therapeutic effect in pungent dispersing. Ironing with a shoe sole was similar to hot packing nowadays for the purpose of evenly distributing the herbal effect. It was believed that this gave superior therapeutic effect.

## XXV.2. JOINT-BENEFITING PILL BY REINFORCING YIN AND RESOLVING DAMPNESS

Joint-benefiting Pill by Reinforcing Yin and Resolving Dampness (Yi Yin Hua Shi Li Jie Wan) was carefully prepared by the imperial physicians Zhang Zhong-yuan and Zhong Xun for Emperor Guangxu on the 10th day of the second month of the lunar calendar, with no information given as to the year.

*Ingredients*

| | |
|---|---|
| Radix Rehmanniae  (Sheng Di) | 12 g |
| Rhizoma Alismatis  (Ze Xie) | 4.5 g |
| Cortex Moudan Radicis  (Dan Pi) | 4.5 g |
| Poria  (Fu Ling) | 9 g |
| Cortex Erythrinae  (Hai Tong Pi) | 6 g |
| Rhizoma Curcumae Longae  (Jiang Huang) | 3 g |
| Radix Angelicae Pubescentis  (Du Huo) | 4.5 g |
| Resina Murrhae  (Mo Yao) | 6 g |
| Radix Gentianae Macrophyllae  (Qin Jiao) | 6 g |
| Pericarpium Citri Reticulatae Viride  (Qing Pi) | 4.5 g |
| Cortex Phellodendri  (Huang Bai) | 4.5 g |
| Rhizoma Anemarrhenae  (Zhi Mu) | 4.5 g |

The original scripts require the Cortex Phellodendri to be prepared with salt, and the Rhizoma Anemarrhenae be roasted before use. The above ingredients were first made into powder, which was mixed with honey to make fine pills. The pills were taken twice daily with boiled water.

*Comments*

Emperor Guangxu had a poor body constitution since early childhood. Conditions such as excessive seminal emissions and chronic lumbar pain greatly damaged his kidney *qi*. Although he complained of painful joints, it was definitely related to his kidney deficiency as well as exogenous pathogenic invasion of wind and dampness. The ingredients in this prescription were therefore determined in an attempt to deal with both the clinical manifestations and root cause. According to the health records of Emperor Guangxu, he "often had a deep wiry pulse on the left, but a deep slippery one on the right." Such a pulse generally "indicated deficiency of kidney water and certain derangement of liver Yang." Therefore, "he would get pounding pain even on the spinal column." This prescription was based on modified Radix Rehmanniae Pill with Six Ingredients (Liu Wei Di Huang Wan) in order to reinforce kidney Yin. Besides, Cortex Erythrinae and Radix Gentianae Macrophyllae were used to eliminate wind and dampness. Cortex Phellodendri and Rhizoma Anemarrhenae were used to sedate fire and reinforce Yin. The combined use of all these ingredients would achieve the effect of reinforcing Yin, eliminating dampness and promoting the motor function of joints, hence the name of the prescription.

# XXVI. PRESCRIPTIONS FOR DERMATOLOGICAL CONDITIONS

## XXVI.1. FACIAL REMEDY FOR CLEARING HEAT AND STOPPING ITCHING

Facial Remedy for Clearing Heat and Stopping Itching (Qing Re Zhi Yang Mian Yao Fang) was carefully prepared by the imperial physician Quan Shun for Emperor Guangxu on the 11th day of the 12th month of the lunar calendar. The year in which it was made remains unknown.

*Ingredients*

| | |
|---|---|
| Herba Schizonepetae (Jin Jie Sui) | 3 g |
| Herba Menthae (Bo He) | 3 g |
| Bombyx Batryticatus (Jiang Can) | 9 g |
| Cortex Erythrinae (Hai Tong Pi) | 6 g |
| Radix Coptidis (Huang Lian) | 2.4 g |
| Borneoleum Syntheticum (Bing Pian) | 1.5 g |

The above ingredients were made into powder which was mixed with tea to be spread on the affected area of the face.

*Comments*

The ingredients in this prescription have the effect of eliminating heat, dispersing cold, clearing dampness and stopping pain. Cortex Erythrinae, bitter and bland in flavour and cool in property, was used to treat patients for severe itching. Pharmaceutical studies prove that one portion of Cortex Erythrinae and three portions of water have the effect of restricting dermal fungus infection caused by Trichophyton Violaceum and Achorion Schoenleini. Its external application is effective in severe chronic itching. Mixed with the liquid from pickled vegetables, it has enhanced effect in stopping itching.

## XXVI.2. FACIAL REMEDY

Facial Remedy (Mian Yao Fang) was made known among the imperial physicians on the 11th day of the ninth month of the lunar calendar. Neither the year nor the imperial physician who made it is known.

*Ingredients*

| | |
|---|---|
| Spica Prunellae (Xia Ku Cao) | 3 g |
| Bombyx Batryticatus (Jiang Can) | 3 g |
| Rhizoma seu Radix Notopterygii (Qiang Huo) | 3 g |
| Sargassum (Hai Zao) | 3 g |
| Radix Angelicae Dahuricae (Bai Zhi) | 3 g |

The above ingredients were processed into fine powder together with a small proportion of Borneolum Syntheticum. The powder was mixed with honey to make the remedy in paste form to spread on a piece of cloth for external application on the affected area of the face.

### Comments

The remedy in plaster form was carefully prepared for Emperor Guangxu for his facial boils. Radix Angelicae Dahuricae has the action of eliminating purulent substance from the boils, relieving swelling and stopping pain. It is conventionally an important ingredient applied externally in the treatment of boils. It contains a fragrant flavour and rich oily substance. *The Original Classics* (*Ben Jing*) claims that it helps the growth and lustre of the skin and may be applied as facial cream. This was done in very ancient times. Sargassum also has the effect of restricting the growth of dermal fungi in addition to softening masses in the body. This remedy would best be applied for the treatment of wind-heat type of boils, furuncles and carbuncles.

## XXVI.3. ALUMEN-REALGAR POWDER

Alumen-Realgar Powder (Xiong Fan San) was carefully prepared for Emperor Guangxu by the imperial physician Zhuang Shouhe on the 11th day of the third month of the lunar calendar, with no information given as to the year.

### Ingredients

| | |
|---|---|
| Realgar (Xiong Huang) | 60 g |
| Alumen (Bai Fan) | 60 g |

The above ingredients were processed into powder of very fine quality to be packed into a cloth bag which was used to scratch the itching areas of the body.

### Comments

This remedy was actually known as Two-ingredient Detoxicating Powder (Er Wei Ba Du San) in the book *Golden Mirror of the Medical Tradition* (*Yi Zong Jin Jian*). The difference was that the dose for Realgar was doubled. It was mainly applied in the treatment of boils, carbuncles, furuncles and tinea as well as insect bites. According to published reports, Realgar has the effect of relieving toxication, killing insects and stopping itching. The external application of Alumen has the effect of relieving toxication, killing insects, drying out dampness and stopping itching. The combination of both can be applied in the treatment of eczema, boils and even tinea. In recent years reports have indicated that doctors in China applied this remedy in the treatment of more than one hundred cases of eczema and herpes zoster with good effects. The aim of the imperial physician Zhuang Shouhe in preparing this remedy for Emperor Guangxu was to help him cope with his dermatological conditions.

## XXVI.4. SCROTUM ECZEMA FORMULA

Scrotum Eczema Formula (Tang Xi Lang Shi Zhi Yang Fang)was carefully prepared for Emperor Guangxu by the imperial physicians Zhuang Shouhe and Li Dechang on the 20th day of the eighth month of the lunar calendar in order to eliminate the dampness in the scrotum and stop itching due to eczema. The year in which it was made was not provided in the original records.

### Ingredients

| | |
|---|---|
| Cortex Dictamni Radicis (Bai Xian Pi) | 15 g |
| Fructus Kochiae (Di Fu Zi) | 15 g |
| Ramulus Cinnamomi (Gui Zhi) | 15 g |
| Fructus Litseae Cubebae (She Chuan Zi) | 15 g |
| Radix Angelicae Pubecentis (Du Huo) | 12 g |
| Fructus Meliae Toosendan (Chuan Lian Zi) | 12 g |
| Fructus Evodiae (Wu Zhu Yu) | 12 g |
| Fructus Foeniculi (Xiao Hui Xiang) | 15 g |
| Pericarpium Zanthoxyli (Chuan Jiao) | 9 g |
| Alumen (Bai Fan) | 6 g |
| Realgar (Xiong Huang) | 6 g |
| Radix Glycyrrhizae (Gan Cao) | 9 g |

The above ingredients were ground into rough powder and packed in a cloth bag to be boiled in water. The warm liquid was used to warm and wash the scrotal area.

### Comments

Ingredients in this prescription are basically those for clearing heat, eliminating dampness and wind. The remedy, applied in the treatment of scrotal eczema, should be effective. Studies show that Cortex Dictamni Radicis, Fructus Kochiae, Fructus Litseae Cubebae and Fructus Meliae Toosendan all have the effect of restraining the growth of dermatological fungi. The combination of the above ingredients should be effective in the treatment of skin conditions.

## XXVI.5. HERBAL WASH REMEDY FOR WARMING THE KIDNEY TO ELIMINATE DAMPNESS AND STOP SWEATING TO RELIEVE ITCHING

Herbal Wash Remedy for Warming the Kidney to Eliminate Dampness and Stop Sweating to Relieve Itching (Wen Shen Shen Shi Lian Han Zhi Yang Teng Xi Fang) was carefully prepared for Emperor Guangxu by the imperial physicians Zhuang Shouhe, Yang Jihe and Quan Shun on the eighth day of the 12th month of the lunar calendar. The year in which the prescription was made remains unknown.

### Ingredients

| | |
|---|---|
| Fructus Litseae Cubebae (She Chuan Zi) | 15 g |
| Ramulus Cinnamomi (Gui Zhi) | 15 g |
| Rhizoma Typhonii Gigantei (Bai Fu Zi) | 15 g |
| Radix Euphorbiae Ebracteolatae (Lang Du) | 9 g |
| Powdered Concha Ostreae (Mu Li Fen) | 15 g |
| Semen Citri Reticulatae (Ju He) | 15 g |
| Fructus Meliae Toosendan (Chuan Lian Zi) | 15 g |
| Fructus Foenoiculi (Xiao Hui Xiang) | 15 g |
| Rhizoma Atractylodis Macrocephalae (Bai Zhu) | 15 g |

| Poria (Fu Ling) | 18 g |
| Fructus Kochiae (Di Fu Zi) | 18 g |
| Radix Stephaniae Tetrandrae (Fang Ji) | 15 g |

The above ingredients were processed into rough powder and packed in a cloth bag to be well boiled in water. The warm bag was used p.r.n. for local hot packing.

### Comments

According to the health records of Emperor Guangxu, he suffered from serious damage of kidney *qi* due to long-standing seminal emission. In the late years of his life, he sometimes had joint attacks of pain in the hip and lumbar region together with scrotal itching and eczema, conditions that caused him tremendous suffering. In order to treat both the symptomatic Biao and the root cause Ben and to combine internal and external therapies for the health of the Emperor, the imperial physicians prescribed Ever-spring Remedy for Longevity and Reproduction (Chang Chun Guang Si Yi Shou Gao) taken internally for reinforcing the kidney. The remedy introduced here was applied externally in combination with the internal remedy. In the prescription, the Radix Euphorbiae Ebracteolatae, mildly pungent and extremely toxic, is believed to have special therapeutic effect in the treatment of psoriasis and neurological dermatitis. It was used as the main ingredient in the treatment of tinea according to *Peaceful Holy Benevolent Prescriptions* (*Sheng Hui Fang*) and *Everlasting Categorization of Seal Formulas* (*Yong Lei Qian Fang*). It was also applied in this remedy for its effect in eliminating dampness and stopping itching in the treatment of tinea and fungal infection.

## XXVI.6. HARMONIZING OINTMENT

It is not known when the prescription for the Harmonizing Ointment (Chong He Gao) was made nor by whom it was formulated.

### Ingredients

Lignum Cercis Chinensis (Zi Jing Pi)
Resina Olibani (Ru Xiang)
Radix Glycyrrhizae (Gan Cao)
Radix Angelicae Dahuricae (Bai Zhi)
Resina Murrhae (Mo Yao)

The above ingredients were mixed together in equal portions and ground into very fine powder.

### Comments

This remedy, consisting of ingredients functioning to activate blood and resolve blood stasis, was applied externally for boils, and internally for damp Bi-syndrome. It was best indicated in the types of boils that would soon ulcerate, known as semi-Yin and semi-Yang condition in TCM. This prescription used in the Imperial Hospital is different from the Harmonizing Ointment as recorded in *True Linage of External Medicine* (*Wai Ke Zheng Zong*). It does not contain Radix Angelicae Pubescentis, Radix Paeoniae Rubra and Rhizoma Acori Graminei, but does contain Resina Olibani, Resina Murrhae and Radix Glycyrrhizae. It is less effective in eliminating dampness, but more effective in activating blood circulation and removing obstruction from channels and collaterals. This difference in therapeutic effect is the main characteristic of the prescription. Pharmaceutical experiments have shown that Lignum Cercis Chinensis had the effect of resisting the growth of staphylococci and JK68-1 virus. It produces certain therapeutic effect in the treatment of Bi-syndrome due to wind, cold and dampness invasion, amenorrhea, boils, tinea and traumatic injuries. Powdered Lignum Cercis Chinensis was used for Emperor Guangxu externally for his open skin lesions.

## XXVI.7. HERBAL WASH REMEDY FOR ACTIVATING BLOOD AND STOPPING JOINT PAIN

Herbal Wash Remedy for Activating Blood and Stopping Joint Pain (Huo Xue Shu Jing Zhi Tong Xi Yao Fang) was carefully prepared for Emperor Guangxu by the imperial physician Fan Yimei on the 16th day of the fourth month of the lunar calendar, with no information given as to the year.

*Ingredients*

| | |
|---|---|
| Radix Angelicae Sinensis (Dang Gui) | 9 g |
| Radix Paeoniae Rubra (Chi Shao) | 6 g |
| Cortex Moudan Radicis (Mu Dan Pi) | 6 g |
| Resina Olibani (Ru Xiang) | 3 g |
| Spica Prunellae (Xia Ku Cao) | 9 g |
| Resina Murrhae (Mo Yao) | 3 g |
| Radix Auchlandiae (Mu Xiang) | 3 g |
| Flos Carthami (Hong Hua) | 3 g |

According to the original recipe, the Radix Angelicae Sinensis and Flos Carthami should be prepared in wine before use, while the Radix Paeoniae Rubra should be roasted, and the Resina Olibani, Resina Murrhae and Radix Auchlandiae should be ground into powder. The above ingredients were well boiled for local washing and hot compress.

*Comments*

The pain in the muscle and joint complained by Emperor Guangxu was caused largely by the deficiency of blood. Though containing chiefly the ingredients to activate *qi* and blood and remove obstruction from the channels and collaterals, this prescription also aimed at nourishing blood. Only by removing stagnant blood can fresh blood be produced. Radix Auchlandiae was added to the formula in an attempt to treat *qi* and blood at the same time. Local washing or hot compress may help dilate the vessels in the affected areas and improve microcirculation, thus enhancing the effect of activating blood circulation, soothing the tendons and stopping pain.

## XXVI.8. EXTERNAL RUBBING REMEDY I

External Rubbing Remedy I (Cha Yao Fang Yi) was carefully prepared for Emperor Guangxu by the imperial physician Tong Chenhai late at night on the

27th day of the fifth month of the lunar calendar. The year in which it was made remains unknown.

### Ingredients

| | |
|---|---|
| Bombyx Batryticatus (Jiang Can) | 3 g |
| Herba Menthae (Bo He) | 2.4 g |
| Realgar (Da Huang) | 3 g |
| Sal (Shi Yan) | 6 g |
| Six-One Powder (Liu Yi San) | 3 g |

According to the original recipe, the Bombyx Batryticatus should be roasted before use. All the ingredients were prepared in powder form and packed into a cloth bag for local rubbing.

### Comments

Ingredients in this remedy have pungent cooling and cold bitter properties, functioning in eliminating wind and heat. The combination of Talcum and Realgar may help treat patients for carbuncles and furuncles. Gentle rubbing in the local area may help dry out the dampness and drain purulent substance. It should be appropriate to treat the Emperor for his eczema and other skin conditions with oozing fluid. However, the remedy may not have been very effective due to its small dosage and insufficient number of ingredients.

## XXVI.9. EXTERNAL RUBBING REMEDY II

External Rubbing Remedy II (Cha Yao Fang Er) was prepared late at night on the 11th day of the sixth month of the lunar calendar. Information concerning when it was made and who made it was not recorded.

### Ingredients

| | |
|---|---|
| Flos Lonicerae (Jin Yin Hua) | 6 g |
| Herba Menthae (Bo He) | 3 g |
| Rhizoma Angelicae Dahuricae (Bai Zhi) | 4.5 g |
| Radix Ledebouriellae (Fang Feng) | 3 g |
| Radix Paeoniae (Chi Shao) | 6 g |
| Fructus Forsythiae (Lian Qiao) | 6 g |
| Six-One Powder (Liu Yi San) | 9 g |
| Radix Rhei (Da Huang) | 3 g |
| Fructus Kochiae (Di Fu Zi) | 4.5 g |
| Sal (Shi Yan) | 4.5 g |
| Bombyx Batryticatus (Jiang Can) | 6 g |
| Ramulus Mori (Sang Zhi) | 6 g |

Three grams of Periostracum Cicadae were added to the prescription, and all the ingredients were prepared in powder form and packed into a cloth bag for gentle local rubbing.

### Comments

This prescription was expanded on the basis of the previous one. It was assumed that Emperor Guangxu had severe itching due to wind-heat invasion. A light dose for a more severe condition might not help achieve the expected therapeutic effect. Therefore, ingredients that have the function of eliminating heat, clearing dampness and wind, and stopping itching such as Flos Lonicerae, Rhizoma Angelicae Dahuricae, Radix Ledebouriellae, Radix Paeoniae, Fructus Forsythiae and Fructus Kochiae were used to ease itching. What deserves mentioning is that both External Rubbing Remedy I and II were prepared late at night, indicating that the Emperor suffered from very severe itching at that time. This also suggested that the pathogenic factors had affected the Pericardium Channel. Such TCM doctrines as "Heat, carbuncles and furuncles are all related to the heart," and "the pericardium will initially bear the pathogenic invasion instead of the heart" also prove the therapeutic principle applied here. It shows at the same time that imperial physicians did work very carefully in light of the theory, principle, prescription and administration when making a formula. They followed the syndrome differentiation in TCM rather than assembling several ingredients into a remedy.

## XXVI.10.  HERBAL PLASTER FOR ACTIVATING COLLATERALS

Herbal Plaster for Activating Collaterals (Huo Luo Tie Yao Fang) was prepared for Emperor Guangxu by the imperial physicians Quan Shun and Zhong Xun on the 26th day of the 11th month of the lunar calendar. No information was given as to the year.

*Ingredients*

| | |
|---|---|
| Resina Olibani  (Ru Xiang) | 3 g |
| Resina Murrhae  (Mo Yao) | 1.5 g |
| Radix Clematis  (Wei Ling Xian) | 1.5 g |
| Rhizoma Curcumae Longae  (Jiang Huang) | 1.5 g |
| Acacia Catechu  (Er Cha) | 9 g |
| Radix Angelicae Pubescentis  (Du Huo) | 1.5 g |
| Rhizoma Cyperi  (Xiang Fu) | 1.5 g |

According to the original recipe, the Rhizoma Cyperi was used raw. The above ingredients were prepared in powder form and mixed with liquid from preserved vegetables. This mixture was spread onto a piece of cloth to be further heated over low fire. The plaster was placed on the painful area.

*Comments*

This prescription is characterized by adding wind-clearing and pain-relieving ingredients to those for promoting blood circulation in the channels and collaterals. The use of a larger dose of Acacia Catechu was to help eliminate dampness and dry the oozing furuncles. Modern pharmaceutical studies prove that Acacia Catechu with water in the ratio of one to two has the effect of restricting the growth of many kinds of skin fungi. In this prescription, the use of Acacia Catechu not only helped Resina Olibani and Resina Murrhae to activate blood circulation, but also assisted Radix Clematis and Radix Angelicae Pubescentis to eliminate wind and dampness. In this external remedy, Rhizoma Cyperi was applied as well largely for its effect of removing obstruction from channels and collaterals. This was to stop pain. The internal therapeutic principle was followed to some degree in the application of this external plaster.

## XXVI.11. EXTERNAL HERBAL TINCTURE I

External Herbal Tincture I (Fu Yao Fang Yi) was carefully prepared for the Emperor by the imperial physician Ren Xigen late at night on the 16th day of the fourth month of the lunar calendar, with no information given as to the year.

At that time, the Emperor was suffering from painless skin rash in the chest area, caused by damp-heat. Three grams of Radix Stemonae were mixed with 50 grams of alcohol and the tincture applied to the affected area.

Reddened rash in the chest area without much pain or itching sensation would not mean onset of boils. The reddened rash, even with slight pain, should be related to stagnant heat. Vinegared Purple Tincture (ingredients of the vinegared tincture include Meretrix, Galla Chinensis, soap, Resina Olibani and Resina Murrhae) was also applied to the rash.

*Comments*

Radix Stemonae is generally considered the principal ingredient for stopping cough in the case of tuberculosis. However, it is also effective in the treatment of urticaria, dermatitis and tinea. Pharmaceutical experiments proved that Radix Stemonae could wipe out skin fungi, pinworms and pediculosis in addition to its effect in restricting the growth of human bacillus tubercle, bacillus dyseneriae, Pseudomonas aeruginosa, staphylococcus and Diplococcus pneumoniae. The book entitled *Complete Works on External Therapies* (*Yang Yi Da Quan*) contains a patent remedy known as Radix Stemonae Paste (Bai Bu Gao)for treating psoriasis. Radix Stemonae was used as its prinicipal ingredient. Alcohol was used to mix with Radix Stemonae powder for rubbing with the underlying mechanism that alcohol could help dilate capillary vessels in the local areas so as to let the active ingredients in the remedy permeate the lesions. Emperor Guangxu at that moment had sudden onset of red rash on his chest area, believed to be caused by heat retention. The imperial physician Ren Xigen was good at surgery. On the one hand, he was applying Radix Stemonae Tincture (Bai Bu Ding), while on the other he was using Vinegared Purple Tincture (Zi Jin Cu Ding) on the local area. This is because Vinegared Purple Tincture (Zi Jin Cu Ding)could be used to treat patients for swollen boils and relieve the toxicity. Vinegar could also help disperse the swelling and mass. The method is therefore both safe and effective.

## XXVI.12. EXTERNAL HERBAL TINCTURE II

External Herbal Tincture II (Fu Yao Fang Er) was carefully prescribed for Emperor Guangxu by the imperial physician Ren Xigen on the 14th day of the sixth month of the lunar calendar, with no information given as to the year.

Half a gram of powdered Scorpio tail was mixed with the Vinegared Purple Tincture (Zi Jin Cu Ding) for external application p.r.n.

*Comments*

This remedy was formed by adding powdered Scorpio tail to the previous Vinegared Purple Tincture, which suited the Emperor's condition and helped relieve some of his symptoms, but not completely. The same method was therefore continued, but adding another ingredient in order to achieve greater therapeutic effect. Scorpio also has the effect of softening mass and relieving toxicity besides calming internal wind, releasing spasm, clearing exogenous wind and stopping pain. According to modern pharmaceutical studies, Scorpio contains scorpion poison, a toxic protein of such multi-chemical elements as carbon, hydrogen, oxygen and sulphur. It is similar to neurotoxin in snakes. The effect of scorpio in softening mass and relieving toxicity could be related to its toxic protein. Imperial physicians used this in light of the principle of "detoxicating poison with poison."

## XXVI.13. BAMBOO LEAF PASTE

Bamboo Leaf Paste (Zhu Ye Gao) was presented for imperial use on the 21st day of the seventh month of the lunar calendar. Information concerning who made it was not given, nor was the year.

*Ingredients*

| | |
|---|---|
| Folium Phyllostachyos Recens  (Xian Zhu Ye) | 480 g |
| Rhizoma Zingiberis Recens  (Sheng Jiang) | 120 g |
| Sal  (Bai Yan) | 180 g |

The original prescription requires clean fresh bamboo leaves containing no stems to be used. The bamboo leaves were first boiled to obtain a concentrated liquid which was mixed with ginger juice to be further decocted. The residue was separated out and salt was added to the bamboo and ginger liquid for further concentrating until dry, the end product being used on the affected area.

*Comments*

This was one of the secret remedies in the Qing Dynasty Imperial Hospital. Bamboo leaves, light in quality, have bland sweet flavour and cold property. Many books of Chinese herbal prescriptions claim to have the function of cooling the heart, moderating the spleen, clearing phlegm and easing thirst. These belong to ingredients of clearing and dispersing property. Such ancient prescriptions as Folium Lophatheri and Gypsum Fibrosum Decoction (Zhu Ye Shi Gao Tang) and Pathogenic Heat Eliminating Powder (Dao Chi San) included Folium Phyllostachyos. Bamboo leaves may be fresh or dried, though both have the effect of clearing heart heat, relieving restlessness and promoting urination. However, the fresh leaves have the stronger effect in clearing heat from the heart while also cooling heat from the stomach. They are mainly used to clear heat from the Upper Jiao. The dried leaves, on the other hand, offer better effect in eliminating dampness and heat. Pharmaceutical studies prove that they may resist the growth of yellow staphylococcus and Pseudomonas aeruginosa. Emperor Guangxu himself suffered from a number of these infections. This paste, applied externally, should deal with carbuncles and furuncles due to the retention of damp-heat. The use of ginger juice, whose pungent flavour offers dispersing effect, was to enhance the effect of bamboo leaves in eliminating dampness and heat.

## XXVI.14. GARDENIAE EXTERNAL REMEDY

Gardeniae External Remedy (Shan Zhi Wai Yong Fang) was prepared for Emperor Guangxu late in the afternoon on the 27th day of the second month of the lunar calendar, the year being not noted.

### Ingredient

Fructus Gardeniae (Shan Zhi)                                          30 g

Powdered Fructus Gardeniae was mixed together with alcohol and wheat flour to be made in the form of small cakes to be applied to the affected areas of the body.

### Comments

Fructus Gardeniae, bitter in flavour and cold in property, can clear heat and sedate fire, cool blood and relieve toxicity. Physicians in ancient times believed that it could clear fire from the triple burner and was therefore used in such formulae as Diaphragm Cooling Powder (Liang Ge San), Detoxicating Decoction with Rhizoma Coptidis (Huang Lian Jie Du Tang), and Fructus Gardeniae Decoction with Rhizoma Rhei (Zhi Zi Da Huang Tang). Its external application is indicated in traumatic injuries, for it has the effect of relieving swelling and stopping pain. Mixing powdered Fructus Gardeniae with wheat flour and alcohol is known as "Tendon Stretching Remedy" in folk medicine, having actions to circulate blood, relieve swelling and soothe tendons. It can be applied in the treatment of traumatic injuries, sprain and bruises, especially such conditions in the four limbs. Contemporary reports also claim its effectiveness in treating twisting of the four limbs. The recommendation of this prescription for the use of Emperor Guangxu suggests that imperial physicians at that time also paid attention to collection of folk and simple remedies aside from their efforts in learning ancient prescriptions.

## XXVI.15. PANACEAN EXTERNAL LOZENGE

Panacean External Lozenge (Wang Ying Ding Tu Yao Fang) was carefully prepared by the imperial physician Ren Xilian on the 21st day of the fourth month of the lunar calendar, with no information given as to the year.

Ten panacean lozenges were mashed into fine powder and mixed with 30 grams of vinegar for external rubbing of the swollen areas. The so-called Panacean External Lozenge contains the following ingredients: Rhizoma Coptidis, Rhizoma Picrorhizae, Resina Olibani, Resina Murrhae, Acacia Catechu, Radix Rhei, Rhizoma Corydalis, Rhizoma Gastrodiae, Fel Ursi, gold powder, natural copper, Borneoleum Syntheticum and Moschus.

### Comments

This prescription was made by the imperial physician Ren Xilian for Emperor Gaungxu for the red boils on his chest. The basic intention was to clear toxic heat, and relieve swelling and masses. Its therapeutic mechanism is similar to that of Panacean Lozenge (Wang Ying Ding).

# XXVI.16. BLOOD-PROMOTING AND HEAT-DISPELLING PASTE

Blood-promoting and Heat-dispelling Paste (Qing Re He Xue Hua Du Gao) was carefully prepared for Emperor Guangxu by the imperial physician Yang Shifen late in the afternoon of the 23rd day of the third month of the lunar calendar. The year remains unknown.

*Ingredients*

| | |
|---|---|
| Resina Olibani  (Ru Xiang) | 1.5 g |
| Fructus Xanthii  (Cang Er Zi) | 1.5 g |
| Radix Glycyrrhizae  (Gan Cao) | 1.5 g |
| Borneoleum Syntheticum  (Bing Pian) | 1 g |

The above ingredients were made into powder and mixed with six grams of Rhizoma Coptidis Paste for clinical application.

*Comments*

The Rhizoma Coptidis in this prescription was used to clear heat, and the Resina Olibani to promote blood circulation. Fructus Xanthii has the action of eliminating wind and dampness. Its internal or external use may be suggested for the treatment of skin rash with itching, and also leprosy. In folk remedies it was mashed for external application to treat carbuncles and furuncles due to dampness retention and bites by bees and insects. It means that Fructus Xanthii has a detoxicating effect. Pharmaceutical studies prove that Fructus Xanthii can help restrain the growth of yellow staphylococci. It was in fact used as the principal ingredient in the prescription. Judging from the ingredients applied here, this prescription was formed to cope with the skin boils of Emperor Guangxu, not for any chronic rhinitis.

# XXVI.17. OINTMENT FOR RELIEVING STASIS AND SWELLING

Ointment for Relieving Stasis and Swelling (Xiao Zhong Huo Yu Gao) was carefully prepared by the imperial physician Zhao Wenkui for Emperor Guangxu on the second day of the intercalary fifth month of the lunar calendar, with no information given as to the year.

*Ingredients*

| | |
|---|---|
| Caulis Spatholobi Paste  (Ji Xue Teng Gao) | 0.9 g |
| Moschus  (She Xiang) | 0.9 g |
| Squama Manitis  (Chuan Shan Jia) | 0.6 g |
| First Fairy Boat  (Di Yi Xian Zhou) | 0.9 g |
| Radix Tinosporae  (Jin Guo Lan) | 0.6 g |

The above ingredients were ground into fine powder and sifted through silk. The powder was mixed with honey to make a paste for local plastering. The original recipe says the quantity of each ingredient should be in balance.

*Comments*

This prescription is also one for activating blood, resolving blood stasis, clearing heat and eliminating swelling. Judging from the actual time, the intercalary fifth month of the lunar calendar, when the remedy was made by Zhao

Wenkui, it should be a prescription formed in 1903. At that time, the Emperor was possibly suffering from severe tuberculosis of the lumbar vertebrae. This prescription could merely relieve his symptoms.

## XXVI.18. POWDER FOR RELIEVING SWELLING AND PAIN

Powder for Relieving Swelling and Pain (Xiao Zhong Ding Tong San) was carefully prepared for Emperor Guangxu by the imperial physicians Yang Jihe and Fan Shaoxiang at noon on the 14th day of the second month of the lunar calendar. The year was not mentioned.

*Ingredients*

| | |
|---|---|
| Radix Tinosporae  (Jin Guo Lan) | 9 g |
| Rhizoma Curcumae Longae  (Jiang Huang) | 9 g |
| Resina Olibani  (Ru Xiang) | 3 g |
| Resina Murrhae  (Mo Yao) | 3 g |
| Flos Mume  (Mei Hua Pian) | 1.2 g |

The original recipe calls for the Flos Mume to be ground into fine powder to be added last. The above ingredients were ground together to make fine powder which was mixed with prepared green tea. This was applied warm to the affected area. When the area was dry, diluted herbal liquid was used as a wash.

*Comments*

Swelling could be caused by either *qi* stagnation or blood stasis. Judging from the prescription, it was mainly suggested to deal with the condition caused by blood -stasis. This coincides with the TCM doctrine that "The disorderly nutrient *qi* causes stasis in the muscle, leading to rise of boils or swellings" from "Vital Energy Communicating with Heaven" in *Plain Questions* ("Sheng Qi Tong Tian Lun," *Su Wen*). The majority of the ingredients function in activating blood circulation, resolving blood stasis, and warming the nutrient blood. They were assisted by the use of Radix Tinosporae and Borneoleum Syntheticum to deal with the damp heat type of skin boils by means of clearing heat and stopping pain.

# XXVII.  BATHING REMEDIES

## XXVII.1.  Herbal Bath Remedy

Herbal Bath Remedy (Mu Yu Xi Fang) was carefully prepared by the imperial physician Fan Yimei on the 29th day of the 12th month of the lunar calendar, with no year given.

*Ingredients*

| | |
|---|---|
| Fructus Chaenomelis  (Mu Gua) | 30 g |
| Radix Ledebouriellae  (Fang Feng) | 9 g |
| Radix Paeoniae Rubra  (Chi shao) | 9 g |
| Cortex Moudan Radicis  (Mu Dan) | 6 g |
| Cortex Phellodendri  (Huang Bai) | 9 g |
| Fructus Kochiae  (Di Fu Zi) | 12 g |

Pericarpium Zanthoxyli  (Chuan Jiao)                                     6 g
Fructus Forsythiae  (Lian Qiao)                                           12 g

According to the original records, the Radix Paeoniae Rubra should be roasted before use, then all the ingredeints were boiled in water for bathing.

## Comments

This prescription, with the effect of cooling blood and eliminating wind and dampness, was applied to deal with painful joints of the four limbs.

# XXVII.2.  HERBAL BATH REMEDY FOR STOPPING DIZZINESS

Herbal Bath Remedy for Stopping Dizziness (Qing Shang Zhi Yun Fang) was prepared carefully by the imperial physician Zhao Wenkui for Emperor Guangxu on the ninth day of the 11th month of the lunar calendar, with no year given.

## Ingredients

Rhizoma Gastrodiae  (Tian Ma)                                           6 g
Herba Menthae  (Bo He)                                                   6 g
Flos Chrysanthemi  (Ju Hua)                                             6 g
Folium Mori  (Sang Ye)                                                   3 g
Fructus Viticis  (Man Jing Zi)                                          9 g
Rhizoma Ligustici Chuanxiong  (Chuan Xiong)                             6 g
Rhizoma Ligustici  (Hao Ben)                                            6 g

The original recipe calls for the Fructus Viticis to be roasted before use. All ingredients were boiled in water for herbal bathing.

## Comments

The ingredients in this prescription are predominantly for eliminating heat and dispersing cold. It is a remedy for dealing with the dizziness and headache due to deficiency of liver Yin accompanied by invasion of wind-heat. The Fructus Viticis and Rhizoma Ligustici in combination were used for treating pain in the vertex and in the temporal regions.

# XXVII.3.  HERBAL BATH REMEDY I FOR CLEARING WIND

Herbal Bath Remedy I for Clearing Wind (Hua Feng Qing Shang Mu Fang Yi) was carefully prepared by the imperial physician Zhao Wenkui on the 18th day of the 11th month of the lunar calendar, with no year given.

## Ingredients

Herba Menthae  (Bo He)                                                   6 g
Radix Ledebouriellae  (Fang Feng)                                       4.5 g
Radix Angelicae Dahuricae  (Bai Zhi)                                     6 g
Radix Puerariae, powdered  (Ge Gen)                                     4.5 g
Fructus Viticis  (Man Jing Zi)                                          6 g
Rhizoma Ligustici Chuanxiong  (Chuang Xiong)                            6 g
Flos Mori  (Sang Ye)                                                    3 g

The original records require that the Herba Menthae grown in south China should be selected, and the Fructus Viticis roasted before use. The above ingredients were boiled in water for herbal bathing.

### Comments

This prescription, containing Radix Angelicae Dahuricae and powdered Radix Puerariae but not Rhizoma Ligustici, was mainly applied to treat the Emperor for his frontal headache, while the combination of Fructus Viticis and Rhizoma Ligustici Chuanxiong should activate blood, eliminate wind and stop pain.

## XXVII.4. HERBAL BATH REMEDY II FOR CLEARING WIND

Herbal Bath Remedy II for Clearing Wind (Hua Feng Qing Shang Mu Fang Er) was carefully prepared by the imperial physician Zhao Wenkui on the 22nd day of the 11th month of the lunar calendar, with no year given.

### Ingredients

| | |
|---|---|
| Herba Menthae  (Bo He ) | 6 g |
| Radix Ledebouriellae  (Fang Feng) | 6 g |
| Radix Angelicae Dahuricae  (Bai Zhi) | 6 g |
| Folium Perillae  (Su Ye) | 3 g |
| Rhizoma Gastrodiae  (Tian Ma) | 6 g |
| Fructus Ligustici  (Hao Ben) | 6 g |
| Flos Chrysanthemi  (Ju Hua) | 6 g |

The original records state that the Herba Menthae grown in south China should be used. The ingredients were boiled in water for herbal bathing.

### Comments

Compared with Herbal Bath Remedy I for Clearing Wind (Hua Feng Qing Shang Mu Fang Yi), this has a stronger effect in dispersing as manifested by the combined use of Folium Perillae and Fructus Ligustici. Also, it was made during winter, and Emperor Guangxu might have been invaded by cold, so the cooling remedy was mixed with pungent warming ingredients. The underlying mechanism was that cold could be eliminated only by warming.

## XXVII.5. HERBAL BATH REMEDY FOR ELIMINATING DAMPNESS

Herbal Bath Remedy for Eliminating Dampness (Qing Shang Qu Shi Mu Fang) was carefully prepared by the imperial physician Zhao Wenkui on the 25th day of the 11th month of the lunar calendar, with no information given as to the year.

### Ingredients

| | |
|---|---|
| Rhizoma Gastrodiae  (Tian Ma) | 6 g |
| Herba Menthae  (Bo He) | 6 g |
| Radix Paeoniae Rubra  (Chi Shao) | 6 g |
| Rhizoma Ligustici  (Hao Ben) | 6 g |
| Flos Chrysanthemi  (Ju Hua) | 6 g |
| Folium Mori  (Sang Ye) | 6 g |
| Bombyx Batryticatus  (Jiang Can) | 6 g |

The original records require the Bombyx Batryticatus to be roasted before use. All ingredients were boiled in water for herbal bathing.

*Comments*

The ingredients in this prescription do not directly have the effect of eliminating dampness, so how did it get its name? It was probably because it contained many wind-eliminating ingredients. According to TCM classics, "Wind takes away dampness." Eliminating wind meant eliminating dampness. Pathogenic dampness could not exist should the function of the liver in maintaining free flow of *qi* and that of the spleen in transforming and transporting be normal.

## XXVII.6. HERBAL BATH REMEDY FOR CLEARING HEAT AND DAMPNESS

Herbal Bath Remedy for Clearing Heat and Dampness (Qing Shang Yi Shi Mu Fang) was carefully prepared by the imperial physician Zhao Wenkui on the 27th day of the 11th month of the lunar calendar.

*Ingredients*

| | |
|---|---|
| Rhizoma Gastrodiae  (Tian Ma) | 6 g |
| Herba Menthae  (Bo He) | 6 g |
| Radix Paeoniae Rubra  (Chi Shao) | 6 g |
| Flos Chrysanthemi  (Ju Hua) | 6 g |
| Folium Mori, frosted  (Sang Ye) | 3 g |
| Rhizoma Ligustici  (Hao Ben) | 6 g |
| Bombyx Batryticatus  (Jiang Can) | 9 g |

The original records state that the Bombyx Batryticatus should be roasted before use.

*Comments*

This prescription was the same as that prescribed on the 25th day of the same month except for a slight variation of doses and the change of nomenclature. It would appear that a great deal of thought had been given to forming this remedy, while in fact it was a simple repetition of the one outlined above.

## XXVII.7. Herbal Bath Remedy for Controlling Fire

Herbal Bath Remedy for Controlling Fire (Qing Shang Yi Huo Mu Fang) was carefully prepared by the imperial physician Zhao Wenkui on the 13th day of the second month of the lunar calendar, while the year was not given.

*Ingredients*

| | |
|---|---|
| Flos Chrysanthemi  (Ju Hua) | 6 g |
| Herba Menthae  (Bo He) | 6 g |
| Folium Mori  (Sang Ye) | 6 g |
| Rhizoma Ligustici  (Hao Ben) | 6 g |
| Rhizoma Gastrodiae  (Tian Ma) | 6 g |
| Bombyx Batryticatus  (Jiang Can) | 9 g |
| Radix Paeoniae Rubra  (Chi Shao) | 9 g |
| Radix Angelicae Sinensis  (Dang Gui) | 9 g |

The original records state that the Bombyx Batriticatus should be roasted before use. All the ingredients were boiled in water for herbal bathing.

### Comments

To the previous prescription, Radix Angelicae Sinensis was added to control fire, and this is the rationale of the remedy. The underlying mechanism was to disperse the pathogenic heat that was retained in the body. The Emperor was supposed to bathe while it was still warm. Pungent warming ingredients were used in an attempt to bring out the heat together with the process of sweating. Dispersing fire would also mean to control it. Pungent warming and cooling ingredients were used at the same time, hence the name fire-controlling.

# XXVIII. ANTI-PERSPIRANT PRESCRIPTION

## XXVIII.1. REMEDY AGAINST PERSPIRATION

Remedy Against Perspiration (Pu Han Fang) was carefully prepared by the imperial physicians Zhuang Shouhe and Yang Jihe for Emperor Guangxu on the 18th day of the 11th month of the lunar calendar, with no year given.

### Ingredients

| | |
|---|---|
| Concha Ostreae, powdered  (Mu Li Fen) | 30 g |
| Aluminum Potassium Sulfate  (Ku Bai Fan) | 30 g |

The above ingredients were ground into extremely fine powder and sifted through a silk cloth. This was followed by purifying and washing the powder before it was ready to be spread on the scrotum to dry the local perspiration.

### Comments

Concha Ostreae, salty, astringent, and cold in property, is often used in the clinic as an astringent for constraining in the treatment of seminal emission, sweating due to Yin deficiency, and leukorrhea. Records concerning the use of anti-perspirant Concha Ostreae powder can be found in TCM classics. Aluminum Potassium Sulfate is often used in external application to dry sweat of the scrotum. Firing the sulfate makes it lose crystal water. Therefore, Aluminum Potassium Sulfate prepared in fire can absorb wetness on the body surface. It is often used in treating dermatitis, eczema and oozing skin. It should be effective when imperial physicians made a combination of the two for Emperor Guangxu to dry the sweat on the scrotum. Such a sweat-absorbing substance, being both simple and clean, deserves further study in application.

# XXIX. PRESCRIPTIONS FOR MALARIA

## XXIX. 1. SHAOYANG HARMONIZING PRESCRIPTION FOR MALARIA

Shaoyang Harmonizing Prescription for Malaria (He Jie Hua Nue Tang) was carefully prepared for Emperor Guangxu on the 21st day of the ninth month of the lunar calendar. Neither the name of the imperial physician who made it nor the year was given.

### Ingredients

| | |
|---|---|
| Radix Puerariae (Ge Gen) | 6 g |
| Radix Stellariae (Yin Chai Hu) | 4.5 g |
| Rhizoma Coptidis prepared in Fructus Evodiae (Yu Lian) | 4.5 g |
| Fructus Tsaoko, powdered (Cao Guo Ren) | 4.5 g |
| Semen Arecae (Bing Lang) | 9 g |
| Herba Agastachis (Huo Xiang) | 6 g |
| Pericarpium Citri Reticulatae (Chen Pi) | 6 g |
| Cortex Magnoliae Officinalis (Hou Po) | 6 g |
| Polyporus Umbellatus (Zhu Ling) | 9 g |
| Herba Artemisiae Capillaris (Yin Chen) | 6 g |

The original records state that the Cortex Magnoliae Officinalis should be prepared before use. Nine grams of Fructus Viticis should also be added to the remedy.

### Comments

TCM classics hold that "onset of malaria is always the affected condition of Shaoyang channels." Prescriptions for malaria were historically based on the Little Radix Bupleuri Decoction (Xiao Chai Hu Tang). Later on, experts worked out three different methods, respectively known as harmonizing, malaria-halting and deficiency-reinforcing, to treat malaria patients. They also found herbal ingredients specifically for wiping out malaria, e.g. Fructus Tsaoko and Radix Dichroae. Among these three methods, harmonizing is often the first choice. The prescription introduced here was formed by the imperial physicians with reference to ancient formulae. It is a combination with modification of the Little Radix Bupleuri Decoction and the Seven Treasures Decoction for Halting Malaria (Jie Nue Qi Bao Yin). Harmonizing Shaoyang means to relieve the pathogenic factors that are semi-internal and semi-external so as to balance the Upper, Middle and Lower Jiao. It can be of some significance in establishing a therapeutic principle of malaria.

## XXIX.2. SECRET EXTERNAL APPLICATION FOR MALARIA

Secret External Application for Malaria (Zhi Nue Ji Wai Fu Pian Fang) was carefully prepared for Emperor Guangxu by the imperial physicians Zhang Zhong-yuan and Yang Shibao on the 29th day of the intercalary fifth month of the lunar calendar, with no information given as to the year.

### Ingredients

| | |
|---|---|
| Gunpowder (Huo Yao) | 7 |
| Sulphur (Liu Huang) | 7 |
| White pepper (Bai Hu Jiao) | 5 |

The original records state that the quantities were determined by proportions. All ingredients were ground into fine powder and mixed with long-preserved vinegar to be prepared in the form of small cakes which were placed in the centre of the umbilicus and sealed with Umbilicus-warming Plaster (Nuan Qi Gao). But this was not done until the fourth malaria attack was over. Earlier use of the cake could lead to malpractice.

### Comments

The use of gunpowder and sulphur in the treatment of malaria was not recorded in any other formula books in China. Zhang Zhongyuan, who served as an imperial physician for a long time, was promoted from an ordinary physician to physician-in-chief in the Imperial Hospital due to his rich clinical experience. He must have had certain proof when he worked out this prescription. Sulphur also contains some arsenicum. In formula books prior to the Qing Dynasty, arsenicum was used in the treatment of malaria. The use of sulphur here was probably related to that.

The whole prescription is characterized by its predominant warming property. The cake was put in the center of umbilicus and further sealed with Umbilicus-warming Plaster (Luan Qi Gao). It is estimated that the malaria was of the most severe type, pertaining to the cold-natured malaria. Therefore, this Yang-warming remedy was applied in order to invigorate Yang *qi* to fight against the pathogenic factors. For this reason Dr. Zhang Zhongyuan warned that it should not be used in the early stage of malaria. This was to prevent anything unexpected to happen due to using Yang-invigorating ingredients in the early stage of malaria. According to the book *Essence of Superb Remedies* (Dan Fang Jing Hua), malaria plaster was used for all sorts of severe malaria cases. It consists of Fructus Crotonis, white pepper and Fructus Tsaoko. It was often placed on the lower border of the third thoracic vertebra. The underlying mechanism was similar to the Secret External Remedy for Malaria (Zhi Nue Ji Wai Fu Pian Fang). The striking difference is that no particular ingredients for halting malaria were used. Whether it should be effective to treat malaria by means of external application or not will require proof from further studies.

# XXX. MISCELLANEOUS PROVED PRESCRIPTIONS

## XXX.1. PILL FOR CLEARING EPIDEMICS AND DISPELLING TOXIN

There was only the recipe for Pill for Clearing Epidemics and Dispelling Toxin (Qing Wen Jie Du Wan) recorded with no information given concerning the date and name of the imperial physician who formulated it.

### Ingredients

| | |
|---|---:|
| Radix Scutellariae  (Huang Qin) | 60 g |
| Radix Dipsaci  (Xuan Shen) | 90 g |
| Radix Platycodi  (Jie Geng) | 60 g |
| Pericarpium Citri Reticulatae  (Chen Pi) | 60 g |
| Rhizoma Coptidis  (Huang Lian) | 6 g |

| | |
|---|---|
| Rhizoma Cimicifugae  (Sheng Ma) | 15 g |
| Lasiophaera seu Calvatia  (Ma Bo) | 45 g |
| Fructus Arctii  (Niu Bang Zi) | 45 g |
| Radix Bulpeuri  (Chai Hu) | 30 g |
| Fructus Forsythiae  (Lian Qiao) | 60 g |
| Radix Isatidis  (Ban Lan Gen) | 45 g |
| Bombyx Batryticatus  (Jiang Can) | 60 g |
| Urine Sediment, prepared  (Ren Zhong Huang) | 45 g |
| Fructus Gardeniae  (Chao Zhi Zi) | 60 g |
| Semen Sojae Praeparatum  (Dan Dou Chi) | 60 g |
| Cornu Rhinoceri Asiatici  (Xi Jiao) | 30 g |
| Herba Menthae  (Bo He) | 30 g |

The original records state that the Fructus Gardeniae should be roasted before use. All ingredients were ground into extremely fine powder which was processed into honey pills.

## Comments

This prescription was formed by adding more ingredients into Toxic Heat Eliminating Decoction for Sick Masses (Pu Ji Xiao Du Yin) initiated by Li Dongyuan. The original remedy, made to clear toxic heat and eliminate wind, was suggested for the treatment of facial swelling and sore throat. However, the prescription introduced here contains a heavy dose of Cornu Rhinoceri Asiatici for cooling the heat in blood and relieving toxicity. Prepared human urine sediment was also used to clear toxic heat. Both can be applied in severe heat syndrome with skin eruptions, toxic heat invasion affecting the blood system or onset of dark purplish skin rash.

## XXX.2. STYPTIC POWDER FOR DISPELLING TOXIN

Styptic Powder for Dispelling Toxin (Xiao Du Zhi Xue San) was prepared for Emperor Guangxu on the fourth day of the 12th month of the lunar calendar, with no year given.

### Ingredients

| | |
|---|---|
| Calculus Bovis  (Niu Huang) | 1.5 g |
| Concha Margaritifera Usta  (Zhen Zhu Mu) | 1.5 g |
| Resina Draconis  (Xue Jie) | 1.5 g |
| Rhizoma Coptidis  (Huang Lian) | 3 g |
| Radix Notoginseng  (San Qi) | 1.5 g |
| Resina Olibani  (Ru Xiang) | 2.1 g |
| Resina Murrhae  (Mo Yao) | 2.1 g |
| Borneoleum Syntheticum  (Bing Pian) | 0.6 g |

The above ingredients were ground into extremely fine powder.

## Comments

This prescription, modified on the basis of Calculus Bovis and Cornu Rhinoceri Asiatici Pill (Xi Huang Wan), has the action of clearing toxic heat, dispersing masses and stopping bleeding. Calculus Bovis and Concha Margaritifera were used to clear heart fire, tranquilize the mind, relieve toxicity and protect the heart from fire invasion. Radix Coptidis also clears toxic heat. Resina Olibani, Resina Murrhae and Resina Draconis were used to activate blood circulation. Radix Notoginseng was used to stop bleeding. Since toxic heat may move via the channels to attack the heart, many ingredients working on blood were selected. For example, Calculus Bovis and Radix Coptidis were introduced into the blood system to clear the toxin. Such an application would be effective in the treatment of toxic heat-related carbuncles, furuncles, skin rash and toxic heat attacking the heart. Judging from the case record of the Emperor and the time, the last month in the lunar year, this prescription was probably prepared to treat the Emperor for his oozing boils.

## XXX.3. NINE-*QI*-CAUSED PAIN RELIEVING PILL

Nine-*qi*-caused Pain Relieving Pill (Jiu Qi Nian Tong Wan) was carefully prepared for the Emperor by the imperial physicians Zhuang Shouhe and Zhong Xun on the 17th day of the seventh month of the lunar calendar, with no year given.

Emperor Guangxu had pain in the left upper chest area, probably caused by poor circulation of lung *qi* and stagnation of liver *qi*. Only six grams of Nine-*qi*-caused Pain Relieving Pill were made for him to take with boiled water.

### Ingredients

| | |
|---|---|
| Radix Angelicae Sinensis  (Dang Gui) | 120 g |
| Rhizoma Alpiniae Officinalis  (Liang Jiang) | 120 g |
| Faeces Trogopterorum  (Wu Ling Zhi) | 120 g |
| Rhizoma Zedoariae  (E Zhu) | 120 g |
| Semen Arecae  (Bing Lang) | 120 g |
| Pericarpium Citri Reticulatae Viride  (Qing Pi) | 120 g |
| Rhizoma Corydalis  (Yuan Hu Suo) | 60 g |
| Radix Curcumae  (Yu Jin) | 60 g |
| Radix Auchlandiae  (Mu Xiang) | 60 g |
| Pericarpium Citri Reticulatae  (Chen Pi) | 60 g |
| Rhizoma Curcumae Longae  (Jiang Huang) | 60 g |
| Rhizoma Cyperi  (Xiang Fu) | 150 g |
| Radix Glycyrrhizae  (Gan Cao) | 45 g |

The above ingredients were ground into fine powder and made into pills with vinegar for application.

### Comments

This prescription already appears in Part One of this book. However, it was prepared for Emperor Guangxu to treat the pain in the area above his left nipple that also radiated to his back. Although the imperial physicians believed that the condition was caused by stagnation of liver *qi* and poor circulation of lung *qi*, the location and the nature of the pain as well as the recipe suggested that the remedy could also be applied for angina pectoris and epigastric pain.

## XXX.4. TRANQUILIZING PILL

Data concerning the preparation of this prescription were not available from the original records.

### Ingredients

| | |
|---|---|
| Lignum Santali  (Tan Xiang) | 60 g |
| Lignum Aquilaridiae  (Luo Shui Chen) | 60 g |
| Radix Auchlandiae  (Mu Xiang) | 60 g |
| Flos Caryophylli  (Ding Xiang) | 60 g |
| Fructus Amomi Kravanh  (Bai Kou Ren) | 60 g |
| Semen Myristicae  (Rou Kou Ren) | 60 g |
| Fructus Galangae  (Hong Kou) | 60 g |
| Semen Alpiniae Katsumadai  (Cao Kou) | 60 g |
| Pericarpium Citri Reticulatae  (Chen Pi) | 60 g |
| Cortex Magnoliae Officinalis  (Hou Po) | 60 g |
| Rhizoma Atractylodis  (Cang Zhu) | 60 g |
| Radix Glycyrrhizae  (Gan Cao) | 60 g |
| Massa Fermentata Medicinalis  (Shen Qu) | 60 g |
| Fructus Hordei Germinatus  (Mai Ya) | 60 g |
| Fructus Crataegi  (Shan Zha) | 60 g |

According to the original records, the Cortex Magnoliae Officinalis should be prepared before use, while the Rhizoma Atractylodis should be roasted with earth. Both the Massa Fermentata Medicinalis and Fructus Hordei Germinatus should be roasted before use, and the Fructus Crataegi should be roasted until yellow. The above ingredients were ground into extremely fine powder and made into honey pills of two grams each.

### Comments

This prescription was formed on the basis of adding ingredients to Stomach Appeasing Powder (Ping Wei San). It has the actions of strengthening the spleen, pacifying the stomach, regulating *qi* and stopping nausea. It has been considered as an important formula for spleen and stomach conditions, being already seen in the prescriptions prepared for Empress Dowager Cixi. It was one of the secret prescriptions in the Qing imperial palace that covered a wide range of indications. According to medical records of the Qing palace, Emperor Qianlong occasionally granted the permission for this prescription to be used by his chancellors as a gesture in praise of their contributions in running state affairs. Emperor Guangxu himself had severe liver and kidney disorders. Why should such a formula be prescribed for him? This is because it is held in TCM that the spleen and stomach form the source for acquired energy. A healthy condition of the spleen would enable a person to enjoy long life expectancy without ailments. There is a saying in TCM, "An effort made in tonifying the spleen would be superior to one made in reinforcing the kidney." It is apparent that Emperor Guangxu had it for the purpose of tonifying.

## XXX.5. REINFORCED THREE SAGES PILL

Data concerning the year and name of the imperial physician who made this Reinforced Three Sages Pill (Jia Wei San Shen Wan) were not available from the original records.

### Ingredients

| | |
|---|---|
| Rhizoma Atractylodis Macrocephalae (Bai Zhu) | 60 g |
| Rhizoma Coptidis (Chuan Huang Lian) | 75 g |
| Fructus Citri Reticulatae (Ju Hong Guo) | 15 g |
| Cornu Antelopis (Ling Yang Jiao) | 9 g |
| Arisaema cum Bile (Dan Nan Xing) | 6 g |
| Fructus Aurantii Immaturus (Zhi Shi) | 15 g |
| Folium Perillae (Su Ye) | 9 g |
| Pericarpium Trichosanthis (Gua Lou Pi) | 12 g |

According to the original records, the Rhizoma Atractylodis Macrocephalae, Rhizoma Coptidis and Fructus Aurantii Immaturus should be roasted. All the ingredients together with Massa Fermentata Medicinalis were ground into fine powder and made into pills the size of Chinese mung beans. 150 pills were taken orally every day with boiled water.

### Comments

The Three Sages Pill (San Shen Wan) was first recorded in *Therapeutic Standards for the Six Medical Departments* (*Liu Ke Zhun Sheng*) by Wang Kentang. The original prescription contained Rhizoma Coptidis (15 g), Rhizoma Atractylodis Macrocephalae (120 g) and Pericarpium Citri Reticulatae (30 g). Having the function of strengthening the spleen and pacifying the stomach, it is indicated in discomfort in the epigastric region. It is mentioned in Part I of this book. Here, the Cornu Antelopis was added to sedate liver fire. Arisaema cum Bile, Fructus Aurantii Immaturus and Pericarpium Trichosanthis were used to clear heat and resolve phlegm. Folium Perillae was used to promote the function of the lung in dispersing *qi*, pacifying the stomach and stopping vomiting. This prescription was modified to treat conditions of the liver and kidney simultaneously. It is also applicable for patients suffering from poor spleen and stomach functions due to retention of phlegm-damp, apart from its clinical use in many other areas. It shows that imperial physicians would not simply copy a read-to-follow remedy when they were working out a formula. Rather, they modified the set prescriptions in accordance with the actual disease condition in order to achieve far wider therapeutic effects.

## XXX.6. PRESCRIPTION FOR CLEARING HEAT AND RESOLVING FLUID

Prescription for Clearing Heat and Resolving Fluid (Qing Re Hua Yin Fang) was prepared by the imperial physician Fan Chengshun on the 20th day of the first month of the lunar calendar, with no year given.

The previous remedy, known as Peony Prescription (Mu Dan Fang), caused heat retention in the interior leading to dryness in the mouth and nose, and phlegm-fluid retention. Prescription for Clearing Heat and Resolving Fluid was therefore substituted.

### Ingredients

| | |
|---|---|
| Radix Scutellariae (Huang Qin) | 3 g |

| | |
|---|---|
| Radix Scrophulariae (Yuan Shen) | 6 g |
| Radix Ophiopogonis (Mai Dong) | 6 g |
| Flos Chrysanthemi (Ju Hua) | 3 g |
| Rhizoma Atractylodis Macrocephalae (Bai Zhu) | 3 g |
| Poria (Fu Ling) | 3 g |

*Comments*

This prescription was made in an attempt to adjust the overriding effect of the previous remedy. Radix Scutellariae and Flos Chrysanthemi were used to clear wind-heat. Radix Scrophulariae and Radix Ophiopogonis were used to nourish Yin and moisten the dryness. Rhizoma Atractylodis Macrocephalae and Poria were used to strengthen the spleen in dissolving dampness. The combined use of the above ingredients was aimed to treat the Emperor for his dry mouth and nose and retention of phlegm-fluid due to his previous use of Peony Prescription. The prescription also copes with residual manifestations.

## XXX.7. MODIFIED SYRUP FOR CLEARING DAMP-HEAT

Modified Syrup for Clearing Damp-Deat (Jia Jian Qing Re Chu Shi Gao) was carefully prepared by the imperial physician Li Dechang on the 14th day of the seventh month of the lunar calendar in 1876.

*Ingredients*

| | |
|---|---|
| Fructus Forsythiae (Lian Qiao) | 18 g |
| Radix Gentianae (Long Dan Cao) | 12 g |
| Red Poria (Chi Fu Ling) | 18 g |
| Radix Ledebouriellae (Fang Feng) | 15 g |
| Cortex Mori Radicis (Sang Pi) | 12 g |
| Semen Phaseoli (Chi Xiao Dou) | 15 g |
| Fructus Crataegi (Shan Zha) | 10 g |
| Massa Fermentata Medicinalis (Shen Qu) | 10 g |
| Fructus Hordei Germinatus (Mai Ya) | 10 g |
| Flos Chrysanthemi (Ju Hua) | 15 g |
| Herba Artemisiae Capillaris (Yin Chen) | 18 g |
| Radix Scutellariae (Huang Qin) | 12 g |
| Bombyx Batryticatus (Jiang Can) | 12 g |
| Radix Glycyrrhizae (Gan Cao) | 6 g |

The above ingredients were well decocted in water and the residue was separated out. Refined honey was added to make a syrup. Two grams of the syrup were infused in boiled water for oral administration.

On the 21st day of the seventh month of the lunar calendar in 1878, the original prescription, minus Radix Scutellariae and Bombyx Batryticatus, was again given. But Poria (18 g), Rhizoma Atractylodis Macrocephalae (15 g), Pericarpium Citri Reticulatae (12 g) and Rhizoma Dio (18 g), all roasted, were added to the original.

*Comments*

TCM holds that the liver, gallbladder, spleen and stomach would be the most likely to suffer from damp-heat syndrome. This remedy has the action of clearing heat from the liver and dissolving dampness from the spleen. Honey was added to make a syrup so that it would appear to be a mild remedy, acquiring a semi-regulating and semi-dispersing property. Perhaps similar symptoms and signs recurred four years later, so the same prescription was followed in principle. But technically speaking, it would be easier to clear the heat, whereas it would be more difficult to dissolve the dampness. This was the reason why ingredients for clearing heat were decreased while those for dissolving dampness were increased, showing how careful the imperial physicians were when working out a prescription for the Emperor.

## XXX.8. ANGELICAE DAHURICAE POWDER WITH BULBUS FRITILLARIAE CIRHOSAE

Angelicae Dahuricae Powder with Bulbus Fritillariae Cirhosae (Zhi Bei San) was prepared early in the evening on the 14th day of the second month of the lunar calendar, with no information given as to the year.

### Ingredients

| | |
|---|---|
| Radix Angelicae Dahuricae  (Bai Zhi) | 30 g |
| Bulbus Fritillariae Cirhosae  (Chuan Bei Mu) | 30 g |

These two ingredients were ground into extremely fine powder and sifted through a silk net. One gram of the powder was taken orally together with warm millet wine after breakfast and dinner.

### Comments

This prescription has the action of eliminating wind, relieving swelling, clearing heat and softening masses. Radix Angelicae Dahuricae, pungent warm, helps dispel the superficial cold and relieve swelling. According to *Collection of Highly Recommended Prescriptions* (*Bai Yi Xuan Fang*), pills made only of Radis Angelicae Dahuricae were called the Pivot Beam Pill (Du Liang Wan) as applied in the treatment of wandering headache. Bulbus Fritillariae Cirhosae may also clear heat and disperse masses in addition to its effect in resolving phlegm and stopping cough. Warm millet wine was used for taking the powder because it has the effect of activating blood and resolving blood stasis.

# APPENDIX

## Index of Medicinal Ingredients in Chinese, Chinese Phonetic Alphabet, and Latin

**A**

| | | |
|---|---|---|
| 阿魏 | A Wei | Resina Ferulae |
| 艾绒 | Ai Rong | Folium Artemisiae Argyi (moxa wool or moxa down) |
| 艾叶 | Ai Ye | Folium Artemisiae Argyi (dried leaf of artemisiae argyi) |
| 安息香 | An Xi Xiang | Benzoinum |

**B**

| | | |
|---|---|---|
| 巴豆 | Ba Dou | Fructus Crotonis |
| 巴戟天 | Ba Ji Tian | Radix Morindae Officinalis |
| 百部 | Bai Bu | Radix Stemonae |
| 百草霜 | Bai Cao Shuang | Fuligo Plantae |
| 白矾 | Bai Fan | Alumen |
| 白附子 | Bai Fu Zi | Rhizoma Typhonii Gigantei |
| 白芨 | Bai Ji | Rhizoma Bletillae Striatae |
| 白蒺藜 | Bai Ji Li | Fructus Tribuli Terrestris |
| 白蔹 | Bai Jian | Radix Ampelopsis |
| 白僵蚕 | Bai Jiang Can | Bombyx Batryticatus |
| 败酱草 | Bai Jiang Cao | Herba cum Radice Patrimiae |
| 白降丹 | Bai Jiang Dan | Medicinal powder mainly consisting of Cinnabari, Realgar, Alumen, Mercurous chloride, etc. |
| 白芥子 | Bai Jie Zi | Semen Sinapis Albae |
| 白菊花 | Bai Ju Hua | Flos Chrysanthemi Morifolii |
| 白蔻仁 | Bai Kou Ren | Fructus Amomi Kravanh |
| 白莲子 | Bai Lian Zhi | Semen Nelumbinis |
| 白梅花 | Bai Mei Hua | Flos Mume Albus |
| 白前 | Bai Qian | Radix et Rhizoma Cynanchi Baiqian |
| 白牵牛 | Bai Qian Niu | Semen Pharbitidis |
| 白芍 | Bai Shao | Radix Paeoniae Lactiflorae |
| 白薇 | Bai Wei | Radix Cynanchi Atrati |
| 白藓皮 | Bai Xian Pi | Cortex Dictamni Dasycarpi Radiciis |
| 白盐 | Bai Yan | Salt |
| 百药煎 | Bai Yao Jian | An empirical remedy consisting of more |

311

| | | than a dozen of ingredients |
|---|---|---|
| 白芷 | Bai Zhi | Radix Angelicae Dahuricae |
| 白术 | Bai Zhu | Rhizoma Atractylodis Macrocephalae |
| 柏子仁 | Bai Zi Ren | Semen Biotae |
| 板兰根 | Ban Lan Gen | Radix Isatidis |
| 斑蝥 | Ban Mao | Mylabris |
| 半夏 | Ban Xia | Rhizoma Pinelliae |
| 半夏曲 | Ban Xia Qu | Pinelliae Fermintata Medicinalis |
| 荜拨 | Bi Bo | Fructus Piperis Longi |
| 蓖麻子 | Bi Ma Zi | Semen Ricini |
| 荸荠 | Bi Qi | Bulbus Eleocharis Tuberosae |
| 萆薢 | Bi Xie | Rhizoma Dioscoreae Septemlobae |
| 扁豆 | Bian Dou | Semen Dolichoris |
| 扁蓄 | Bian Xu | Herba Polygoni Avicularis |
| 鳖甲 | Bie Jia | Carapax Trionycis |
| 槟榔 | Bing Lang | Semen Arecae |
| 冰硼散 | Bing Peng San | Medicinal powder mainly consisting of Borneoleum Syntheticum, Cannabari, Matrii Sulfas Exsiccatus and Borax |
| 冰片 | Bing Pian | Borneoleum Syntheticum |
| 冰糖 | Bing Tang | Sacchrum Sinensis |
| 薄荷 | Bo He | Herba Menthae |
| 勃荠 | Bo Qi | Bulbus Eleocharis Tuberosae |
| 补骨脂 | Bu Gu Zhi | Fructus Psorleae |

**C**

| | | |
|---|---|---|
| 蚕沙 | Can Sha | Droppings |
| 苍耳子 | Cang Er Zi | Fructus Xanthii |
| 苍术 | Cang Zhu | Rhizoma Atractylodis |
| 草豆蔻 | Cao Dou Kou | Alpiniae Katsumadai |
| 草果 | Cao Guo | Fructus Tsaoko |
| 草河车 | Cao He Che | Radix Bistortae |
| 草决明 | Cao Jue Ming | Semen Cassiae (Jue Ming Zi) |
| 草蔻仁 | Cao Kou Ren | Semen Alpiniae Katsumadai |
| 草霜 | Cao Shuang | Fuligo Plantae |
| 草乌 | Cao Wu | Radix Aconiti Kusnezoffii |
| 侧白叶 | Ce Bai Ye | Cacumen Biotae |
| 茶叶 | Cha Ye | Folium Camelliae Sinensis |
| 柴胡 | Chai Hu | Radix Bupleuri |
| 蟾蜍 | Chan Chu | Venenum Bufonis |
| 蝉蜕 | Chan Tui | Periostracum Cicadae |
| 常山 | Chang Shan | Radix Dichroae |
| 车前子 | Che Qian Zi | Semen Plantaginis |
| 陈皮 | Chen Pi | Pericarpium Citri Reticulatae |
| 沉香 | Chen Xiang | Lignum Aquilariae Resinatum |

| 橙子 | Chen Zi | Fructus Citrus Junos |
|------|---------|---------------------|
| 赤茯苓 | Chi Fu Ling | Red Poria |
| 赤金 | Chi Jin | Aurum |
| 赤芍 | Chi Shao | Radix Paeoniae Rubra |
| 赤石脂 | Chi Shi Zhi | Halloysitum Rubrum |
| 赤小豆 | Chi Xiao Dou | Semen Phaseoli |
| 茺蔚子 | Chong Wei Zi | Fructus Leonuri |
| 川贝 | Chuan Bei | Bulbus Fritillariae Cirhosae |
| 川椒 | Chuan Jiao | Pericarpium Zanthoxyli |
| 川楝子 | Chuan Lian Zi | Fructus Meliae Toosendan |
| 穿山甲 | Chuan Shan Jia | Squama Manitis |
| 川乌 | Chuan Wu | Radix Aconiti |
| 川芎 | Chuan Xiong | Rhizoma Ligustici Chuanxiong |
| 茨菇 | Ci Gu | Rhizoma Pleionis |
| 刺疾黎 | Ci Ji Li | Fructus Tribuli |
| 磁石 | Ci Shi | Magnetitum |
| 刺猬皮 | Cei Wei Pi | Corium Erinacei |

# D

| 大葱头 | Da Cong Tou | Fructus Allii Fistulosi |
|------|-------------|------------------------|
| 大风子 | Da Feng Zi | Semen Hydnocarpi |
| 大腹皮 | Da Fu Pi | Pericarpium Arecae |
| 大黄 | Da Huang | Radix et Rhizoma Rhei |
| 大回香 | Da Hui Xiang | Fructus Illicii Veri/Fructus Anisi Stellati |
| 大麦面 | Da Mai Mian | Hordeun Vulgare |
| 大青叶 | Da Qing Ye | Folium Isatidis |
| 代赭石 | Dai Zhe Shi | Haematitum (Ochra) |
| 淡豆豉 | Dan Dou Chi | Semen Sojae Praeparatum |
| 胆南星 | Dan Nan Xing | Arisaema cum Bile |
| 丹参 | Dan Shen | Radix Salviae Miltiorrhizae |
| 当归 | Dang Gui | Radix Angelicae Sinensis |
| 当门子 | Dang Men Zi | Moschus |
| 党参 | Dang Shen | Radix Codonopsis Pilosulae |
| 灯芯草 | Deng Xin Cao | Medulla Junci Effusi |
| 地别虫 | Di Bie Chong | Eupolyphagaseu Steleophaga |
| 地肤子 | Di Fu Zi | Fructus Kochiae |
| 地骨皮 | Di Gu Pi | Cortex Lycci Radicis |
| 地龙 | Di Long | Lumbricus |
| 地榆 | Di Yu | Radix Sanguisorbsae |
| 丁香 | Ding Xiang | Flos Caryophylli (Flos Syzygii Aromatici) |
| 冬虫夏草 | Dong Chong Xia Cao | Cordyceps |
| 独活 | Du Huo | Radix Angelicae Pubescentis |
| 杜仲 | Du Zhong | Cortex Eucommiae |

## E

| 鹅儿不食草 | E Er Bu Shi Cao | Herba Centipedae |
| 阿胶 | E Jiao | Colla Corri Asini |
| 莪术 | E Zhu | Rhizoma Zedoariae |
| 二宝花 | Er Bao Hua | Flos Lonicerae |
| 儿茶 | Er Cha | Acacia Catechu |

## F

| 防风 | Fang Feng | Radix Ledebouriellae |
| 防己 | Fang Ji | Radix Stephaniae Tetrandrae |
| 榧子 | Fei Zi | Semen Torreyae |
| 风化硝 | Feng Hua Xiao | Mirabilitum |
| 伏龙肝 | Fu Long Gan | Ignited Yellow Earth |
| 复盆子 | Fu Pen Zi | Fructus Rubi |
| 浮萍草 | Fu Ping Cao | Herba Spirodelae |
| 茯神 | Fu Shen | Radix Poria |
| 茯苓 | Fu Ling | Poria |
| 抚芎 | Fu Xiong | Rhizoma Ligustici Chuanxiong |
| 附子 | Fu Zi | Radix Aconiti Praeparatae |

## G

| 甘草 | Gan Cao | Radix Glycyrrhizae |
| 甘草梢 | Gan Cao Shao | Glycyrrhiza Uralensis Fish |
| 干姜 | Gan Jiang | Rhizoma Zingiberis |
| 甘松 | Gan Song | Rhizoma Nardostachyos |
| 甘遂 | Gan Sui | Radix Euphorbiae Kansui |
| 藁本 | Gao Ben | Rhizoma et Radix Ligustici |
| 高良姜 | Gao Liang Jiang | Rhizoma Alpiniae Officinari |
| 蛤蚧粉 | Ge Jie Fen | Gecko |
| 蛤粉 | Ge Fen | Powdery Concha Meretricis seu Cyclinae |
| 葛根 | Ge Gen | Radix Puerariae |
| 鸽条白 | Ge Tiao Bai | Pigeon waste |
| 粳米 | Geng Mi | Semen Oryzae Sativae |
| 公丁香 | Gong Ding Xiang | Flos Syzygii Aromatici |
| 枸杞子 | Gou Qi Zi | Fructus Lycii |
| 钩藤 | Gou Teng | Ramulus Uncariae cum Uncis |
| 谷精草 | Gu Jing Cao | Flos Eriocauli |
| 古墨 | Gu Mo | Chinese calligraphy ink |
| 壳砂 | Gu Sha | Fructus Amomi |
| 骨碎补 | Gu Sui Bu | Rhizoma Drynariae |
| 谷芽 | Gu Ya | Fructus Oryzae Germinature |
| 瓜蒂 | Gua Di | Pedicellus Melo |
| 瓜蒌 | Gua Lou | Fructus Trichosanthis |
| 瓜蒌皮 | Gua Lou Pi | Pericarpium Trichosanthis |
| 瓜蒌子 | Gua Lou Zi | Semen Trichosanthis |

| 贯众 | Guan Zhong | Rhizoma Qsmundae |
| 广红 | Guang Hong | Exocarpium Citri Grandis |
| 广陵 | Guang Ling | Herba Lysimachia Foenum-graecum |
| 龟板 | Gui Ban | Plastrum Testudinis |
| 鬼箭羽 | Gui Jian Yu | Herba Huchnera Cruciata |
| 桂园 | Gui Yuan | Arillus Longan |
| 桂枝 | Gui Zhi | Ramulus Cinnamomi |

## H

| 蛤蟆草 | Ha Ma Cao | Herba Plantaginis |
| 海风藤 | Hai Feng Teng | Caulis Piperis Futokadurae |
| 海桐皮 | Hai Tong Pi | Cortex Erythrinae |
| 海藻 | Hai Zao | Sargassum |
| 汉防己 | Han Fang Ji | Radix Stephaniae Tetrandrae |
| 旱莲草 | Han Lian Cao | Herba Ecliptae |
| 旱三七 | Han San Qi | Radix Notoginseng |
| 寒水石 | Han Shui Shi | Calcitum (Fang Jie Shi) |
| 合欢枝 | He Huan Zhi | Ramulus Albiziae |
| 诃子 | He Zi | Fructus Chebulae |
| 黑丑 | Hei Chou | Semen Pharbitidis |
| 黑豆 | Hei Dou | Glycine Max |
| 黑矾 | Hei Fan | Melanterite |
| 何首乌 | He Shou Wu | Radix Polugomi Multifori |
| 核桃仁 | Hei Tao Ren | Semen Juglandis |
| 黑芝麻 | Hei Zhi Ma | Semen Sesami Nigrum |
| 红大戟 | Hong Da Ji | Radix Knoxiae |
| 红花 | Hong Hua | Flos Carthami |
| 红蔻 | Hong Kou | Fructus Galangae |
| 红曲 | Hong Qu | Monascus Purpureus |
| 红玉膏 | Hong Yu Gao | Medicinal cream made from Radix Angelicae Sinensis, Flos Carthami, Radix Ledebouriellae, Radix Paeoniae Rubra, Resina Olibani, etc. |
| 红枣 | Hong Zao | Fructus Ziziphi Jujubae |
| 厚朴 | Hou Po | Cortex Magnoliae Officinalis |
| 厚朴花 | Hou Po Hua | Flos Magnoliae Officinalis |
| 虎骨 | Hu Gu | Os Tigris |
| 胡黄连 | Hu Huang Lian | Rhizoma Picrorhizae |
| 虎胫骨 | Hu Jing Gu | Tiger tibia |
| 胡芦巴 | Hu Lu Ba | Semen Trigonella |
| 琥珀 | Hu Po | Succinum |
| 胡桃肉 | Hu Tao Rou | Semen Juglandis |
| 滑石 | Hua Shi | Talcum |
| 槐花 | Huai Hua | Flos Sophora Immaturus |
| 槐角 | Huai Jiao | Fructus Sophorce |

| 槐条 | Huai Tiao | Petiolus Sophorce |
| 黄柏 | Huang Bai | Cortex Phellodendri |
| 黄丹 | Huang Dan | Red lead |
| 黄腊 | Huang La | Cera Flava |
| 黄连 | Huang Lian | Rhizoma Coptidis |
| 黄连炭 | Huang Lian Tan | Carbonized Radix Coptidis |
| 黄芪 | Huang Qi | Radix Astragali seu Hedysari |
| 黄芩 | Huang Qin | Radix Scutellariae |
| 霍香 | Huo Xiang | Herba Agastachis |
| 火硝 | Huo Xiao | Niter |

## J

| 蒺藜 | Ji Li | Fructus Tribuli |
| 鸡内金 | Ji Nei Jin | Endothlium Corneum Gieriae Galli |
| 寄奴 | Ji Nu | Herba Artemisia Anomala |
| 鸡血藤 | Ji Xue Teng | Caulis Spatholobi |
| 鸡血藤膏 | Ji Xue Teng Gao | Caulis Spatholobi cream |
| 伽南香 | Jia Nan Xiang | Lignum Aguilariae Resinatum |
| 僵蚕 | Jiang Can | Bombyx Batryticatus |
| 姜黄 | Jiang Huang | Rhizoma Curcumae Longae |
| 姜连 | Jiang Lian | Radix Coptidis prepared with ginger |
| 江米 | Jiang Mi | Semen Oryzae Glutinosae |
| 降香 | Jiang Xiang | Lignum Dalbergiae Odoriferae |
| 椒目 | Jiao Mu | Semen Zanthaxylum |
| 焦三仙 | Jiao San Xian | Charred triplet |
| 桔梗 | Jie Geng | Radix Platycodi |
| 金珀 | Jin Bo | Amber |
| 金大戟 | Jin Da Ji | Radix Euphorbiae Pekinesis |
| 金狗毛 | Jin Gou Mao | Rhizoma Cibotii |
| 金果榄 | Jin Guo Lan | Radix Tinosporae |
| 金银花 | Jin Yin Hua | Flos Lonicerae |
| 金樱子 | Jin Ying Zi | Fructus Rosae Laevigata |
| 精草 | Jing Cao | Flos Eriocauli |
| 荆芥 | Jing Jie | Herba Schizonepetae |
| 荆芥穗 | Jing Jie Sui | Herba Schizonepetae |
| 韭菜 | Jiu Cai | Allium Tuberosum |
| 韭菜籽 | Jiu Cai Zi | Semen Allii/Semen Allis Tuberosi |
| 菊花 | Ju Hua | Flos Chrysanthemi |
| 桔红 | Ju Hong | Pericarpium Citri Reticulatae Rubra |
| 橘络 | Ju Luo | Retinervus Citri Fructus |
| 橘皮 | Ju Pi | Exocarpium Citri Grandis |
| 决明子 | Jue Ming Zi | Semen Cassiae |

## K

| 枯矾 | Ku Fan | Dried Alum |

| 苦梗 | Ku Gen | Radix Platycodi |
|---|---|---|
| 苦参 | Ku Shen | Radix Sophorae Flavescentis |
| 苦石莲 | Ku Shi Lian | Semen Caesalpiniae |
| 款冬花 | Kuan Dong Hua | Flos Farfarae |

**L**

| 莱菔子 | Lai Fu Zi | Semen Raphani |
|---|---|---|
| 狼毒 | Lang Du | Radix Euphorbiae Ebractedatae |
| 老鹳草 | Lao Guan Cao | Herba Erodii seu Geranii |
| 鲤鱼胆 | Li Yu Dan | Fel Cyprinus Carpio |
| 连翘 | Lian Qiao | Fructus Forsythiae |
| 莲子 | Lian Zi | Semen Nelumbinis |
| 两头尖 | Liang Tou Jian | Radix Anemone Raddeana |
| 零陵草 | Ling Ling Cao | Herba Lysimachia |
| 羚羊角 | Ling Yang Jiao | Cornu Antelopis |
| 刘寄奴 | Liu Ji Nu | Herba Artemisia Anomala |
| 柳条 | Liu Tiao | Ramulus Salix Babylonica |
| 龙齿 | Long Chi | Dens Draconis |
| 龙胆草 | Long Dan Cao | Radix Gentianae |
| 龙骨粉 | Long Gu Fen | Os Draconis |
| 蝼蛄 | Lou Gu | Gryllotalpa Africana |
| 芦根 | Lu Gen | Rhizoma Phragmitis |
| 绿豆 | Lü Dou | Semen Phaseoli Radiatus |
| 稆豆皮 | Lu Dou Pi | Glycine Max |
| 鹿角 | Lu Jiao | Cornu Cervi |
| 鹿角胶 | Lu Jiao Jiao | Colla Cornu Cervi |
| 路路通 | Lu Lu Tong | Fructus Liquidambaris |
| 鹿茸 | Lu Rong | Cornu Cervi Pantotrichum |
| 芦荟 | Lu Hui | Aloe |
| 萝卜子 | Luo Bo Zi | Semen Raphani |
| 落水沉 | Luo Shui Chen | Lignum Aquilariae Resinatum |

**M**

| 马勃 | Ma Bo | Lasiophaera seu Calvatia |
|---|---|---|
| 麻黄 | Ma Huang | Herba Ephedrae |
| 玛瑙 | Ma Nao | Achates |
| 马齿苋 | Ma Chi Xian | Herba Portulacae |
| 马前子 | Ma Qian Zi | Semen Strychni |
| 麻叶 | Ma Ye | Folium Cannabis Sativa |
| 麻油 | Ma You | Oil Oleum Sesami |
| 芒硝 | Mang Xiao | Natrii Sulphas |
| 麦冬 | Mai Dong | Radix Ophiopogonis |
| 麦芽 | Mai Ya | Fructus Hordei Germinatus |
| 蔓荆子 | Man Jing Zi | Fructus Viticis |
| 玫瑰花 | Mei Gui Hua | Flos Rosae Rugosae |

| 玫瑰花 | Mei Gui Hua | Pian Rose petals |
| 梅花片 | Mei Hua Pian | Flos Mume |
| 蒙花 | Meng Hua | Flos Buddlejae |
| 礞石 | Meng Shi | Chlorite |
| 蜜柑 | Mi Gan | Fructus Citrus Chachiensis |
| 米壳 | Mi Ke | Pericarpium Papaveris |
| 密陀僧 | Mi Tuo Seng | Lithargyrum |
| 明矾 | Ming Fan | Alumen |
| 没药 | Mo Yao | Resina Murrhae |
| 木鳖花 | Mu Bi Hua | Flos Momordica Cochinchinensis |
| 木鳖子 | Mu Bie Zi | Semen Momordica Cochinchinensis |
| 牡丹皮 | Mu Dan Pi | Cortex Moudan Radicis |
| 母丁香 | Mu Ding Xiang | Fructus Cinnamomi |
| 木瓜 | Mu Gua | Fructus Chaenomelis |
| 牡蛎 | Mu Li | Concha Ostreae |
| 木通 | Mu Tong | Caulis Akebiae |
| 木樨 | Mu Xi | Osmanthus Fragrans |
| 木香 | Mu Xiang | Radix Auchlandiae |
| 木贼 | Mu Zei | Herba Equiseti Hiemalis |

### N

| 南星 | Nan Xing | Rhizoma Arisaematis |
| 年健 | Nian Jian | Rhizoma Homalomenae |
| 牛蒡子 | Niu Bang Zi | Fructus Arctii |
| 牛黄 | Niu Huang | Calculus Bovis |
| 牛膝 | Niu Xi | Radix Achyranthis Bidentatae |
| 女贞子 | Nü Zhen Zi | Fructus Ligustri Lucidi |
| 糯米 | Nuo Mi | Semen Oryzae Glutinosae |

### O

| 藕 | Ou | Nodus Nelumbinis Rhizomatis |
| 藕粉 | Ou Fen | Nodus Nelumbinis Rhizomatis |

### P

| 排草 | Pai Cao | Herba Lysimachia Capillipes |
| 佩兰 | Pei Lan | Herba Eupatorii |
| 盆糖 | Pen Tang | Solid sugar |
| 硼砂 | Peng Sha | Borax |
| 皮胶 | Pi Jiao | Colla Coria Asini |
| 枇杷叶 | Pi Pa Ye | Folium Eriobotryae |
| 破故纸 | Po Gu Zhi | Fructus Psoraleae |
| 朴硝 | Po Xiao | Mirabilite |
| 蒲公英 | Pu Gong Ying | Herba Taraxaei |
| 蒲黄 | Pu Huang | Pollen Typhae |

**Q**

| 蕲艾 | Qi Ai | Folium Artemisiae Argyi |
| 蕲蛇 | Qi She | Agkistrodon |
| 茜草 | Qian Cao | Radix Rubiae |
| 前胡 | Qian Hu | Radix Peucedani |
| 千金子 | Qian Jin Zi | Semen Euphorbiae Lathyridis |
| 芡实 | Qian Shi | Semen Euryales |
| 羌活 | Qian Huo | Rhizoma seu Radix Notopterygii |
| 秦艽 | Qin Jiao | Radix Gentianae Macrophyllae |
| 秦皮 | Qin Pi | Cortex Fraxini |
| 青茶 | Qing Cha | Green tea |
| 青黛 | Qing Dai | Indigo Naturalis |
| 轻粉 | Qing Fen | Calomel |
| 青风藤 | Qing Feng Teng | Caulis Sinomenii |
| 青果 | Qing Guo | Fructus Canarit |
| 青木香 | Qing Mu Xiang | Radix Aristolochiae |
| 青皮 | Qing Pi | Pericarpium Citri Reticulatae Viride |
| 青箱子 | Qing Xiang Zi | Semen Celosiae |
| 青盐 | Qing Yan | Halite |
| 蚯蚓 | Qiu Yin | Lumbricus |
| 瞿麦 | Qu Mai | Herba Dianthi |
| 全蝎 | Quan Xie | Scorpio |

**R**

| 忍冬藤 | Ren Dong Teng | Caulis Lonicerae |
| 人参 | Ren Shen | Radix ginseng |
| 人中白 | Ren Zhong Bai | Human urine sediment |
| 人中黄 | Ren Zhong Huang | Radix Glycyrrhizae in Taeniam soaked in human waste |
| 肉丛蓉 | Rou Cong Rong | Herba Cistanchis |
| 肉豆蔻 | Rou Dou Kou | Semen Myristicae |
| 肉桂 | Rou Gui | Cortex Cinnamomi |
| 肉蔻仁 | Rou Kou Ren | Semen Myristicae |
| 乳香 | Ru Xiang | Resina Olibani |
| 蕤仁 | Rui Ren | Nux Prinsepiae |

**S**

| 三棱 | San Leng | Rhizoma Sparganii |
| 三奈 | San Nai | Rhizoma Kaempferiae |
| 桑白皮 | Sang Bai Pi | Cortex Mori Radicis |
| 桑椹子 | Sang Shen Zi | Fructus Mori |
| 桑寄生 | Sang Ji Sheng | Ramulus Loranthi |
| 桑叶 | Sang Ye | Folium Mori |
| 桑枝 | Sang Zhi | Ramulus Mori |
| 砂仁 | Sha Ren | Fructus Amomi |

| | | |
|---|---|---|
| 沙参 | Sha Shen | Radix Adenonhorae Strictae |
| 沙菀子 | Sha Wan Zi | See Tong Ji Li |
| 山茨菇 | Shan Ci Gu | Bulbus Cremastrae |
| 珊瑚 | Shan Hu | Corallium Japonicum |
| 山奈 | Shan Nai | Rhizoma Kaempferiae |
| 山羊血 | Shan Yang Xue | Goat blood |
| 山楂 | Shan Zha | Fructus Crataegi |
| 山楂核 | Shan Zha He | Semen Crataegi |
| 山茱萸 | Shan Zhu Yu | Fructus Corni |
| 山药 | Shan Yao | Rhizoma Dio |
| 蛇床子 | She Chuang Zi | Fructus Litseae Cubebae |
| 射干 | She Gan | Rhizoma Belamcandae |
| 蛇蜕 | She Tui | Periostracum Serpentis |
| 麝香 | She Xiang | Moschus |
| 伸筋草 | Shen Jin Cao | Herba Lycopodii |
| 神曲 | Shen Qu | Massa Fermentata Medicinalis |
| 生地黄 | Sheng Di Huang | Radix Rehmanniae |
| 生姜 | Sheng Jiang | Rhizoma Zingiberis Recens |
| 升麻 | Sheng Ma | Rhizoma Cimicifugae |
| 石菖蒲 | Shi Chang Pu | Rhizoma Acori Graminei |
| 石膏 | Shi Gao | Gypsum Fibrosum |
| 石斛 | Shi Hu | Herba Dendrobii |
| 石决明 | Shi Jue Ming | Concha Haliotidis |
| 石榴枝 | Shi Liu Zhi | Pericarpium Granati |
| 石南 | Shi Nan | Photimia |
| 柿子霜 | Shi Zi Shuang | Powder on the suface of a dried persimmon |
| 熟地黄 | Shu Di Huang | Radix Rehmanniae Praeparatae |
| 水银 | Shui Yin | Hydrargyrum |
| 丝瓜络 | Si Gua Luo | Retinervus Luffae Fructus |
| 松罗茶 | Song Luo Cha | Usonea |
| 松枝 | Song Zhi | Ramulus Pinus Tabulaeformis |
| 松子 | Song Zi | Pini Nodi |
| 苏梗 | Su Geng | Ganlis Perillae |
| 苏合油 | Su He You | Resina Liquidambar Orientalis |
| 苏木 | Su Mu | Lignum Sappan |
| 苏叶 | Su Ye | Folium Periilae |
| 酸枣仁 | Suan Zao Ren | Semen Ziziphi Spinosae |
| 缩砂仁 | Suo Sha Ren | Fructus Amomi |

**T**

| | | |
|---|---|---|
| 苔乌 | Tai Wu | Radix Linderae |
| 檀香 | Tan Xiang | Lignum Santali |
| 桃条 | Tao Tiao | Ramulus Prunus Persica |
| 桃仁 | Tao Ren | Semen Persicae |

| 藤黄 | Teng Huang | Resina Garciniae |
| 天冬 | Tian Dong | Radix Asparagi |
| 天花粉 | Tian Hua Fen | Radix Trichosanthis |
| 天麻 | Tian Ma | Rhizoma Gastrodiae |
| 天仙藤 | Tian Xian Teng | Caulis Aristolochia Debilis |
| 天竹簧 | Tian Zhu Huang | Concretio Silicea Bambusae |
| 铁锤柄 | Tie Chui Bing | Iron scale |
| 潼蒺藜 | Tong Ji Li | Semen Astragali Complanati |
| 透骨草 | Tou Gu Cao | Herba Speranskia Tuberculata |
| 土鳖虫 | Tu Bie Chong | Eupolyphaga seu Steleopnaga |
| 菟丝子 | Tu Si Zi | Semen Cuscutae |
| 土茱萸 | Tu Zhu Yu | Fructus Euodiae |
| 团粉 | Tuan Fen | Cooking Starch |

### W

| 煨姜 | Wei Jiang | Rhizoma Zingiberis Praeparatae |
| 威灵仙 | Wei Ling Xian | Radix Clematis |
| 文蛤 | Wen Ge | Meretrix |
| 蜈蚣 | Wu Gong | Scolopendra |
| 五倍子 | Wu Bei Zi | Galla Chinensis |
| 五加皮 | Wu Jia Pi | Cortex Acanthopanacis Radicis |
| 五灵脂 | Wu Ling Zhi | Faeces Trogopterorum |
| 乌梅肉 | Wu Mei Rou | Fructus Mume |
| 乌梢蛇 | Wu Shao She | Zaocys |
| 午时茶 | Wu Shi Cha | Noontime tea |
| 乌头 | Wu Tou | Radix Aconiti |
| 五味子 | Wu Wei Zi | Fructus Schisandrae |
| 乌药 | Wu Yao | Radix Linderae |
| 吴茱萸 | Wu Zhu Yu | Fructus Evodiae |

### X

| 犀角 | Xi Jiao | Cornu Rhinoceri Asiatici |
| 细麹 | Xi Qu | Massa Fermentata Medicinalis |
| 希莶草 | Xi Xian Cao | Herba Siegesbeckiae |
| 细辛 | Xi Xin | Herba Asari |
| 西洋参 | Xi Yang Shen | Radix Panacis Quiquefloii |
| 夏枯草 | Xia Ku Cao | Spica Prunellae |
| 香附 | Xiang Fu | Rhizoma Cyperi |
| 香薷 | Xiang Ru | Herba Elsholtzia |
| 线胶 | Xiang Jiao | Colla Corii Huso Dauricus |
| 小茴香 | Xiao Hui Xiang | Fructus Foeniculi |
| 新会皮 | Xin Hui Pi | Pericapium Citrus Chachiensis |
| 辛荑 | Xin Yi | Flos Magnoliae |
| 杏仁 | Xing Ren | Semen Armenicacae |
| 熊胆 | Xiong Dan | Fel Ursi |

| 熊骨 | Xiong Gu | Os Ursi |
|---|---|---|
| 雄黄 | Xiong Huang | Realgar |
| 熊油 | Xiong You | Oleum Ursi |
| 续断 | Xu Duan | Radix Dipsaci |
| 旋覆花 | Xuan Fu Hua | Flos Inulae |
| 玄明粉 | Xuan Ming Fen | Natrii Sulfas Exsiccatus |
| 玄参 | Xuan Shen | Radix Scrophulariae |
| 血竭 | Xue Jie | Resina Draconis |
| 血珀 | Xue Po | Amber |
| 血余 | Xue Yu | Crinis Carbonisatus |

### Y

| 鸭梨 | Ya Li | Pyrus |
|---|---|---|
| 牙硝 | Ya Xiao | Mirabilitum |
| 牙皂 | Ya Zao | Spina Gleditsiae |
| 阳起石 | Yang Qi Shi | Actinolitum |
| 羊腰 | Yang Yao | Goat kidney |
| 野於术 | Ye Yu Shu | Rhizoma Atractylodis Macrocephalae |
| 益母草 | Yi Mu Cao | Herba Leonuri |
| 薏苡仁 | Yi Yi Ren | Semen Coicis |
| 一枝蒿 | Yi Zhi Hao | Herba Achillea Alpina |
| 益智仁 | Yi Zhi Ren | Fructus Alpiniae Oxyphylla |
| 银柴胡 | Yin Chai Hu | Radix Stellariae |
| 茵陈 | Yin Chen | Herba Artemisiae Capillaris |
| 萤火虫 | Yin Huo Chong | Luciola Vitticollis |
| 银朱 | Yin Zhu | Sulphur-mercury |
| 罂粟壳 | Ying Su Ke | Pericarpium Papaveris |
| 郁金 | Yu Jin | Radix Curcumae |
| 萸连 | Yu Lian | Rhizoma Coptidis baked with Fructus Evodiae |
| 榆条 | Yu Tiao | Ramulus Ulmus Pumila |
| 玉竹 | Yu Zhu | Rhizoma Polygonati Odorati |
| 元胡索 | Yuan Hu Suo | Rhizoma Corydalis |
| 芫花 | Yuan Hua | Flos Genkwa |
| 远志 | Yuan Zhi | Radix Polygalae |
| 云连 | Yun Lian | Rhizoma Coptidis |

### Z

| 皂角刺 | Zao Jiao Ci | Spina Gleditsiae |
|---|---|---|
| 枣树根 | Zao Shu Gen | Radix Ziziphus Jujuba |
| 泽兰 | Ze Lan | Herba Lycopi |
| 泽泻 | Ze Xie | Rhizoma Alismatis |
| 獐胆 | Zhang Dan | Fel Hydropotes Inermis |
| 獐脑 | Zhang Nao | Camphora |
| 浙贝母 | Zhe Bei Mu | Bulbus Fritillariae Thunbergii |